D0722824

WITHDRAWN

The Health Care "Safety Net" in a Post-Reform World

Critical Issues in Health and Medicine

Edited by Rima D. Apple, University of Wisconsin–Madison,
and Janet Golden, Rutgers University, Camden

Growing criticism of the US health care system is coming from consumers, politicians, the media, activists, and health care professionals. Critical Issues in Health and Medicine is a collection of books that explores these contemporary dilemmas from a variety of perspectives, among them political, legal, historical, sociological, and comparative, and with attention to crucial dimensions such as race, gender, ethnicity, sexuality, and culture.

For a list of titles in the series, see the last page of the book.

The Health Care "Safety Net" in a Post-Reform World

Edited by
Mark A. Hall and Sara Rosenbaum

Rutgers University Press
New Brunswick, New Jersey, and London

Library of Congress Cataloging-in-Publication Data

The health care "safety net" in a post-reform world / edited by Mark A. Hall and Sara Rosenbaum.
    p. ; cm. — (Critical issues in health and medicine)
    Includes bibliographical references and index.
    ISBN 978–0–8135–5305–4 (hardcover : alk. paper) — ISBN 978–0–8135–5306–1 (pbk. : alk. paper) — ISBN 978–0–8135–5317–7 (e-book)
    I. Hall, Mark A., 1955– II. Rosenbaum, Sara. III. Series: Critical issues in health and medicine.
    [DNLM: 1. Medically Uninsured—United States. 2. Community Health Services—economics—United States. 3. Health Care Reform—United States. 4. Hospitals, Public—economics—United States. 5. Insurance, Health—United States. 6. Medically Underserved Area—United States. W 250 AA1]
    368.38′200973—dc23

                                                            2011037585

A British Cataloging-in-Publication record for this book is available from the British Library.

Work on this book was funded by the Robert Wood Johnson Foundation through its Investigator Awards in Health Policy Research Program and its Coverage Program. Jan Lawlor and Emily Hoppes provided extensive editorial assistance. Patricia Perrier prepared the index.

Visit our website: http://rutgerspress.rutgers.edu

Manufactured in the United States of America

To the memory of Alison Snow Jones, our colleague and friend who devoted her career and considerable passion and intellect to advancing true social and personal welfare

Contents

Part III   Safety-Net Systems

Figures

Tables

The Health Care "Safety Net" in a Post-Reform World

The Health Care Safety Net in the Context of National Health Insurance Reform

The Patient Protection and Affordable Care Act (Affordable Care Act, or ACA) is expected to extend public and private insurance to about thirty million more people, more than half of those who are currently uninsured. Experts estimate that when fully implemented in 2019 the ACA will increase coverage from about 83 percent to 94 percent of the total US population. This is a monumental achievement.

As with all major leaps forward, this one comes with challenges because of who the law includes and excludes, the levels of subsidies that will be available, and the retention of multiple insurance markets that individuals must traverse as income, work, and family circumstances change. The first and perhaps most important limitation is that more than twenty million people—about 8 percent of the nonelderly population—will remain uninsured. Some will be excluded because they will be unable to satisfy the act's requirement of legal US status to receive premium subsidies or nonemergency Medicaid benefits, the two principal forms of direct federal aid under the law for low- and moderate-income populations. Others will be individuals for whom coverage will remain unaffordable, as defined by the law. Still others will be individuals who experience interruptions in coverage because of lapses in Medicaid or subsidy eligibility, as well as enrollment barriers that persist despite the relatively aggressive enrollment assistance efforts that the law requires.

A second challenge arises from the fact that insurance coverage alone does not cure nonfinancial barriers to health care. Millions of Americans live in urban and rural communities officially designated as medically underserved because of a serious shortage of primary care providers coupled with lower population income. While the expansion of health insurance may ultimately attract more health care providers into these communities, medical practice remains challenging because underserved patients may be more clinically complex. Also, the proportion covered by subsidized insurance is far higher and thus provider compensation is lower. Resources ultimately may improve in these communities, but this shift inevitably will be slow to come, especially given the overall primary care shortage.

A third challenge can be found in the nature of the health insurance coverage under health reform. The ACA's nondiscrimination provisions make coverage available to millions of people that insurers previously excluded because of preexisting conditions, and the ACA's elimination of lifetime and annual caps and coverage of "essential health benefits" promise to strengthen the scope of coverage available in the individual and small-group insurance markets. At the same time, to keep premiums affordable, the actuarial value of coverage for which the insurer is responsible will remain relatively low, leaving individuals with potentially significant cost-sharing exposure (deductibles, copayments, coinsurance) for covered benefits. In addition, the definition of essential health benefits excludes some items and services (such as vision and dental care for adults) or limits others to less than what some patients need (such as therapy interventions for a disabled child that exceed plan limits). Thus, even with cost-sharing assistance, financial exposure will remain significant for lower-income people covered through insurance exchanges.

For these reasons, safety-net providers, programs, and systems will remain essential in a postreform world, for newly insured and uninsured alike (Hall 2011a, 2011b; Katz 2010). The safety net consists primarily of publicly funded and community-supported clinics as well as public hospitals and mission-driven nonprofit hospitals that take all patients regardless of ability to pay (Lewin and Altman 2000). From one perspective, insurance reform will be a boon for these organizations. Expansion of Medicaid and private insurance coverage will reduce the collective burden of uncompensated care by over half and will increase the revenues that safety-net organizations receive from well-insured patients. Also, the ACA contains large funding increases for community health centers. However, the ACA also reduces other safety-net investments, most notably, funding for hospitals that serve a disproportionate number of low-income persons. Furthermore, dependence on the health care safety net may increase for the remaining uninsured population as providers that previously might have provided uncompensated care seek out the newly insured. These policy realities mean that some safety net providers will continue to experience significant gaps in geographic availability, scope of services, and capacity as well as a perception that safety nets are no longer necessary components of the health care system, even as the need for safety net services continues to remain significant for those left out of insurance reforms as well as individual and families who continue to face barriers to health care because of geographic, language, and cultural barriers.

This book arose from our collective interest in and concern about these competing forces. We aim to better understand what role various components of the safety net can and should have following health insurance reform, and what policies and resources are needed to best facilitate adaptation to these evolving roles. In this overview chapter, we first outline the changing composition of the uninsured and highlight key needs that safety net providers and institutions can help to meet for underserved populations in the reformed environment, regardless of insurance status. We then summarize how each chapter addresses its piece of the larger picture that is painted by this book as a whole.

The Changing Composition of the Uninsured

The vulnerable populations served by safety-net providers and programs include both insured and uninsured patients, but the proportion of patients who are uninsured vastly exceeds the uninsured proportion outside safety-net care settings. Thus an important development in the evolution of the safety net is the change in composition of the uninsured that can be expected as a result of ACA passage. This change will not occur overnight; full implementation of health reform will take several years. But over time the ACA can be expected to alter the composition of uninsured people even as it increases demand for care from newly insured populations.

Safety-net providers historically have served the uninsured without regard to questions of legal status. Undocumented residents will rise as a proportion of the uninsured population because the ACA reforms principally benefit lower-income citizens and legal residents. The uninsured will continue to include Medicaid-eligible individuals who simply are not enrolled in the program or who are between enrollment periods. Also among the postreform uninsured will be individuals who cannot afford coverage under the law's affordability test (set at 8 percent of income); those whose inability to secure coverage is, for other reasons, deemed by the Secretary of Health and Human Services to be a hardship; or those who refuse to purchase coverage despite the mandate.

According to estimates by the Urban Institute using its sophisticated microsimulation model (Buettgens and Hall 2011), more than a third of uninsured adults will be eligible for Medicaid, a quarter will be undocumented immigrants, and a quarter will have affordable insurance available to them (and thus probably will be in violation of the individual mandate). Only 16 percent of uninsured adults will be legal residents exempt from the mandate for failing to have an affordable option.

The one-quarter of uninsured who do not purchase insurance despite having an affordable option will not be as irresponsible as might first appear. Included in this number are individuals who experience lapses in coverage because of movement in and out of Medicaid and movement from Medicaid to the exchange system. This group will be concentrated among lower-income people who historically have been uninsured. Recognizing the difficulty in remaining seamlessly insured across transitions in jobs and eligibility, the ACA does not penalize lapses in coverage of up to three months' duration. Furthermore, some people who refuse premium subsidies will do so because of the significant risk of having to repay excess subsidies. It is often difficult or impossible to know one's eventual income bracket later in the year at the time insurance is purchased at the start of a year. Rather than waiving good-faith errors, legislation enacted in late 2010 greatly increases the repayment obligation for receiving a premium subsidy overpayment, from a $400 maximum to as much as $2,500 (Pub. L. 111–309).

Insurance reform will also affect the economic profile of the uninsured. Prior to reform, more than half of the uninsured not eligible for Medicaid had family incomes below 200 percent of poverty, and only about a third of these were undocumented immigrants. After reform less than 15 percent of the uninsured not eligible for Medicaid will be legal residents below 200 percent of poverty (Buettgens and Hall 2011). Among uninsured adults who decline affordable subsidized insurance options, incomes will be moderately low (median of 280 percent of the federal poverty level [FPL]), but most (61 percent) will be singles without children, and younger (median age of thirty-three). Those uninsured adults who are not eligible for either subsidies or an affordability exemption will have fairly high incomes (median of 490 percent of the FPL). These estimated figures offer only a snapshot and thus do not capture the longitudinal effects of churning among lower-income, previously uninsured persons that can threaten coverage, plan enrollment, and continuity of care. Nonetheless, these figures suggest an important long-term shift in the socioeconomic profile of the uninsured.

Naturally, these numbers will vary considerably among states and localities according to their economic and demographic characteristics and other factors, such as their preform Medicaid eligibility criteria. For example, the overall uninsured rate is projected to vary regionally from about 5 percent in New England to more than 10 percent in the west-south-central region (Buettgens and Hall 2011), and the composition of uninsured also will vary. For instance, the proportion of uninsured projected to be undocumented immigrants ranges from 12 to 32 percent among regions of the country, and the proportion of uninsured adults with no affordable insurance option is estimated to range from 14 to 25 percent.

Safety-Net Roles Following Reform

Despite the reduced number and changing composition of the uninsured, the safety net will remain critically important to meeting the ACA's core goals of improving access, and to moving beyond those immediate goals to achieve something approaching universal access. There are several crucial roles for safety-net providers, programs, and systems. First, expanded health insurance coverage will not translate to improved access to care without additional investments in the existing safety net. Empirical evidence drawn from past insurance expansions, such as Massachusetts's reform, suggests that expanded insurance in fact intensifies the need for the health care safety net because of heightened expectations among newly insured who are still medically underserved (Ku et al. 2009). Insurance reforms will cover more low-income people, but because of their personal characteristics, the clinical challenges they present, their places of residence, and the characteristics of their coverage, newly covered people may continue to experience significant access problems that in turn will lead to avoidable suffering, disability, and death. With some ninety-six million US residents estimated to be living in communities classified as medically underserved, the health care safety net will continue to play a crucial role in translating coverage into care.

Second, the reform law's subsidies are not available to undocumented immigrants, and legal immigrants are eligible for Medicaid only after residing in the United States for five years. Serving noncitizen residents is a traditional role for most safety-net organizations, but this role will likely become more visible and thus more controversial. Safety-net programs will need to remind constituents that their inclusive policies are based not only on undocumented immigrants' being a major component of the needy population but also on the reality that demanding documentation from all patients, including citizens, is both impractical and offensive.

Among legal residents, some middle-income people will face insurance premiums greater than the affordability threshold. This will be particularly true for older people since insurers will be permitted to vary premium rates threefold based on age under the ACA's modified community rating requirements. Accordingly, uninsured adults who are eligible for an afford-ability exemption will have a median age of fifty-one, their incomes will be moderately low (median of 250 percent FPL), and half will have dependents. Given their age and incomes, many of the people who remain uninsured because of affordability problems can be expected to have significant unmet needs.

Third, people are not subject to a mandate penalty if they are uninsured for only three months or less. Observing the similar reform measures in Massachusetts (Hall 2010), we learn that gaps in coverage are difficult to avoid when people switch from public to private coverage. This is because private insurance, even when highly subsidized, is not designed for immediate or retroac-tive enrollment. Also, once the new insurance exchanges are operational, it is entirely possible that open enrollment will not be continuously available but instead will be limited to certain times of the year. Employers may still impose a three-month waiting period before covering new workers, and lower-income workers and their families will face considerable problems in smoothly transi-tioning between Medicaid and exchange coverage. Accordingly, insurance gaps caused by transitions between jobs and between public and private cov-erage and by movement between the Medicaid and exchange markets will be fairly common. Half of people below 200 percent of poverty each year have a shift in income that will change their eligibility for Medicaid or private insur-ance, and roughly a fifth of working people change jobs each year (varying widely by sector) (Sommers and Rosenbaum 2011; Short et al. 2011). The result-ing gaps in coverage can disrupt continuity of care. Therefore, an important safety-net role is to maintain access for an entire family regardless of different types of insurance within the same family or changes in coverage over time. Providing a medical home regardless of type or source of payment will go a long way to making seamless the complex patchwork of ACA coverage options. Furthermore, the safety net possesses unique expertise in serving patients who traditionally have faced financial and nonfinancial barriers to care.

Seamless access is facilitated by an ACA provision that requires health insurers who want to sell through the new insurance exchanges to include in their provider networks any "essential community providers" in their service areas who are willing to accept the insurer's standard rates. Whether by invok-ing this provision or otherwise, participating in insurers' networks will be an important step for safety-net providers to broaden their enrollment. But becom-ing more mainstream and more fully integrating with local delivery systems will entail managerial and operational shifts that may be challenging for many safety-net providers, particularly free clinics and health centers. Until now, most have been operated independently from major delivery systems and governed by specially composed boards. They also have encountered significant barriers in referring uninsured and publicly insured patients. These institutional cultures and legal structures could form barriers to the forms of affiliation and integration needed for health centers to be most effective.

Fourth, some people who qualify for subsidies and purchase insurance will still face high premiums or out-of-pocket costs. The ACA subsidizes cost-sharing for people below 250 percent of the federal poverty level, but even some of these people can still face catastrophic levels of expense relative to their modest incomes. Certainly this will be true for people above 250 percent of poverty who receive no cost-sharing reduction. Many analysts view 10 percent of income as a rough gauge for affordability. The Urban Institute estimates that for people above 300 percent of poverty, the most costly decile covered by nongroup insurance will incur costs that exceed twice this affordability threshold— 20 percent of household income. This is because the insurance premium alone for people with family incomes at or above 250 percent of poverty amounts to between 8 and 9.5 percent of household income for each covered person. When added to out-of-pocket payments for covered and uncovered services, the financial burden of health care even after health reform will surpass 10 percent of income for many newly insured persons. Thus, the need for providers who discount their care in accordance with ability to pay and who are sources of lower-cost care for uncovered services will remain considerable.

Finally, safety-net organizations will have a major role to play in helping people navigate the complex and changing system in 2014. The insurance exchanges and subsidy structures will be new and unfamiliar, and Medicaid eligibility will be substantially revamped. Even though the ACA calls for a system of navigators to provide assistance in enrollment and establishing and using plan benefits, the process will be complex. This will be particularly true for those for whom insurance is a new experience. Furthermore, people can be expected to be distressed about the tax penalty consequences for noncompliance and will need help avoiding recoupment in the event of premium credit overpayments. Therefore, a great deal of assistance and encouragement from entities known and trusted in their communities will be necessary for people to know what they are supposed to do and how to go about doing it. Many safety-net organizations already are adept at screening and referring people for Medicaid or other public program eligibility. This puts them in an excellent position to be part of the navigation system that the ACA funds to facilitate eligibility screening and enrollment.

In sum, despite comprehensive health insurance reform, the effort to achieve truly universal coverage has only begun. This book assesses the role of the safety net as an integral component of health insurance reform and as an ongoing and essential component of the health care system for those who are currently insured, those who are newly insured, and those who will remain uninsured when the Affordable Care Act is fully implemented. This collection, written by some of the country's best thinkers on the health care safety net and vulnerable populations, offers an in-depth, interdisciplinary understanding of health reform's challenges and the opportunities for safety-net providers and programs. The book's authors are drawn mostly from current and former researchers supported by the Robert Wood Johnson Foundation, principally through its Investigator Awards in Health Policy Research program, which also supported production of this book, for which we are grateful. In three basic parts, summarized below, the book surveys the organizational structures and social policies needed to sustain and build an adequate access system for uninsured persons as well as for socially disadvantaged populations as a complement to health reform's insurance expansions.

Community Health Centers

Part I addresses the primary care backbone of the safety net: community health centers and free clinics. In chapter 2, political scientist Robert W. Mickey traces the political evolution of the federal community health centers program, a critical component of America's health safety net. From its inception as a War on Poverty demonstration program until the late 1990s, the health centers program grew steadily but slowly. The author points out that, from a practical point of view, the need for such a program in medically underserved communities was never in doubt. But the program was viewed through the political lens of each party at various points in time. During the 1970s and 1980s, Republicans objected to the program (indeed, Congress in 1981 went so far as to block-grant the health centers, reversing itself in 1985) because it represented a direct incursion by the federal government into the health care system, an "alternative health care delivery system," in the words of one high-ranking Reagan administration official. While health centers survived the 1981 legislation (in fact, four years later, they were able to persuade Congress to do the unimaginable and repeal the block grant and reinstate a federally administered program), federal appropriations for the program essentially stagnated thereafter when adjusted for inflation.

The enactment of the Medicare and Medicaid federally qualified health centers (FQHC) payment system several years after the block grant reversal signaled the political strength of the health centers movement in Congress. At the same time, however, the Clinton administration essentially ignored health centers, seeking no major growth in their capacity and providing no supplemental funding for their expansion in the 1993 health reform legislation. Although health centers continued to have a wide circle of political supporters (legislation to expand the program as part of the Clinton reform plan was introduced separately, for example), they were ignored by a Democratic White House in the 1990s, which judged them to be a blunting influence on the urgency of health reform itself. Ironically, the same "alternative delivery system" feared by the Republicans a decade earlier was this time, with a different spin, rejected by Democrats. In surprising contrast, President George W. Bush launched a health centers initiative that essentially doubled their capacity in the 2000s.

In Mickey's view, the political trajectory of the program over its first three and a half decades can be understood through the prism of political learning. Democrats and Republicans essentially learned lessons during the long battle over national health insurance and adapted their positions on many health policies in light of these lessons. Beginning in the 1970s, Republicans came to see the national expansion of the health centers program as a conscious strategy to facilitate Democratic proposals for universal coverage. National health insurance proponents would, conservatives feared, be able to point to the existence of a delivery network of facilities for the poor already in place, thus reducing some of the practical difficulties of moving toward a workable system. By the 1990s some progressives devoted to the attainment of universal health coverage had developed a strange ambivalence toward programs for the underserved. Many came to see them, in Leninist "one step forward" fashion, as weakening pressures for systemic reform of the health care system. Over time, conservatives came to agree with them. Mickey explains that the early conservative attack, the subsequent conservative embrace, and many progressives' puzzling ambivalence toward health centers are explicable in terms of learning and adaptation. The chapter closes with a brief discussion of the program's future in light of the 2010 ACA.

Picking up the narrative where Mickey leaves off, Sara Rosenbaum explores in chapter 3 the investment in health centers as a core and multifaceted aspect of 2010's health reform. She starts by examining the combination of permanent authorization; the capital investment in health center growth and operations; and the dramatic Medicaid eligibility, coverage, and payment expansions during 1984–1990, which in turn fueled health center growth beginning in the 1990s. This growth has lasted into the present and has received a further dramatic boost under 2010 health reform. What demarcates this reform effort from earlier reforms, as Rosenbaum notes, is congressional willingness to grapple directly with the issues of access in medically under-served communities as a core aspect of coverage reform. Some of this evolution can be ascribed to the enormous changes in public and private health insurance that have taken place since the early 1990s. At the dawn of the Clinton reform era, networked health insurance products were still not the norm; today they are. This is particularly true for the more than half of all Medicaid beneficiaries enrolled in managed care, whose access to care depends entirely on the capacity of their plan networks. Families of modest income enrolled in subsidized exchange plans will be similarly dependent on plan networks because they will lack the discretionary income to seek out-of-network care.

The increased prominence of disparities in health and health care repre-sents another factor driving Congress's willingness to tackle access as part of health reform. Attention to disparities in health and health care became a signature Clinton administration initiative of the late 1990s—one shared by nationally known researchers, foundations, and prestigious bodies such as the Institute of Medicine. The impact of this focus has been far reaching and has served to propel forward investment in community assets such as health cen-ters, whose services have been shown to reduce disparities while improving patient health outcomes.

A final factor that accounts for the emphasis on health centers in health reform has been the political evolution of the program. Far from being dis-missed as a distraction from or a nose under the tent of national health insur-ance, health centers have come into their own politically over the past decade and have been embraced by champions ranging from the G. W. Bush adminis-tration (which doubled the number of health centers) to the Congressional Black Caucus and the Senate's lone socialist (Vermont's Bernie Sanders).

Health reform will bring a new insurance market to connect with, a restructured Medicare payment system, and millions of new Medicaid beneficiaries. But in Rosenbaum's view, an equally important challenge that lies ahead is the full clinical integration of health centers into the new delivery arrangements and financing structures established under the law. As she notes, clinical integration is a requirement of the program and has been for decades. At the same time, integration has been hard to achieve because of the characteristics of patients served by health centers, the unique corporate structure of FQHCs (governed by community and patient board), and the fed-eral legal interest in the program, which makes FQHCs more highly regulated than other primary care practice groups. These considerations all make the integration pathway complex, and yet affiliations are increasingly common even as health centers face the challenge of primary allegiance to their statutory mission—location and service to medically underserved communities, acceptance of "all comers" regardless of ability to pay, and a unique governance structure. The chapter examines opportunities such as preferred payment rates, risk adjusted premiums, continuing grant support, and joint venture capabilities that together present the basis for propelling health centers into a postreform era.

Dayna Bowen Matthew, the author of chapter 4, considers the crucial issue of undocumented immigrants and their place in American society. Borrowing from the Group Identity Model formulated by social psychologists, health law professor Matthew explores the root cause of the social and political reactions to the problem, reactions sufficiently harsh to make efforts to find a reasonable and ultimately unifying solution difficult. The effects of this visceral social reaction—and efforts to politically capitalize on it—can be seen in the total exclusion of individuals without legal status not merely from health reform's federal subsidy system (following the parallel Medicaid exclusionary policy in place since 1996) but also from the ability to purchase private coverage in health insurance exchanges at any price. The spillover health policy effects of this exclusion are numerous: a permanently uninsured class of US residents without much hope of coverage; an insurance industry empowered to argue for the importance of retaining the individual-insurance market outside of state health insurance exchanges where products are less likely to be overseen for their performance and quality; a continuing high uncompensated care burden on the health care safety net along with heightened political exposure; and entire communities at higher health risk as undocumented residents go without care.

Matthew argues for broad social and political engagement to realign group identities in order to reduce the types of conflicts that have led to these results. She contends that arriving at a place that supports constructive immigration reform will require a conscious employment of the types of lessons learned in the Group Identity Model. Of particular interest to her is use of the model to extend the health care safety net to undocumented immigrants, in stark contrast to the recent trend to isolate and punish, as her numerous examples illustrate. In her view, it is this realignment of identity—the effort to describe undocumented persons in ways that are inclusive rather than exclusionary—that ultimately will make it possible to change the underlying social consciousness from which the political order springs.

In chapter 5, political scientist Thomas R. Oliver and physicians Richard E. Rieselbach, Byron J. Crouse, and John G. Frohna address gaps that will exist in the US health care system regardless of the scope of national reform efforts

now under way. They focus on primary care physician shortages and the associated problems of limited access for underserved segments of the population
and suboptimal primary care graduate medical education. The authors propose
a linkage between primary care graduate medical education and care for
the underserved in community health centers, which must expand to absorb
the anticipated surge in care-seeking among those who are newly insured. The
authors advocate for the establishment of primary care teaching health centers
as a companion to the community health centers program in order to create
focused residency training opportunities and expand workforce capacity and
recruitment. Under their model (a version of which was included in the ACA),
residents would receive their final year of training in specially designated
health centers, followed by the incentive of National Health Service Corps
debt repayment for subsequent practice in an underserved area. Primary care
residents being trained in this setting would immediately increase the clinical
capacity of community health centers and ultimately expand the primary care
physician workforce.

Despite health care reform's support for some safety-net organizations, it
also presents substantial challenges in the form of increasing patient demand
and waning financial resources. In chapter 6, public health law professor
Peter D. Jacobson and his colleagues broadly examine the current organizational
models that FQHCs and community-based organizations are using and assesses
whether the organizational and operational structures are adequate to meet
the primary care needs of the target populations. These needs include acute
care, triage, referrals to specialists, chronic care management, and access to
pharmaceuticals. The ability of safety-net organizations to remain financially
viable while maintaining their mission of providing health care to uninsured
and underinsured populations (the target populations), depends on developing
innovative and efficient health care delivery strategies to meet these needs.
Until now, some federally qualified health centers and most community-based
organizations such as free clinics have viewed themselves as mission oriented;
at best, attention to sound business practices has been a secondary consideration. But as financial pressures and growing unmet need threaten their survival, many safety-net clinics have recognized the need to operate as small
businesses with greater attention to efficiency. What they collectively lack,
however, is the means to identify what those operational and organizational
strategies should be and how they might be implemented.

Drawing from detailed qualitative research of Michigan clinics and a thor-
ough literature review, the chapter addresses a range of important questions:
Are FQHCs, free clinics, or hybrids (clinics that take insurance but are also

committed to serving those without insurance) capable of acting as medical homes? To what extent are connections to larger health care systems necessary to sustain safety-net clinics? To what extent have changes in target population groups (undocumented immigrants and newly unemployed individuals) resulted in new organizational and delivery arrangements? The chapter offers policy recommendations that focus on alternative organizational strategies that could best serve the target populations and ensure a sustainable health care safety net, along with innovative policies that states can adopt.

Safety-Net Hospitals

Under the logic that there will be substantially fewer uninsured people, an important funding source for insurance expansion is to reduce and redirect funds previously aimed at safety-net care for the uninsured. Accordingly, the ACA cuts existing federal payments to hospitals that serve a disproportionate share of uninsured and low-income patients (so-called disproportionate share hospital payments, or DSH payments), just as the Massachusetts reform did with its state safety-net pool. At the same time, hospitals can expect their Medicaid patient load to roughly double, and the ACA does nothing to require or encourage states to increase their current hospital payment rates under Medicaid. These rates average roughly 10 percent below hospitals' costs and a third less than private insurer rates, with rates in some states considerably lower. Unlike physicians, most hospitals have no realistic option to refuse Medicaid patients, but their ability to make up for Medicaid shortfalls will not increase commensurate with their increasing Medicaid patient load. In Massachusetts, this combination of factors caused safety-net hospitals to experience increased financial strain following reform. Part II thus addresses the critical issue of how insurance reform will affect safety-net hospitals.

In chapter 7, political scientists Michael K. Gusmano and Frank J. Thompson assay the evolution of DSH policy and its implementation since the initiative's birth in 1981. DSH provides a particularly vivid example of what social scientists call path dependence; its first decade established the tone for this grant program—one rooted in federal suspicion that states relied on fiscal gimmicks in spending their allotments. The early years also led to the concentration of Medicaid DSH monies in a relatively small number of states. The chapter then explores the degree to which Medicaid DSH effectively targets funds among and within states. Comparing Medicare DSH to Medicaid, the authors conclude that Medicaid targeting suffers from serious limitations—a circumstance that may well shortchange the neediest states and safety-net hospitals. Congressional testimony and debate in the months leading to passage of comprehensive health reform anticipated four challenges that safety-net hospitals will face in the future: they will need to assist eligible patients with enrolling and remaining enrolled; Medicaid payment rates will remain below market levels; attempts to improve targeting of DSH funds will disadvantage some hospitals more than others; and hospitals will be asked to account more clearly for how DSH funds are used. Analyzing these four problem areas, the authors conclude that there is a need to rethink Medicaid DSH as a policy tool.

In chapter 8, health economist Gloria J. Bazzoli and health system administrator Sheryl L. Garland examine the historical context that has led public hospitals and academic medical centers (AMCs) to serve as an important component of the health safety net and how their role in the safety net has been shaped by the stresses they faced. These institutions frequently offer outreach services to uninsured populations, provide primary care services through their emergency departments or affiliated clinics, coordinate referral and specialty services, and collaborate with local agencies to address social and behavioral issues and provide follow-up care. Public hospitals and AMCs have faced many stresses and challenges over the years in maintaining these safety-net roles, including growing numbers of uninsured individuals, changing reimbursement policies and insurance programs, uncertain funding for programs to help offset uncompensated care costs, and growing competition for profitable services that once allowed them to cross-subsidize indigent care. Over time many public hospitals and AMCs have shown their resilience to these stresses in part through the development of collaborative provider networks to address local problems.

The chapter then explores how the ACA will likely affect safety-net hospitals and their ongoing roles in the community, including how these institutions will likely build upon their prior efforts to address future challenges and what questions and concerns remain given the future that could unfold through health reform.

Health care reform presents both challenges and opportunities to public hospitals. To set these in context, public policy researcher Jack Needleman and physician Michelle Ko in chapter 9 review evidence of changes in public hospital capacity and factors that drive both closure/conversions and new openings and investments. Previous literature has noted that the decline in public hospitals has been greater than the overall decline in hospital capacity generally. Little noted, however, is a countertrend, with some new public hospitals opening or private hospitals converting to public status during the 1990s and early 2000s. This chapter analyzes data on the numbers and characteristics of the hospitals and communities in which this countertrend has occurred, and augments this finding with several limited case studies of the reasons for public investment in these facilities. Possible applications of these insights are suggested for shifts in funding anticipated by health insurance reform.

Safety-Net Systems

Earlier sections of this book consider particular parts, providers, and aspects of the safety net. Part III, in contrast, considers the potential for safety-net providers and programs to organize into systems of access and care. In most places safety-net providers are underfunded and experience limited integration with the broader health care system. However, in some parts of the country the safety net serves as a functioning model for clinical integration, with a high presence of medical-home-styled primary health care services linked to specialists and hospitals willing to take referrals on a sliding-scale charity-care basis for patients with greater medical needs. Where this is the case or is possible, we should consider if an adequately funded and structured system of safety-net providers can do a decent job of filling remaining coverage gaps. The overriding goal of health care reform, after all, is to provide affordable access to adequate health care. To the extent that this cannot be achieved by health insurance, perhaps that safety net itself can provide at least minimally adequate access to a fairly comprehensive range of services.

Most research on the safety net tends to focus on the deficiencies of its interstitial role. Lacking is conceptual and policy mapping of how integrated networks of safety-net providers can be formed and supported to provide decent access to medically underserved populations. Rather than continuing to regard the safety net as a last resort for those who remain uninsured, safety-net providers with better funding and integration potentially can serve as a viable first resort for those who lack good access, whether insured or uninsured. This inquiry turns in part on how one defines "adequate" or "decent" access, either with or without insurance.

In chapter 10, Mark A. Hall reviews the empirical and conceptual literature on access measures in the context of safety-net care. In brief, adequacy can be assessed either subjectively (according to the views of those who receive care) or objectively (according to expert opinion based on system characteristics). Normatively, adequacy can be defined by benchmarking these access measures to the levels provided by conventional insurance to similar populations. This conceptualization provides a set of measures that can evaluate whether safety-net systems in fact convey a level of coverage roughly equivalent to that provided by either public or subsidized private insurance.

One frequently stated concern about improvements to safety-net access for the uninsured is that a better safety net will "crowd out" the purchase of private insurance. The use of the term "crowding out" to describe substitution of public access for private health insurance implies a net societal loss due either to inefficiencies or to erosion of a policy goal of reducing the number of uninsured or those without access to health care. Both conceptualizations imply reductions in societal welfare. In chapter 11, health economist Alison Snow Jones (sadly, who died as she was completing this work) examines crowding out in health insurance markets in contexts of both Medicaid expansion and safety-net access for the uninsured. She provides a review and critique of empirical studies that have examined the issue and their findings. She emphasizes both that major studies are methodologically flawed and that they tend to neglect the larger normative question of whether crowd-out in fact results in a net decrease in social welfare. The chapter concludes with a discussion of the ways in which the concept of crowding-out by health and social safety nets should be refined to ensure that the policy goal of improving social welfare is properly understood and comprehensively measured.

Conclusion

Just as the Affordable Care Act will reshape Medicaid and the private insurance market, it will fundamentally change the landscape of the safety net. Insurance reform presents different opportunities and challenges to each part of the safety net, but all parts will need to adapt their institutional strategies and programs to fit the new composition of the thirty million people who will gain insurance, the twenty-three million people who will remain uninsured, and the many millions more who will remain underinsured and underserved.

Doing so may be disruptive. Free-care institutions may need to start charging sliding-scale fees. Community health centers will need to consider affiliating or integrating with the broader delivery systems in their areas. And all institutions will need to articulate justifications for serving undocumented immigrants or people who are not poor. But in these challenges also lie opportunities. With reduced need for free care and increased sources of payment, safety-net institutions may be able to find the right combination of revised mission and financial support to allow them to serve both the uninsured and newly insured better and more comprehensively. Perhaps we will even come within sight of the holy grail of health policy: access to a decent level of care for everyone.

References

Buettgens, M., and M. A. Hall. 2011. "Who Will Be Uninsured after Health Insurance Reform?" March. Urban Institute and Robert Wood Johnson Foundation. http://www.rwjf.org/files/research/71998.pdf.

Hall, M. A. 2010. "The Costs and Adequacy of Safety Net Access for the Uninsured: Boston, Massachusetts." June. Robert Wood Johnson Foundation, Princeton, NJ. http://www.rwjf.org/files/research/safetynetmass201006.pdf.

———. 2011a. "The Mission of Safety Net Organizations Following National Insurance Reform." *Journal of General Internal Medicine* 26, no. 7: 802–805.

———. 2011b. "Rethinking Safety-Net Access for the Uninsured." *New England Journal of Medicine* 364:7–9.

Katz, M. H. 2010. "Future of the Safety Net under Health Reform." *Journal of the American Medical Association* 304, no. 6: 679–680.

Ku, L., E. Jones, B. Finnegan, and S. Rosenbaum. 2009. "How Is the Primary Care Safety Net Faring in Massachusetts? Community Health Centers in the Midst of Health Reform." Issue Brief No. 7878, March 24. Kaiser Commission on Medicaid and the Uninsured, Washington, DC. http://www.kff.org/healthreform/upload/7878.pdf.

Lewin, M. E., and S. Altman 2000. *America's Health Care Safety Net: Intact but Endangered.* Washington, DC: National Academies Press.

Short, P. F., K. Swartz, N. Uberoi, and D. Graefe. 2011. "Implementing National Health Insurance Reforms: Maintaining Affordability, Shared Responsibility, and Continuity When Life Changes." New York: Commonwealth Fund.

Sommers, B. D., and S. Rosenbaum. 2011. "Issues in Health Reform: How Changes in Eligibility May Move Millions Back and Forth Between Medicaid and Insurance Exchanges." *Health Affairs* 30, no. 2: 228–236.

Part I

Community Health Centers

Dr. StrangeRove; or, How Conservatives Learned to Stop Worrying and Love Community Health Centers

Almost sixty million Americans—about one in five—go without regular primary care (NACHC 2009a; AHRQ 2006). Lack of access is not simply a matter of insurance status; the difficulty of finding a primary care provider is a massive barrier to the use of primary care. Traditionally, charity care for the medically indigent has existed outside of government channels. From the early 1900s, local and county governments experimented with funding, coordinating, and even providing ambulatory care; none of these efforts survived attacks by local physicians. But beginning in the mid-1960s the federal government began funding a new mode of primary care delivery: community health centers.

Community health centers are not-for-profit entities serving residents of areas designated by the Department of Health and Human Services (HHS) as "medically underserved." Subsisting on third-party reimbursements (mainly Medicaid), competitive federal grants and loan guarantees awarded by the HHS, and some state and local governmental support and philanthropic funding, they provide comprehensive ambulatory care, either free or on a sliding scale. Centers also offer different mixes of "enabling" services, from case management and transportation to and from the facility, to translation services, and to substance abuse programs, immunizations, and screenings. In addition, all centers regularly assess community health problems and conduct health education and outreach programming; some target specific populations, such as migrant workers, public housing residents, homeless individuals, and elementary and secondary school children.

Today, more than 1,100 centers provide what is considered cost-effective and high-quality care to more than twenty million Americans at more than

7,900 delivery sites. Health centers improve access and use for the under-served, and reduce ethnic and racial disparities in health outcomes. About one-third of their patients are Hispanic (most of whom rely on bilingual staff), and another quarter are African American. Seventy percent of patients are poor. Fully 60 percent of users have some form of health insurance.[1]

The health centers program constitutes the country's largest primary care system. With annual expenditures of more than $7 billion (not including addi-tional funding through FY 2015 provided through the Patient Protection and Affordable Care Act of 2010 [Affordable Care Act, or ACA]), community health centers now occupy a central role in America's safety net of health care provi-sion. Combining primary care with some public health functions—a departure from the traditional bifurcation of medical care from public health—health cen-ters also feature a quite radical governance structure begun during the program's origins during the War on Poverty: a majority of each center's governing board must consist of active patients residing nearby (Brandt and Gardner 2000).

Excluding state and local sources, patient payments, and third-party reimbursements, HHS spends more than $2 billion per year on the program (figure 2.1). Relying more than other health facilities on nurse practitioners, physicians' assistants, and other non-MD health professionals, health centers are also heavily dependent on the National Health Service Corps and other federal medical workforce programs. Just over one-half of health centers are in rural areas while just over one-half of all patients reside in urban areas. Health centers exist in every state, in more than 90 percent of congressional districts, but in only about one-quarter of those areas designated by HHS as medically underserved (Iglehart 2010, 343). The program is managed by HHS's well-regarded Health Resources and Services Administration (HRSA), and for more than three decades a highly effective national lobby and its state affiliates have played a critical role in the program's survival and its recent, strange expansion.

Begun as a demonstration project during the War on Poverty, the program has until recently remained in the shadows of the health care system. Uncon-troversial and of low salience to members of Congress, it muddled through for three decades. Targeted by Republican administrations and conservatives for reduction or elimination through budget cuts or conversion into block grants, it survived but never experienced the massive expansion for which its propo-nents long hoped. The Clinton administration was also strangely uninterested in it, and it grew during the 1990s only due to the initiative of a bipartisan coalition in Congress and improved financing arrangements. In the past decade, a massive expansion has occurred, but under the unlikely stewardship of the George W. Bush administration. While many other programs for the poor

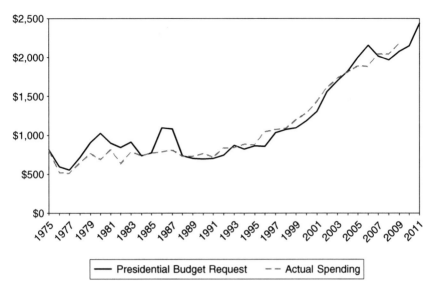

Figure 2.1 Federal Spending on Community Health Centers, 1975 to 2011 (millions, in constant 2010 dollars)

Source: The Budget of the US Government, Appendix, 1975–2009

or medically underserved were slashed or eliminated during the Bush years, the number of delivery sites has tripled since 2000 and the number of patients served has more than doubled. Plans folded into the ACA are even bolder; funding commitments call again for these centers to double their patients served to *forty* million by 2015, or fully two-thirds of America's medically underserved (Ku et al. 2010).

This bizarre trajectory, I argue, cannot be explained simply by shifts in party control of Congress or the White House, ideological trends, or the vagaries of distributive politics. Rather, the ebbs and flows of this program are best understood as the product of political learning. I argue that Democrats and Republicans learned lessons during the long battle over national health insurance (NHI), that they adapted their positions on health policies in light of these lessons, and that these adaptations help explain the trajectory of the health centers program. Beginning in the 1970s Republicans came to see the health centers program, and particularly its national expansion, as part of a strategy to facilitate Democratic proposals for universal coverage. NHI proponents would, Republicans feared, be able to point to the existence of a network of facilities for the poor already in place, thus reducing some of the practical difficulties of creating a workable system. Republican attempts to eliminate the program are best viewed in the context of their efforts to tear down the welfare state through a frontal assault. Meanwhile, by the 1990s many progressives devoted to the attainment of universal health coverage had developed a strange ambivalence toward programs for the underserved. They came to see them, in Leninist "one step forward" fashion, as weakening pressures for systemic reform of the health care system.

Over time, conservatives came to agree with them. This chapter explains the Bush administration's embrace of the program as an adaptation to conservatives' earlier failures to retrench the US welfare state head on, and as part of a renewed effort by conservatives to "limit—or, more often, refocus and redirect—activist government." The Bush health centers expansion was consistent with other federal interventions into health care, education, and pensions. These interventions, while angering many fiscal conservatives, grow out of their adaptation to lessons learned: a longer-term strategy to build some government programs in order to shrink other larger programs (Pierson and Skocpol 2007, 3; Glenn and Teles 2009). Bush's health centers initiative reflected this new understanding as well as lessons that Karl Rove and others learned about the electoral consequences of their party's vilification during budget battles with President Bill Clinton in the mid-1990s. The response to this second set of lessons helped produce "compassionate conservatism."

Thus, the early conservative attack, many progressives' puzzling ambivalence toward health centers, and the subsequent conservative embrace are, I argue, explicable in terms of learning and adaptation. I describe the origins and development of the health centers program amidst the War on Poverty, and I chart how the program muddled through from the Nixon years until 2001. Of particular importance here is the ambivalence shown toward the program by the Clinton administration. I offer an explanation of the puzzling Bush health centers initiative. The chapter closes by discussing some challenges facing the program in the aftermath of the landmark ACA.[2]

The Prehistory of the Federal Community Health Centers Program

Traditionally, public health and medical care in the United States were squarely the concern of local communities, especially their private actors. States and the federal government evinced little interest in these matters, save for episodic outbreaks of cholera and other infectious diseases (Duffy 1990). During the first three decades of the twentieth century, a health centers movement emerged in America's cities, growing out of similar circumstances, organizational forms, and objectives as those that would appear in the 1960s—in particular, recent demographic changes in American cities. Reformers focused on the medically indigent urban poor, the vast majority of whom were thought culturally different from the mainstream.[3] They sought to rationalize medical care through community health planning and to disperse medical care in stations or clinics at the neighborhood level. By one count, more than 1,500 centers operated in the United States in 1930. But the term "health center" was applied broadly; it referred to child welfare stations, tuberculosis dispensaries, hospital outpatient departments, settlement houses, local health department substations, and so on. Very few of these offered a full range of primary care. They were not meant to supplant the role of doctors but performed diagnoses and made referrals to private physicians. Still, local medical societies strongly objected to them and blocked efforts by state legislatures to assist them. They faded in the 1930s (Davis 1927; Hiscock 1935, 434; Starr 1982).

For most of its history, the federal government was effectively absent from the provision of health care, apart from its efforts on behalf of a few populations (merchant marines, military personnel, federal prisoners, Native Americans, etc.). This situation began to change somewhat in the early 1920s with the provision of grants to states for establishing centers for prenatal and child care and health education.[4] During the New Deal, the federal government began experimenting with other public health grants to states (Stern 1946).[5] In 1946 President Harry S. Truman signed the landmark Hill–Burton Act, and the federal government's involvement in medical care began in earnest. Over the next two decades, federal matching grants for hospital construction and modernization—alongside "urban renewal" development projects—helped reshape the local political economy of health care access. By 1971 more than $60 billion (in 2009 dollars) had been spent on almost eleven thousand projects. Hill–Burton helped construct the modern American hospital. But this and other federal interventions did not much change American primary care, the main features of which had taken shape by the 1920s. Most individuals saw fee-for-service doctors in solo practice. Hospital outpatient departments provided some primary care to means-tested charity patients. While there were networks of health reformers, some of whom challenged this orthodoxy, few communities nurtured critical masses of health professionals calling for new ways to deliver care to the medically indigent (Sardell 1988, 37; Derickson 2002; Hoffman 2003).[6]

While most observers of American primary care may have been confident in the basic arrangements, they began to notice problems. Accelerated by technological advances, federal support of biomedical research, and facilities construction, the share of general practitioners (GP) was in sharp decline.[7] As an older generation of primary care providers began to relocate or retire, the maldistribution of GPs increased in central cities throughout the 1950s. Poorer city residents increasingly sought care in hospital outpatient departments and emergency rooms (Hoffman 2006). Meanwhile, the demographics of these central cities were changing quickly. At the time of the consolidation of the "second ghetto" in non-Southern cities in the 1930s, the average black city dweller lived in a neighborhood that was about 40 percent black; by 1970 this would rise to 68 percent. Poverty was becoming much more concentrated, and white residents as well as health professionals began to exit central cities in larger and larger numbers in the 1950s. As the quality of care increased for many Americans, it declined in many cities. By 1965 majority-black neighborhoods numbering tens of thousands of residents relied on sometimes no more than five or six doctors, most semiretired (Lashof 1968; Richmond 1969, 94).

On the eve of the development of the community health centers program, observers could reflect back on a recent history in which public health functions remained isolated from the provision of medical care, and local medical establishments had defeated or deterred local and state governments from developing coordinated institutions of subsidized care for the medically indigent. Those interested in developing new arrangements had a good sense of the barriers facing them.

The Origins of the Community Health Centers Amid the War on Poverty

The community health centers program emerged from the confluence of several factors: structural changes in US politics, savvy policy entrepreneurs, pressures from below, and a search by empowered federal officials for policy alternatives that fit their own goals. Here, I sketch the origins of the program and discuss the politics of its early expansion and performance.

The overarching context in which the health centers program developed was an especially propitious environment for new social policymaking. President John Kennedy's death provided President Lyndon Johnson with an opportunity to pursue his longstanding interest in attacking poverty. However, Johnson's 1964 landslide victory over Goldwater, coupled with now massive Democratic majorities in Congress, provided the real political opening. In their absence, the Great Society along with its War on Poverty programs would not have been possible.

Besides this structural opportunity, the Johnson administration felt pressured from many quarters to address issues of poverty and inequality, especially as these affected American cities. As early as 1964 the administration perceived the need to craft urban policies that would reduce material deprivation and thereby reduce the likelihood of riots and other threats to social order. And Johnson was himself personally driven to attack poverty in cities and in rural America. With respect to electoral considerations, even after the landslide victory over Goldwater, Johnson and others in his administration were growing worried about the health of the Democratic Party's New Deal coalition. As "white ethnics" streamed out to the suburbs, the White House felt an urgent need to cement the party loyalty of America's increasingly black and brown cities—and, if necessary, to do so by delivering policy benefits to them over and around potentially recalcitrant city halls.[8]

The War on Poverty also provided a favorable institutional setting. In early 1964 the White House began to develop the legislation that came to be known as the Economic Opportunity Act (EOA), as well as plans for the Office of Economic Opportunity (OEO). Johnson preferred that War on Poverty programs be developed and implemented by the OEO, a new agency housed within the Executive Office of the President. This was done partly to facilitate more rapid, innovative programs that would not be slowed or stalled in the federal bureaucracy (Flanagan 2001). The OEO would be staffed by officials highly sympathetic to Johnson's aims. Many of them had been involved in, or witness to, direct action and other campaigns in the South and North beginning in the 1940s.[9] Thus, when the poverty warriors would turn to the health care of the poor, they did so in communities already marked by episodic organized protest on health issues.[10]

A sustained, federal intervention into the provision of primary care was anything but preordained. Of course, health care was in the forefront of the administration's policy goals. Medicare and Medicaid would become law during the same year that the first health centers were established. Still, the EOA did not suggest that the federal government's antipoverty programs would impinge upon medical care. Nor did OEO staff or White House officials plan on developing health-related programs. However, as other programs such as Head Start and Job Corps conducted physical and dental exams for its participants, OEO staffers were shocked by the magnitude of the health problems they encountered. According to one report, 70 percent of Head Start children had never seen a doctor (Geiger 1984). This led OEO staff and, later, community action agencies to develop health delivery projects as part of other antipoverty programs, such as Volunteers in Service to America (VISTA).

OEO officials could choose to help local community action agencies develop a range of small projects or they could develop a program that, if successful, could be deployed on a larger scale. Still, they believed that the poor had much more complex health needs than the nonpoor, and that these needs were not being met by current arrangements of uneven charity care and beleaguered city hospitals. Federal bureaucrats and other policymakers located within the executive branch developed key precepts of the War on Poverty—including its emphasis on community participation, enshrined in the EOA—from a variety of sources. The roots of many programs later associated with the War on Poverty began several years earlier in the form of interventions by philanthropic foundations and governments to attack problems of juvenile delinquency and joblessness. Casting about for ideas to develop programs of medical care for the poor, OEO staffers were disappointed with what they found via inquiries to the Department of Health, Education, and Welfare (HEW), and in particular its Public Health Service (Administrative History Papers 1974, 131, 327; Schorr 1988, 130). Thus, even after OEO officials had convinced themselves that an expansion of antipoverty programming into health care was advisable, developing something like a health centers program was still far from likely.

Then, one day in early 1965, Dr. William Kissick, assistant to the Surgeon General of the US Public Health Service, called Lee Bamberger Schorr, an OEO official with a background in health policy. "There's a wild man in my office, and he's got some ideas we can't do much with over here, but I think you people in the War on Poverty would find him pretty interesting. I'm sending him right over." Jack Geiger met with Schorr, and the health centers program soon began (Schorr 1988, 130–131). Geiger, a physician long active in efforts to fight race-based inequalities in the United States, had worked in the 1950s as part of a legendary effort in rural South Africa to craft what public health advocates now call "community-oriented primary care."

Along with a collaborator, Dr. Count Gibson Jr., Geiger developed a funding proposal to establish two community health centers that built on the South Africa model. The first would be in Boston's Columbia Point, a predominantly black housing project. The second, later named the Delta Health Center, would operate in Bolivar County, Mississippi, a rural, predominantly black area. The centers would provide comprehensive ambulatory care to all residents in these severely medically underserved areas (Geiger 2005, 314; Lefkowitz 2007, 35). Like those in South Africa, these centers would conduct aggressive outreach work through the employment of local residents as health workers. They would also provide a range of public health functions. And the centers were to be managed and operated in part by residents themselves.[11]

OEO staff welcomed the proposal, and Geiger and Gibson won approval for grants for both centers in June 1965.[12] The funding source was the research and demonstration authorization of the OEO's Community Action

Program. Both centers were quickly successful in increasing access to primary care, and in developing and implementing public health functions (Administrative History Papers 1974, 346; Geiger 2002, 1715; Geiger 2005, 317; Dittmer 2009).

Through these and a handful of other grants over the next year, the health centers program began to take shape. Several important decisions were made early on. First, the program would continue to develop quietly, without the visibility that would come with its own statutory authorization or budget line. As a research and demonstration project, it would be housed in the research and development office of the Community Action Program.[13] Second, the program would operate by providing grants in a competitive process. Applicants would have to come from a public or private nonprofit organization, and would have to be sponsored by another institution, whether a community action agency, medical school, hospital, or local health department. A sufficient coalition of actors within a community would have to want health centers in order to receive federal funding for them. It is generally agreed that the OEO (and, later, the HEW) kept "politics" out of the grant evaluation process. Third, in keeping with the "maximum feasible participation" directive of the EOA, all centers would have to be either advised or actually governed by nearby residents. Fourth, all residents living in a center's designated catchment area (between ten thousand and thirty thousand) would be eligible for free care. Fifth, centers would provide not just comprehensive ambulatory care but also what would come to be called supplementary services, from health education to substance abuse to transportation arrangement and outreach efforts. Sixth, health workers would explore new ways of using support staff and developing careers for poor residents.

Growth, Eligibility, Financing, and Community Relations

By 1971 there were between eighty and one hundred ongoing projects, three-quarters of them in urban areas (particularly those where black protest had been strong) (Hollister 1974, 2; Hollister, Kramer, and Bellin 1974, 17). The health centers were often thought of as "ghetto medicine," a view that did not change much until the rapid expansion of rural centers during the Carter administration. Some preferred that the program develop slowly and remain small enough so that it did not develop bureaucratic requirements that would stymie the ability of centers to adapt to local needs, conditions, and resources (Administrative History Papers 1974, 326). From this perspective, it was an asset that the program was a demonstration project shielded from congressional oversight and much publicity. Those who sought to revolutionize the provision of primary care, or those who wanted to maximize access to the underserved, wanted a much larger funded program to develop quickly. For instance, an HEW planning document in 1967 called for the establishment of one thousand centers that would serve some twenty-five million poor individuals by 1975. Projected costs were $3.5 billion (or about $15 billion in 2009 dollars) (HEW 1967; Lefkowitz 2007, 10).

Besides budget constraints, there were additional limits on the size of the program on both the supply and demand sides. The OEO lacked the administrative capacity to encourage, review, and help implement many federal grants (Administrative History Papers 1974, 327, 337–338).[14] Moreover, the number and quality of applications depended in part on the number of local health care reformers. A weak infrastructure nationwide limited the number of communities with a critical mass of reform-minded medical professionals who could agitate, advocate, and cajole potential health center sponsors to help develop and sign onto grant proposals.

After a few years of receiving and encouraging grant proposals from maverick, reformist public health activists and medical professionals, it became increasingly difficult for potential applicants to find sponsoring institutions that would accept the required governance structure and other features of the program (Lefkowitz 2007, 12). A successful application required that an organization could demonstrate that it had the potential involvement of health professionals and institutions as well as a physical location, a financial plan, and so on. Local and state networks of health center advocates were vital for encouraging organizations within communities to apply; the communities in greatest need often lacked the resources to craft competitive applications. Of course, in the mid-1960s, these networks had not yet developed. Many communities were prevented from submitting competitive applications often for the same reason they needed health centers: the lack of primary care providers. The program began almost ten years before the first group of National Health Service Corps physicians began arriving at (usually rural) centers (Zwick 1972, 392, 404).

Within the OEO, views differed on key issues such as eligibility. OEO initially imagined that all residents of a health center's designated area would be eligible for free care there, and program guidelines reflected this. However, this preference was based in part on their expectation that some 80 percent of families in designated neighborhoods lived below the federal poverty line. This estimate was significantly off; the actual share was between 40 and 60 percent. If centers came to serve as the regular primary care provider for a higher share of the nonpoor, the program would be open to the same criticism that ultimately killed off the health centers of the 1920s—that the nonpoor abused the public trust as private physicians lost patients to the state. Officials in OEO's legal and political offices therefore opposed a geographic eligibility standard. They were not disappointed, then, when Congress in 1967 restricted free care to "low-income" residents. In the OEO's interpretation of this statutory language, the poverty index or the particular state's Medicaid income eligibility standard was to be used. Thus the program became known as "poor people's medicine." Of course, the near-poor would be shut out of this arrangement. In 1969, spurred on by complaints from local doctors, Congress held that although health centers could serve families above poverty on a partial or full-pay basis, no more than one-fifth of all patients could be served in this manner (Zwick 1972, 410). Observers argued later that these restrictions on health centers' ability to rely on paying patients "guaranteed the almost total dependence of the . . . program on public funds" (Davis and Schoen 1978).

In 1965 OEO officials never envisioned that the centers would become fully federally funded. Indeed, the hope was that local resources, paying patients, and Medicare and Medicaid would develop self-sufficient centers (Schorr and English 1974). Medicare and Medicaid—especially the latter— would be the key to financing the centers. Indeed, Medicaid officials expected that the program would be able to support health centers across all fifty states by 1975. Federal grants, then, would provide resources for establishing centers and perhaps expanding the services they could offer but would not be critical to year-to-year operation.

On this view, the program's fate depended on the reimbursement arrangements that OEO made with HEW (for Medicare and maternal and child health programs), HEW and the states (for Medicaid), and private insurers. By the late 1960s it was clear that the early hopes of financial self-sufficiency would not be fulfilled. State Medicaid programs restricted rather than expanded both eligibility standards and the scope of reimbursable services. Some did not even recognize health centers as facilities qualifying for reimbursement. Adding insult to injury, both Medicaid and Medicare developed much more generous reimbursement systems with hospital outpatient departments. Still, health centers treated many patients not covered by state Medicaid programs. Even worse for their financing, they remained true to their mission. By the early 1970s only about 60 percent of operating expenses went to medical care. Dental care absorbed another 15 percent, as did health education, community organization, and social work—none of which Medicaid reimbursed. By the early 1970s Medicaid and Medicare constituted less than 20 percent of operating revenues (Zwick 1972; GAO 1973, 79; Sardell 1988; Schorr 1988).

Most centers partnered with hospitals and medical schools. This was part of a conscious strategy by OEO staff to prevent local opposition. Reform-minded medical professionals were more likely to be located in these institutions than, say, local health departments; the latter often resented competing for control of services for the medically indigent with others, or were ideologically opposed to the mixture of medical care and public health functions (Colgrove 2007, 15).[15] Indeed, medical schools submitted the best applications. Another motive drove this pattern—because this was a new program initiated by a quickly beleaguered agency, there was a strong desire among OEO staffers that the first wave of centers succeed. Finally, any OEO grants to "limited purpose organizations" such as community action agencies could be vetoed by governors, and OEO officials feared Southern vetoes of health care funds. However, educational institutions such as medical schools were exempt from this rule.

From the start, program administrators leaned on grantees to involve members of the local medical establishment wherever possible in order to tamp down opposition to the centers. Additionally, health centers were directed by hospital staff, medical school faculty, officials from local health departments, and physicians in private practice.

Local (white) medical societies often opposed health centers in their early days. Still, outright battles with local doctors and grant applicants were not very common; doctors rarely intervened in communities where applications had been submitted. Hospitals were at first hesitant about accepting health centers. After all, health centers could be seen as competing with hospitals' own outpatient departments. However, many came to appreciate the presence of health centers for reducing problems of overcrowding. Later still, some saw them as competition as their worries shifted to empty beds, especially given expanding new opportunities for recouping third-party payments (Hollister 1974, 17).

Advocates and Critics

There were early concerns that the American Medical Association (AMA) might kill off the program. Young senator Ted Kennedy (D-MA) was chosen to sell the program on the Hill, and his staff crafted amendments to the EOA.[16] In 1966 Congress provided for the funding of "comprehensive health service programs" for the underserved in both rural and urban areas. Kennedy proposed a budget of $100 million, but about $51 million dollars was authorized (for thirty-three existing centers and eight new ones). Congress nodded at centers' less strictly health-related activities, noting that whenever possible they should furnish "arrangements for providing employment, education, social or other assistance needed by the families and individuals served." Kennedy argued that the program should be viewed separately from other War on Poverty programs; health centers, unlike community action agencies, were apolitical.[17]

At this time Congress began to fund a range of regional health planning projects, formula grants to states for health services, and state comprehensive health planning agencies. Much of this activity came in the form of block grants authorized by the Partnership for Health Act. The legislation also authorized project grants for new types of health services. Vague language provided the surgeon general (then head of the Public Health Service) with discretion to operate many different programs. A small coalition of health center advocates inside the HEW eventually won this budget line as a safe place from which to fund health centers.[18]

In Washington the health centers program engendered little discussion and even less controversy.[19] This was in part a function of the program's small size; in terms of appropriations, it lagged far behind youth programs, Job Corps, Head Start, VISTA, and other programs. Many OEO controversies involved the mobilization of the poor—especially blacks and Hispanics—in central cities. But health centers were effectively framed in congressional hearings as non-political in a way that other OEO programs were not. Still, the appearance of a new generation of "activist MDs" often proved controversial at the local level. In some cities, large conflicts were sparked by health centers and other efforts to introduce community input in the governance of health facilities (including mental health clinics and hospitals) (Mullan 1976).

For the program's first decade, the (white) AMA as a national body vacillated between rejecting almost any federal role in health care delivery and seeking a leadership role in the health centers program for local medical societies.[20] Despite OEO's commitments to AMA representatives that its projects would not compete with local physicians, medical societies sometimes blocked applications, and it is likely that many more individuals and groups were self-deterred by potential opposition. But in 1969, just four years after the program began, the OEO considered the AMA a strong supporter of the program. In the interim, the AMA had become somewhat more image-conscious. Medical schools soon came around, often in part to deflect standard "town/gown" criticisms of their (non)involvement in communities. The black National Medical Association was mostly supportive, but at the local level, groups of black health care professionals and community groups frequently charged that OEO failed to incorporate black doctors into the program (Boyce 1969; Richard 1969).

As oversight of OEO increased and its budget declined, the heat on the program rose. OEO (and later HEW) was pressured to evaluate the program

according to some often-ridiculous standards—such as demonstrating immediate reductions in rates of infant mortality (Tilson 1973; Hollister 1974). Early
assessments suggested that centers increased access and use of health care,
reduced the use of emergency rooms by the poor, and elicited positive assessments by users (Hillman and Charney 1972; Zwick 1972). Serious criticisms
existed on both the left and right. From the right, they were criticized as too
costly and inefficient. In particular, there were often administrative problems,
especially involving recordkeeping, securing reimbursement from third-party
payers, and personnel issues. From the left, there was some concern that the
program merely maintained rather than alleviated a "two-tiered" health care
system, and that they served as a safety valve to relieve pressure on systemic
health care reform (Torrens 1971; Hollister 1974, 3; Marcus 1981). On the eve
of Nixon's inauguration, the future of the program was in doubt.

Health Centers from Nixon through Bush, 1969–1993

What is impressive about the health centers program across this quarter-
century is its stability amid so much change. The program was transferred multiple times across and within cabinet departments and agencies, and survived
attempts to reduce or eliminate it by three Republican presidents. Begun as a
predominantly urban program dispensing what many called "ghetto medicine," community health centers had to weather an abrupt decline in interest
in and attention to America's cities. Moreover, they had to compete for attention amid various proposals for health maintenance organizations (HMO), NHI,
and calls for the retrenchment of Medicare and Medicaid. Meanwhile, the
problems driving the program worsened, among them increasing numbers of
underserved and uninsured individuals and decaying safety-net facilities.
Over this period, the program did develop a means to defend itself in the form
of a federated lobby. But it also developed more serious opponents. As the
program wended its way through the 1970s and 1980s, conservatives began to
see it less as a small, if inefficient program, better administered by the states
and more as one step in a carefully planned incrementalist drive toward NHI.

The Nixon and Ford Years

The rapid expansion of medical costs put cost containment at the forefront of
President Richard Nixon's health agenda (Richmond and Fein 2005, 59–60).
During his first term, Democrats continued to capture the momentum on developing credible NHI proposals, most importantly the Kennedy–Griffiths proposal. In late 1970 Nixon searched for a way to advance his own health reform
as this momentum increased. He asked HEW secretary Elliott Richardson to

prepare a major "presidential health message" describing Nixon's alternative health insurance proposal, with HMOs as its centerpiece. However, OEO director Donald Rumsfeld proposed an alternative restructuring of the health care system: a network of eight hundred to one thousand health centers providing primary care to tens of millions of Americans. The idea was rejected for several reasons, among which were HEW's preference for HMOs and the fact that calling for an expansion of a War on Poverty program would not allow Nixon to leave his own mark on health policy (Nixon 1971).[21]

Perhaps more consequential for the health centers program was Nixon's determination to reverse President Johnson's "creative federalism." For Nixon, an appropriate balance of power between the federal government and the states required for devolution to the states of program administration. Given his proposed massive expansions of income transfers to the poor, his concerns seemed less budgetary than administrative. Plans for several large block grants coupled with revenue sharing would, he hoped, allow states to administer federal funds more effectively. Block grants would reduce the administrative complexity and poor performance of hundreds of federal programs in states and municipalities, each with its own (often contradictory) requirements. Additionally, Nixon sought to shrink the federal bureaucracy he so loathed and distrusted (Conlan 1998).[22]

Nixon's efforts were generally unsuccessful. Proposing six large block grants, he was able to secure passage of two of them through a distrustful Democratic-controlled Congress. Block grants have always been feared by constituencies of discretionary programs. When funds are transferred to states, a mad scramble often ensues to preserve funding for each program. But the situation for health centers was much more difficult than usual. First, the program served social groups who had very little power. Second, states had not come to rely on this new program. Thus, surmised its proponents, it would have to compete for funds with other programs for the disadvantaged and would have to face off against much more politically influential programs (such as those providing funding to hospitals). Health centers, they feared, would be early victims in the budgetary politics that followed a conversion of federal health programs into block grants. For reasons that had little to do with the particularities of the program, Congress defeated proposals to block grant health centers. But the specter of health centers' death-by-block-grants would appear again.

OEO remained supportive of the health centers program, which it saw as generally successful.[23] Nevertheless, Nixon downgraded OEO into an incubator of new programs, as was expected; more stable ones would be moved to relevant agencies. From 1970 operational responsibilities for the health centers program began to be transferred gradually to HEW, a process that ended in

1973 when the OEO was effectively terminated. There was a good deal of concern that the move from OEO to HEW would damage the program. HEW's regional offices oversaw health centers and took over the grant awards process. However, the staff of these regional offices rarely had experience with or taste for health centers (Sardell 1988, 79). More generally, health center advocates feared that the move from OEO to HEW would rob the program of its staunchest allies in the executive branch during its hour of need, and might defang the program of its most provocative features. Most important here were the centers' provision of nonmedical and social services, and their community governance requirements. However, by the time the move occurred, a small but determined group of advocates for the program had developed in HEW's new Bureau of Comprehensive Health Services (which was established in 1972 as part of another reorganization of the Public Health Service).

Besides the danger of block grants, Nixon (and, later, President Gerald Ford) opposed what seemed like runaway growth in federal spending via discretionary grants and sought to attack them directly. (Here, community health centers were not themselves singled out among primary care programs.) The Nixon administration directed the HEW to reduce or eliminate discretionary programs the administration had been unable to block-grant back to the states. HEW had been forced by the White House to cease its communication with congressional supporters of health centers, part of a larger "centralized politicization" of the executive branch during the Nixon years (Nathan 1975). Relatedly, the White House demanded that the program justify its existence in terms of both cost-benefit analysis and financial self-sufficiency. In 1972 and 1973 the HEW published regulations claiming that the health centers' statutory authorization required them to become self-sufficient. Thus, federal grants supporting them would be ending.

Given the financing problems presented by Medicare and Medicaid, self-sufficiency was out of the question unless the health centers were to be converted into the barest of clinics (GAO 1973). The Medicaid situation was dire. In 1973 federal bureaucrats required states to provide outpatient care at hospital "clinics" to Medicaid patients, but payment to health centers were considered "optional." Four years later, only twenty-two states and Washington, DC, recognized health centers as "clinics" and therefore guaranteed their reimbursement. Even when so recognized, only five of these states reimbursed centers for their outreach services. Worse, neither Medicare nor Medicaid reimbursed health centers for the work of nontraditional providers, such as nurse practitioners, physician assistants, and family health workers.[24] Finally, reimbursement rates for Medicaid were often very low. The continued provision of federal grants was thus imperative. Ultimately, HEW decided to guarantee continued financing but demanded that centers rely more heavily on third-party payers (GAO 1973; Sardell 1988, 87, 127–128; Lefkowitz 2007, 20).

The budgetary authority used for health centers remained a vague "projects" line for HEW. The weakness of lacking its own specified budgetary authority was becoming apparent, for Nixon used this same budget line to finance HMO demonstration projects.[25] These projects effectively squeezed out health center funding. In 1971 one hundred OEO centers and about fifty HEW centers were in operation. From 1971 to 1973, no grants were awarded to establish new centers. Still, congressional appropriations each year exceeded Nixon's requests. Members from highly rural and highly urban states were most supportive.

The most serious threat to the program's survival occurred when Nixon (and later Ford) opposed the reauthorization of grants for health centers. At the time, health centers and twelve other health programs were due to expire at the end of fiscal year (FY) 1973. Nixon proposed that health centers and five related programs not be reauthorized, and the remainder reduced in size. Congress balked, extending funding for the threatened six for one more year. Congress did so by veto-proof margins, and Nixon signed this into law in June 1974. Congress then sought to stabilize the program through new legislation that specifically authorized "community health centers" by name and with its own designated funding. It did so by unanimous voice vote in the Senate and by a vote of 359–12 in the House. The program clearly remained uncontroversial, but Ford pocket-vetoed the legislation in December 1974, arguing that it "would result in an unjustified expenditure of federal taxpayers' funds" (Ford 1974). Congress repeated the process in 1975, Ford vetoed the bill, and Congress overrode his veto by huge margins.

Health centers had, for the first time, their own legislative authority.[26] They now also had legislative protection from future Republican presidents who might seek to use HEW rulemaking powers to weaken the centers. Congressional advocates did this by explicitly defining "primary" (required) services and so-called supplementary (recommended) services. Still, Ford continued to fight health centers and major discretionary health programs through low budget requests, another veto, and continued efforts to block-grant these programs. He envisioned replacing not just these small programs but also Medicaid and all health planning funding with revenue sharing (Sardell 1988, 100–101, 111).

Organized Interests

At the national level, the AMA continued to send mixed signals. While ostensibly advocating for the program's continuation, AMA president Carl A. Hoffman,

MD, suggested in 1972 that armed guards be stationed outside "ghetto health centers" in order to overcome doctors' reluctance to work in them (*New York Times*, Nov. 27, 1972). But the AMA did not deploy its still considerable political forces in Washington against the program during congressional deliberations. Rather, it voiced in rather perfunctory fashion its arguments for a more limited federal role in the provision of health care. One observer suggested that serious opposition would develop only "when the program gets bigger." These mixed signals may have reflected ideological and generational conflict within the national organization. Perhaps more important than the lobbying of the national association was the behavior of county medical societies. At the local level its county medical societies seemed to have made their peace with the program; by 1982 they were considered "overwhelmingly positive" toward the health centers. The passage of time convinced many that health centers would not destroy their private practices. And the relative importance of local doctors' preferences vis-à-vis the AMA grew over time as a result both of the waning power of the latter and of the increasing share of congressional districts featuring health centers (Sardell 1988, 94–95, 80–81, 183).

Over this period, the most important development regarding organized interests was the birth and growth of a lobby for health centers. Termed a "health centers movement" by those involved, the National Association of Community Health Centers (NACHC) formed in the early 1970s and played a pivotal role in the program's survival and growth. The federal government also played a critical role in accelerating the development of the NACHC by awarding it training and research grants. OEO staffers were well aware of the need for a "viable political constituency" supporting health centers. By 1973 it had supplanted the regional networks of health centers that had begun in the late 1960s. However, it was not until the late 1970s that the NACHC moved to center stage in health center policymaking. While useful in congressional deliberations and helping advocates within HEW prevent cuts in the list of services required of health centers, the lobby's real impact would be felt a few years later, as it did battle with the Reagan administration.[27]

In another significant development, in the 1980s the Robert Wood Johnson Foundation helped fund efforts by the NACHC to develop state-level primary care associations and nine regional associations (mirroring HEW-designated regions) (Sardell 1988, 190). State-level lobbies were potentially important, especially in congressional deliberations about funding and finance mechanisms. Finally, as health centers became established in their communities, their governing boards became important political supporters. Impressively, the community governance element of health center governance did not fade, even as the mantra of "maximum feasible participation" had been replaced, at least in elite policy circles, with the mocking phrase "maximum feasible misunderstanding." On the contrary, governance requirements grew *more* demanding, not less. By 1973 OEO required that community participation be effected only through governing, not advisory, boards featuring a majority of active consumers. Many of the nonconsumer members were pillars of their communities, knowledgeable about politics, and familiar with their member of Congress. Over time, the duration of health centers thus came to enhance their durability.

The Carter Administration

Health policy during the Carter years is remembered for the failed attempts to contain hospital costs and for the failure of progressives and political leaders to converge behind a single NHI proposal. Even in failure, though, the administration's own NHI proposal confirmed many conservatives' suspicion that the expansion of community health centers was a key part of a long-term plot to secure NHI.

In 1977 the incoming Carter administration gave reason for both health center advocates and proponents of NHI to be optimistic (Iglehart 1978). The 1976 Democratic party platform had urged that the health centers program be "resumed." Unlike Nixon and Ford, Carter and his advisers were likely to be sympathetic toward the program, and he staffed HEW with several individuals who had been instrumental in nurturing the program from the beginning. Carter—unlike Republican presidents—needed to reward traditional Democratic voters, including those in big cities. He could also look out his window and see a Congress controlled by very large Democratic majorities.

Carter called for and won funding increases for both community health centers and migrant health centers. The year 1978 was important for the program. Having finally secured its own legislative authority in 1975, it was now up for reauthorization.[28] Still, the program attracted little attention, positive or negative.[29] The program received a three-year reauthorization and substantially higher funding levels; its FY 1981 authorization was more than double that of FY 1978 (not controlling for inflation). It passed by large margins in both chambers but faced substantial Republican opposition in the House.

Besides securing separate legislative authority in 1975, the most important change in the 1970s was Carter's expansion of the program. Through the Rural Health Initiative, Carter's HEW built on a small program begun by HEW's Bureau of Comprehensive Health Services to target more funding to rural areas—especially those unable to develop competitive grant proposals. This was funded out of the same appropriation as all other centers.[30] Politically, this was advantageous to the health centers program because it greatly widened the number of congressional districts with centers; no longer would it be a "black program" (Sardell 1988, 117). Substantively, the Rural Health Initiative's effects were less clear. On the one hand, it redressed a serious imbalance. One-half of medically underserved individuals lived in rural areas, and yet some 85 percent of grant funding went to cities (ibid., 112). This imbalance had many causes, one of which may have been that urban proposals were more competitive because they were more likely to make credible claims about recruiting health professionals than their rural counterparts. By the end of Carter's term, every state and a majority of congressional districts had at least one of the 862 health centers funded in 1978; of these, 571 were in rural areas (Reynolds 1999, 8).

On the other hand, the Rural Health Initiative also began a tendency to develop a "lean and mean" program. The emphasis was on developing hundreds of additional centers, but smaller ones.[31] Later the "lean and mean" ethos extended to urban centers. Prodded by members of Congress representing large cities, Carter launched an urban health initiative that funded many projects at smaller levels (Sardell 1988, 118). To many HEW officials, the program's expansion meant developing sites of care provision that more closely resembled existing safety-net facilities, such as hospital outpatient clinics, and turning away from the grander visions of the 1960s. While many centers managed to find nonfederal sources to fund environmental and other nonmedical services, or coordinated with other local organizations and agencies, smaller awards for new and existing centers—coupled with inflation—forced many centers to abandon their supplementary services; in fact, HEW enacted rule changes that made it easier for grantees to avoid offering these services (Lefkowitz 2007, 299).[32] Although the program was expanding, by 1978 it still reached fewer than 10 percent of the medically underserved. And while it now had its own legislative authorization, it still remained poorly integrated with Medicaid and therefore remained financially vulnerable. Its next problem, though, was political.

Ronald Reagan and the Threat of Death-by-Block Grant

President Reagan posed the most serious threat to the health centers program thus far in its history (Reynolds 1999). While continuing efforts of his Republican predecessors to kill off discretionary health programs through block grants, he had some important resources that they had lacked. He operated with a perceived mandate to cut taxes and spending and to devolve the role of the federal government. Moreover, he assumed office with this mandate while Republicans held a majority of Senate seats; the Democratic majority in the House had been whittled down to only twenty-six seats. Congressional Republicans had grown much more conservative since the Nixon years, and many Democrats, especially in Reagan's first term, were "running scared" and in a mood to compromise.

It is in the early Reagan administration that we can begin to see more clearly the influence of the conservative movement on Republican domestic policy. This is in part because the Reagan years both were fueled by and further accelerated the development of an infrastructure for conservative policy analysts and political strategists. This is visible most clearly in *Mandate for Leadership*, the Heritage Foundation's famous 1980 effort to assist a victorious conservative candidate. Subtitled *Policy Management in a Conservative Administration*, the 1,093-page book was made available to Reagan's transition team. The chapter on the Department of Health and Human Services (HHS) is instructive, for it articulated the then-predominant view of conservative analysts and officeholders about community health centers and other health care delivery programs. Here the program's national expansion was viewed as a conscious strategy to hasten the passage of Democratic proposals for universal coverage. The prior development of health centers might serve as a "bootstrap" to NHI because proponents would be able to point to the existence of a delivery network of facilities for the poor already in place, thus reducing some of the practical difficulties toward a workable system.[33]

Reagan's first budget (FY 1982) slashed $6.6 billion in grants-in-aid funding, including cuts in funding for health centers of about 25 percent.[34] These cuts forced the Health Services Administration, the agency then administering the health centers program in the new HHS, to alter the metrics used to designate areas as either "medically underserved" or as "health professional shortage areas" in an effort to justify cuts to health center funding. The Bureau of Comprehensive Health Services took back control of the grant-making process so it could manage the cuts, which led to a reduction in patients served and a decline in the nonprimary services that the centers offered. In all, about 187 centers were eliminated.[35]

As with many parts of the federal bureaucracy, the early 1980s were not happy times for health center advocates in the HEW/HHS. Reagan cleaned house, sweeping away many of the more pragmatic appointees, convincing many civil servants to resign, and taking budget-making power away from the agency and installing it in the Office of Management and Budget (OMB). The AMA and the Association of Medical Colleges chose the appointees for the critical positions of assistant secretary for health affairs and his deputy;

these appointees were not enamored with the health centers program. Civil servants who remained in the agency were "severely limited in their ability to make autonomous decisions" (Sardell 1988, 180). Reagan named Richard Schweicker, a former Republican senator from Pennsylvania (home, he reminded, to the nation's largest rural population), to serve as HHS secretary. Schweicker insisted that between 40 to 60 percent of all grants be awarded to rural areas. By 1987, by one estimate, rural grantees operated 825 of 1,264 health centers, and served 2.6 million people, one-half of the national total.

More threatening than the 25 percent cut in federal grant funding was Reagan's attempt to block-grant health programs. His overall proposal was to consolidate eighty-five discretionary grant programs into five large block grants to the states. Congress eventually consolidated fifty-seven of these programs into nine block grants. The community health centers program was among twenty-six health services and research programs that would be combined into two large block grants. States would then decide how to allocate resources across the programs, and decide services provided, eligibility standards, and so on. The only federal restriction was that the monies spent for each block grant had to be one-quarter less than the FY 1981 appropriations level. In this proposal, health centers would be part of the health services block grant. However, due to some impressive politicking, the proposal became a completely unique animal: a "block grant in name only" (Sardell 1988, 166).

The Health subcommittee of the House Committee on Energy and Commerce was ideologically polarized. Members were able to agree that migrant health centers should be spared from a block grant. Migrant workers traveled across states, and thus it made more sense for the program to remain a federal one; moreover, because they did not vote, committee members expected states to neglect their health needs rather than cut another troubled program (*New York Times*, Apr. 3, 1981). Rep. Henry Waxman (D-CA) argued that because states had never been involved in the program or shown much interest in community health centers, the program should remain a discretionary federal program. States would naturally fund those programs that organized interests and state officials had become accustomed to (Reynolds 1999, 18). But Republicans disagreed, and the full committee failed to approve a budget proposal. The Senate considered the health services block grant proposal in the full Labor and Human Resources committee, chaired by Sen. Orrin Hatch (R-UT). This committee finally decided to place community health centers and migrant health centers in a protected block grant. Here existing centers would be funded through FY 1983, and funding had to be maintained by each state at a certain percentage of the FY 1981 appropriation through FY 1985.

In conference committee, the largest conflicts occurred over the National Health Service Corps, family planning projects, and community health centers. Hatch was adamant about the need to block-grant the health centers. He viewed them, along with the National Health Service Corps, as part of Carter's plan to build the "core of a national health insurance scheme," and "a significant portion of the population would receive health services at federally run clinics staffed by federally salaried physicians." For evidence, he pointed to planning papers written by Carter HEW official Karen Davis concerning a rapid expansion in centers over a five-year period. He also argued that many centers served areas that did not need them, and that much of the program's spending was inefficient (Sardell 1988, 175–176; Reynolds 1999). Here Hatch followed the Heritage Foundation's analysis closely. Twenty years later, conservatives would offer precisely the opposite analysis: rather than part of an incrementalist strategy by liberals to build national health insurance, health centers were a benign—even helpful—means of avoiding an incrementalist path to NHI.

In the end, while the Republicans saved face by placing primary care programs in what they called a block grant, they had lost. Health centers would remain a federal program for FY 1982; for FY 1983, states would have to apply to take over their administration. If a state did not do so, the program would remain federal. If it did choose to do so, it would have to fund each existing center at the same FY 1982 grant level, match a share of federal funds, and meet other requirements, including the community governance requirement. It was understood that these and other strings attached served to deter states from accepting the primary care block grant. This was "devolution" in name only, and a key moment for health centers. Fending off the block-granting of the program was much more significant than absorbing budget decreases. There was good reason to think that budgets could recover, but a block grant seemed like a death sentence (Davis 1981, 322). While funding did decline by about one-quarter (from $325 million to about $248 million), the NACHC declared victory.

Reagan was not done. Each year from 1982 to 1986, the administration proposed that health centers be included in a health services block grant. Finally, in 1986, over Reagan's pocket veto and thanks in large part to moderate Republican senators Robert Stafford (VT) and John Chafee (RI), Congress secured legislation authorizing health centers as an independent, discretionary grant program. After five years, the program's bizarre, quasi-block-grant status had ended.[36]

Bush 41 and the Birth of Federally Qualified Health Centers

The atmosphere in Washington for community health centers improved a good deal under the administration of President George H. W. Bush. While many social programs were cut, there were some important expansions of the activist state as well, including the Americans with Disability Act. Bush's attitude toward health centers differed from Reagan's as well. He requested spending increases, and in 1988 and in 1990, the program was reauthorized at a higher level and with his support (Reynolds 1999, 32). Health centers also benefited from drug company discounts and federal liability protection (which greatly reduced malpractice insurance costs). However, the most important change for health centers during this period involved changes in their financing.

In 1990, due in large measure to the persistence of the NACHC and a strong health center advocate, Sen. John Chafee (R-RI), Congress established an official reimbursement category in Medicare and Medicaid for what were termed federally qualified health centers (FQHCs). These provided much higher reimbursement rates based on actual costs. As part of this legislation, FQHCs were legally defined, reimbursable services were enumerated, and reimbursement arrangements specified. Moreover, health centers not receiving federal grants but otherwise fulfilling all legal requirements were termed "look-alikes," and these were also eligible for the same reimbursements from Medicare and Medicaid.

Although these arrangements have undergone several changes—most importantly the move to a prospective-payment system in Medicaid managed care—the FQHC arrangement effectively saved the program. Medicaid eligibility expansions began in the 1980s, but the FQHC arrangement provided the financial footing it needed; health centers would no longer have to rely so heavily on federal grants to cover the underpayments for Medicaid patients. By 1996 Medicaid reimbursements constituted a greater share of operating revenues than federal grants; today Medicaid's share is more than two-and-one-half times higher than it was in 1985.[37] Moreover, Medicaid managed care is credited with forcing health centers to improve their business acumen; this, in turn, has helped them survive and thrive. OEO's health centers program began in 1965, as Medicare and Medicaid were enacted. Twenty-five years later, they were finally integrated.

During the 1970s health centers were seen as complementary with national health insurance, not as a substitute or as a hindrance for winning support for national health insurance. As revealed in its deliberations over health centers and HMOs, the Nixon White House did not perceive them as in tension with NHI. Nor did Senator Kennedy, who saw the two as linked. In the early 1970s his staff even drafted legislation for comprehensive health centers that would merge mental health centers with community health centers and be a key service provider in his NHI proposal (Sardell 1988, 91–92). Carter and congressional supporters expanded the program even as they attempted to hammer out a workable NHI proposal. Besides the program's survival through three hostile Republican administrations, the most important development was the highly belated integration of Medicare and Medicaid financing with health center operations. As the problems of the underserved grew more severe, this integration meant that the centers were poised to assume a more central role in the US health safety net.

The Dog That Didn't Bark: Clinton and the Health Centers

The opposition by Republican administrations to the federal health centers program may seem unsurprising given traditional Republican principled commitments to federalism and limited government and a suspicion that a large health centers program could help pave the way for a national health insurance program. Here I try to understand why the Clinton administration did not push for the expansion of a small program that targeted a Democratic constituency with a typically Democratic redistributive policy. Clinton placed health care access at the center of his 1992 presidential campaign. After the failure of his proposed Health Security Act, why did he not assert himself in attacking problems of primary care access for the underserved? Why were congressional appropriations for health centers larger than the president's budgetary requests for seven of Clinton's eight budgets (see figure 2.1)? It is worth noting that this lack of assertion was not deadly for the program. Given the new surge of Medicaid funding coursing through the network of community health centers, increasing the number and size of federal grants was no longer a matter of survival. Still, the Clinton administration's ambivalence to health centers—referred to by a former HHS official as a "mystery and a scandal" (*Washington Post*, Aug. 26, 1999)—is important and needs to be explained.

The failure of the administration to back health centers was not due to a misunderstanding of the issue. During the efforts in 1993 to develop comprehensive reform proposals, internal deliberations recognized that the need for health centers would not disappear with the arrival of universal coverage (White House 1994, 2–3, 5). As planning proceeded, health center advocates in NACHC and elsewhere worried about some features of the proposed system. In particular, they were concerned about what looked like a block-granting of health centers in the midst of the proposed health alliances. They pushed for and won the designation "essential community provider" for health centers, at least for a transitional period. Concern with the effects on underserved access and safety-net facilities in the wake of national health insurance was not new to the Clinton years, but the health center lobby worried about the administration's downgrading of access issues that were unrelated to insurance status.[38]

After Clinton's failure at comprehensive reform and the Republican land-slide in the 1994 midterm elections, budget constraints seemed to dominate administration thinking on discretionary health programs. Health centers rarely were protected by being placed in "the most highly protected budget cat-egory"; this honor was reserved for, among other programs, AIDS and family planning. HHS secretary Donna Shalala even had the heretical preference for "marrying the health centers to teaching hospitals," thus scrapping their gov-ernance feature (teaching hospitals could not become controlled by patients). This also jeopardized health centers' supplementary services. In fact, "HHS officials . . . questioned whether health centers were 'community friendly,' because they were rarely funded through local health departments." The administration's attitude toward the program drifted further still from that of the Johnson years (Lefkowitz 2007, 22).

In late 1995 Clinton had a classic confrontation with the Republican lead-ership. Clinton seized the initiative by linking Medicare cuts to Republican tax cuts, charging them with a regressive redistribution of income, and dramatiz-ing proposed cuts in popular programs such as school lunches. Gingrich's room for maneuver in these negotiations was hampered greatly by his new House firebrands. After a settlement was reached, conservatives were left caricatured by Clinton and the Democrats (Zelizer 2007, 127).

The administration as well as health reform advocates in Congress con-tinued to pursue incremental advances in insurance expansion, such as the Kennedy–Kassenbaum Health Insurance Portability and Accountability Act of 1996 and the State Children's Health Insurance Program (SCHIP), an amend-ment to the Social Security Act that assisted states in expanding coverage to poor and near-poor children.[39] For the rest of his term, though, Clinton priori-tized reforms that would improve quality and lower the costs of health care, giv-ing little attention to access for the underserved (Richmond and Fein 2005, 149).

Gearing up for the general election in the summer of 1996, top Clinton advisers suggested in a memo to the president how he might claim credit for substantial health policy achievements, and they provided a menu of propos-als to be developed and advanced in a second term. Health centers were not mentioned in the "achievements" section; indeed, improvements in access to care were not mentioned. Looking to a second term, all possible policies were examined through the prism of insurance coverage of children. Health center expansion, perhaps through school-based clinics, was rejected because it would not "significantly increase coverage." Moreover, funding for health centers under a balanced budget imperative was considered impossible without dropping "some other priority," since "investments in community health centers and school-based centers" would cost "something like $15–$20 billion over 7 years." A final concern was that working on health centers might convince Democrats in Congress that the administration had given up on expanding coverage (Rasco and Tyson 1996).

Of course, HHS did not lack for health center advocates. By the mid-1990s, HRSA served as an important lobby for the program within the department. Still, neither HHS leadership nor Clinton's top domestic policy aides placed much attention on the growing problems of the medically underserved. HHS secretary Donna Shalala interpreted the administration's health priorities in terms of the expansion of coverage for children. In addition, Assistant Secretary for Health Phil Lee focused single-mindedly on insurance coverage rather than access and, like Shalala, was drawn more toward the world of academic medical centers instead of community clinics (Shalala 1999, 4, 6). And this is not because the problem was easing. The numbers of uninsured American residents continued to climb throughout the 1990s. Almost one-half of health centers were in "severe fiscal trouble" (*Washington Post*, Aug. 26, 1999). Bonnie Lefkowitz, a long-time HHS policy analyst with expertise in health centers, served on the White House Health Care Interdepartmental Working Group. She notes diplomatically that the administration did not "provide the support health center advocates had hoped for" (Lefkowitz 2007, 21). Why not?

A few answers are possible. First, perhaps the administration viewed the US public as arrayed against any other reforms of the health care system. This was certainly not what his own pollsters must have told Clinton, however. By the end of his first term, the public still favored some sort of comprehensive reform, and a majority of respondents concluded that Clinton's Health Security Act would have left them "better off." Nor was there much support for slashing Medicare and Medicaid, even among Republican groups (Peterson 2000). Additionally, it is unlikely that the administration feared advancing a large expansion in health centers out of fear that the Republican-controlled Congress would attack it.

A second possibility is related: the administration may have sought to avoid, as both a political and a policy matter, discussions of the poor when advocating health care reforms. Its relentless focus on the middle-class and "hardworking" Americans, both during the 1992 campaign and during the push for health savings accounts, is well known and was aimed in part at clarifying to the public the intended beneficiaries of structural reform. However, it is not at all obvious why programs for the poor could not have been folded into the array of smaller initiatives developed after the failure of the Clintons' comprehensive reform proposal. A third possible answer is that the administration—prioritizing budget reductions and cognizant of bipartisan support on the Hill for health centers—decided to keep the president's budget request lower as a political move. It could do so, in this view, without harming the underserved.[40] There is some evidence that this indeed occurred. Still, it leaves unexplained why the White House did not imagine an expansion of the program beyond the moderate increases appropriated by Congress.

Did the administration—or its advocates in Congress who also supported NHI—fear the deleterious political consequences for NHI of a health centers "fig leaf"? In 1994 congressional debates over health insurance, there was an interesting exchange over a Republican bill to increase funding for community health centers. Democrats, led by House Appropriations Committee chair David Obey (D-WI), "denounced the proposal as an effort to undermine any health care reform package that Congress might produce in 1994." "What we have here is a political fig leaf . . . They want to be on the record, somewhere, somehow, on the cheap, in voting for health care. I don't think that's the way to do business." House Minority Leader Robert H. Michel (R-IL) replied that, "regardless of what health care reform we eventually undertake, we still need expansion of the community health center network." (CQ Almanac 1995).[41] Especially after Clinton's defeat of Gingrich over the government shutdown in 1995, Republicans were motivated to adopt a caring posture.

As discussed earlier, during the Reagan years, many conservatives feared an expansion of health centers as laying the groundwork—really, the delivery system—for a nationalized system featuring universal coverage. Democratic proponents of NHI such as Kennedy and Carter, on the other hand, were comfortable seeing health centers and NHI as complementary—maybe even both necessary—for successful systemic reforms. Thus, many progressives' ambivalence about a strong health safety net was not logically entailed in the long struggle for something close to universal coverage.

But the exchange described earlier suggests that both opponents and supporters of NHI might have flipped their strategic assessments of the effects of federal safety-net programs on NHI politics. The Democrat favoring NHI worried that an expansion of health centers would relieve pressure on the system. Meanwhile, perhaps Michel believed the same thing and therefore pushed for this expansion.[42] In this 1990s perspective, an NHI politics of incrementalism had faded, and in its place had arisen on both sides a Leninist "one step forward" conception of NHI politics. Anything that papered over the severity of the problems at hand or reduced the crisis footing set back the cause. Senator Kennedy, the leading defender of health centers since their inception more than forty years ago, over time seemed to articulate just this fear. He said in a

1996 interview that the "more conservative members of Congress view health centers as an alternative way of serving the poor, rather than through universal health care." He continued, "There will never be enough money or enough health centers to truly care for the needs of the underserved. Without universal health care, there will always be people who fall through the cracks." "I'm not prepared at this time to think that [expansion of the program to cover underserved areas] is the way [to] go. . . . This doesn't replace the need for universal health care coverage" (Reynolds 1999, 95, 127, 121).[43]

Additionally, health center advocates report in confidential interviews that they are often confronted with this criticism of their efforts to expand primary care to the underserved. NHI advocates accuse them of "aiding and abetting" conservatives opposed to NHI. Clearly, not everybody "learns" the same lessons. Leading voices in the philanthropic, research, and advocacy communities, such as the Commonwealth Fund, the Robert Wood Johnson Foundation, the Milbank Fund, the Urban Institute, and many others, championed both universal coverage and the expansion of health centers. But over the past two decades, health center advocates have felt the need to reassure others that health centers are a complement to, not a substitute for, universal coverage (Wilensky and Roby 2005). While this is not evidence that the refusal of the Clinton administration to push for safety-net initiatives was motivated by fear of a "one step forward" dynamic, the fact pattern sketched here is not inconsistent with this motivation. I now turn to a different but related puzzle: the Bush health centers initiative.

George W. Bush's Health Centers Initiative

The health centers initiative, which Bush signed into law early in his first term, was rolled out in his 2000 presidential campaign. One stated goal of the initiative was to create twelve hundred new or expanded centers in five years, but the primary goal was to expand health center care to an additional 6.1 million patients. In order to accomplish this goal—which was completed ahead of schedule—funding for the centers more than doubled (see figure 2.1) (Politzer 2005). Moreover, the administration stayed vigilant in meeting its necessary spending goals even as wars, homeland security appropriations, Hurricane Katrina, and other forces impinged on the budget. For instance, in the FY 2006 budget, health center spending continued to increase even as Bush and the Republican Congress eliminated many discretionary programs and cut discretionary spending by 1 percent. This included a reduction in health safety-net programs such as Medicaid disproportionate share hospital payments (*Washington Post*, Feb. 57, 2005). And in FY 2007—the most fiscally conservative of Bush-era budgets—health centers secured an increase of more than $100 million, the largest increase for any HHS discretionary program (Lefkowitz 2007, 24).

Throughout his time in office, Bush highlighted the health centers initiative as a prominent goal, and then a major achievement, of his presidency (*New York Times*, Feb. 28, 2001; White House 2004, 2006). While Clinton mentioned health centers fewer than ten times, Bush mentioned the program—one of only hundreds of HHS programs receiving OMB's top ranking—in countless speeches and settings, even defending it on the *Bill O'Reilly Show*.[44] Additionally, members of Congress regularly publicized—often with high-level HHS political appointees, if they were Republicans representing marginal districts—the opening or expansion of federally funded health centers. The health centers initiative was obviously out of step with three Republican administrations and with Republican and conservative commitments in favor of traditional federalism, against redistribution, against larger discretionary spending programs, and against a strong federal role in health care finance (much less health care delivery). The initiative also seemed to offer a conservative Republican president little; the beneficiaries of the health centers are highly unlikely to become loyal, active, Republican voters.[45] What is going on here?

The 2000 Campaign

Bush rolled out his health centers initiative during the 2000 campaign as part of a plan titled, "Strengthening the Health Care Safety Net." "Under my plan, we would provide $3.6 billion in federal money over a five-year period to create 1,200 new centers from coast to coast," Bush said. This was intended "for those in the most desperate circumstances—a safety net that includes income support, housing assistance, and health services" (Bush 2000a).[46] In calling for a large expansion of health centers, he joined Democratic presidential candidate Sen. Bill Bradley (D-NJ), who called for doubling the capacity of health centers in one to two years. (The Democratic presidential nominee, Vice President Al Gore, did not mention health centers.)

The health centers initiative seemed constructed to help Bush win the election; it did not emerge clearly out of his tenure as governor of Texas from 1995 to 2001. As governor, he did not prioritize health policy, his aides acknowledged (Clymer 2000). He rarely spoke in public about health policy, despite his state's crisis of the uninsured, weak health safety net, and deplorable public health record in its forty-three border counties (including a return of tuberculosis). On the stump in 2000, he took credit for the state's patient's bill of rights, and claimed to have "embraced" Texas's participation in the Children's Health Insurance Program; neither assertion was accurate

(Dubose 1999; Dubose 2000; *New York Times*, Oct. 16 and 18, 2000; *Texas Observer*, Nov. 3, 2000). And he presided over one of the country's most oner-ous and intimidating Medicaid systems. Finally, the uninsured were not a big priority for him; his own commissioner of health downplayed the importance of insurance as a determinant of health outcomes. There is evidence that Bush visited health centers in Texas and thought the program a valuable one; clearly, however, his support of health centers, and the development of his initiative, did not have deep ideological roots.

Bush adviser Karl Rove emphasized six issues during this campaign: tax cuts, federal education standards, military upgrades and a defense shield, federal support for faith-based initiatives, the partial privatization of Social Security, and Medicare reform and prescription drug coverage (Sinclair 2008, 166). The safety-net proposal fit here as "part of a sustained drive by [Bush] to eat into the traditional Democratic advantage on issues like education and health care, which have moved into the forefront of public concern in a time of peace and security" (*New York Times*, Apr. 13, 2000). At the 2000 Republican national convention, Bush spelled out his governing philosophy of "compas-sionate conservatism": "Big government is not the answer, but the alternative to bureaucracy is not indifference. It is to put conservative values and conser-vative ideas into the thick of the fight for justice and opportunity" (Bush 2000b).[47] To describe the health centers initiative as a small, cheap effort that amounted to little more than posturing is to raise the question, why did it take Republican party leaders and presidents thirty-five years to seize on this long-available opportunity? This policy and compassionate conservatism reflect both Republican learning about electoral politics and the conservative movement's learning about how to wield the activist state to achieve privati-zation in several policy areas.

Short-Term and Long-Term Electoral Goals

To a greater degree than any presidential adviser in decades, Bush strategist Karl Rove remained focused on carving a durable partisan majority out of the electorate. Attempting to use domestic policy to induce a realignment, rather than waiting for voters to do it, Rove left normally implacable scholars mar-veling at his audacity (Conlan and Dinan 2007, 18; Green 2007, 56).[48] He and his staff devised policies that would entice additional voters into the party, in particular Catholics, white women, African Americans, and Hispanics.

Like other Republicans, Rove watched and learned from Gov. Pete Wilson's (R-CA) ill-fated embrace of Proposition 187's restrictions on illegal immigrants, as well as the perceived electoral consequences of the "Republican Revolution" of 1994 and Clinton's besting of Newt Gingrich during the government shut-down of 1995–1996. Compassionate conservatism—as it was employed as a frame for domestic policies—can be seen as a direct result of Republican learn-ing from these episodes. Bush's faith-based initiative was intended partly to offer patronage to black religious leaders (especially in the South) (Conason 2003; Wills 2006), while a number of appeals to Hispanics were thought impor-tant in Bush's winning 39–40 percent of the Hispanic vote in 2004 (Leal et al. 2005).[49] In 2000 and 2004 Rove and other Republicans were determined not to repeat the mistakes of the past. As one GOP staffer said, "We're not going to be throwing something out there for liberal to portray as wild-eyed conservatives running amok through the Capitol" (*Washington Post*, Nov. 7, 2002).

Developing and deploying domestic policies for political uses required unusually pliable policymaking institutions. These included a highly central-ized domestic policy apparatus in the White House, which Rove quickly harnessed and eventually housed within his Office of Political Affairs, an unprecedented centralization and merging of electoral politics and governing (Dilulio and Suskind 2002; Green 2007; Rudalevige 2008). Moreover, the White House ran roughshod over both career civil servants and its own political appointees in the federal agencies, and it perfected what came to be called "asset deployment." For example, Rove's office bested all of its predecessors in using announcements of federal grants for electoral purposes. HHS was no exception, focusing its very public rollout of health center awards on swing congressional districts (Solomon, MacGillis, and Cohen 2007).

One of the ways in which the health centers initiative might be considered strange as an electorally useful policy is that, unlike most policies, the admin-istration's vote-seeking targets were not usually the policy's beneficiaries. Rather, the health centers initiative fit into a range of policies that were used to perform "bankshot politics." In the same way that African Americans filling the dais at the Republican national convention were not present to help usher blacks into the Republican party, programs such as health centers can be inter-preted as directed more toward suburban white women worried that "Repub-licanism with a Human Face" is an oxymoron. Programs such as SCHIP are simply too expensive to be deployed as a tool of electoral politics, but pro-grams of the size of health centers work nicely.[50] On the view sketched here, the health centers program was viewed by Bush and by many in his party as electorally useful for more than seven years. Of course, the health centers ini-tiative was a fairly small, so it was useful only at the margins. However, in an era when the partisan balance in Congress, state legislatures, and presidential elections sat on a knife's edge, all of the era's politics were on the margins.

Long-Term Policy Goals

The Bush administration's policy goals meshed fairly well—but not perfectly—with an emerging consensus among conservatives to retrench many tasks of the state. Building on insights developed by conservative politicians and the ideational infrastructure developed on the right over the past few decades, the Bush administration, some argue, embraced longer time-horizons, and a controversial statism to pursue retrenchment across various policy arenas. Not only did the administration and leading conservatives back away from the goals of the 1980s and 1990s to shrink government directly, but their own policy ideas also became increasingly statist. In current dollars, total federal outlays from 2001 to 2007 increased 49 percent, and 18 percent in constant dollars (Conlan and Dinan 2007, 13).[51] Federal grants—not including so-called entitlements—increased from $55 billion to $93 billion, mainly for education, Homeland Security, and other programs. Even in 2006, as the administration made some attempts to rein in its spending, federal grants amounted to 16 percent of total federal spending, a higher share than in any year from 1980 to 2000 (Bartlett 2007, 14).

From No Child Left Behind to his yearlong attempt to privatize Social Security, Bush proposed several large new public policies in what many saw as an effort to shrink the state. As many policy analysts have argued, No Child Left Behind, which would typically be an offense to conservative mores, might actually be useful in developing a metric of school quality, shining a spotlight on poor school performance, and hastening public support for vouchers (Butler and Germanis 1983; Derthick and Teles 2003; Henig 2009; Teles and Derthick 2009). Additionally, Medicare reform emerged as a clear long-term policy goal of conservatives. Here, though, the goal was not a short-term frontal assault on the program but a policy of gradually drawing down Medicare spending in order to fund tax credits for the purchase of private insurance. Of course, the Medicare Modernization Act of 2003 entailed huge federal expenditures. Usually reliable small-government conservatives such as Newt Gingrich, though, urged Republican congressional support (Gingrich 2003). Democrats and progressives lamented that "their" issue had been co-opted by Republicans even as the latter's long-term policy goals diverged greatly from progressives' understanding of public opinion regarding Medicare.

All of these policies seemed to have both short- and long-term electoral benefits because they struck at the heart of the major policies that have provided the glue between Democratic candidates and voters over the past several decades. Bush's health centers initiative is consistent with this overall project. Republicans and conservatives have realized over the past few decades that a frontal assault on the welfare state has not worked, whether defunding, block-granting, or attacking the federal agencies that implemented social policies. And they realized, consistent with compassionate conservatism (or what Bush White House courtiers such as Fred Barnes termed "big-government conservatism" [Barnes 2003]), that there are electoral benefits to doing redistribution on the cheap.

Of course, the Bush administration's embrace of statism and massive tax cuts managed to anger many conservatives, and some skillful messaging was needed to limit this anger (Tanner 2007). To this end, Bush, Rove, Republicans on Capitol Hill, and conservative commentators spread the gospel of "starve the beast." This notion holds that if tax cuts are piled one atop another, deficit imperatives will emerge before long and will force spending cuts. Bush sometimes justified his 2001 tax cuts in these terms. Regardless of its validity, the idea was politically very useful for the Bush White House in that it provided conservatives with a rationalization for the Bush era's combination of tax cuts and spending increases (Bartlett 2006, 50, 157–174).

Witness the convergence from the 1970s to the 1990s of Senators Kennedy and Hatch on the "lesson" that expanded health centers may not hasten the coming of national health insurance. As recently as the Heritage Foundation's 1980 *Mandate for Leadership*, a sophisticated conservative health analyst had learned the very different "lesson" that an expanded network of health centers amounted to a stage-setting for NHI. It is unclear why health centers constitute an "incremental" move accelerating or slowing momentum toward universal coverage (depending on the lessons one thinks one has learned since the 1960s). Health centers may or may not stall momentum toward universal coverage, but they are properly understood *not* as incremental progress toward universal coverage. After all, they have little or no impact on the share of the population that is insured.[52] Rather, they are meant to alleviate some of the negative consequences—for individuals as well as the health care system—of uninsurance and the maldistribution of primary care providers. Conservative fears about health centers were therefore not really fears about a politics of incrementalism. Rather, the fear was that the prior existence of an infrastructure to implement universal coverage might weaken arguments about the doability of universal coverage. There is, of course, a wide range of views about incrementalism, and advocates of NHI have offered a number of possible ways by which incremental gains in health care access might stall progress toward their goal (Oliver 1999; Jacobs 2007).

Whether there *are* lessons to learn about incrementalism is beside the point; rather, we must understand what lessons about the political effects of public policies that politicians *think* they have learned in order to explain their choices. The (admittedly highly suggestive) argument made here is not that Bush did not himself sincerely like health centers. There is evidence that he does, as did (and do) many Republicans. But presidents like many policies that they do not enact. Rather, the argument here is that the health centers initiative was consistent with both shorter-term and longer-term electoral and policy goals of the Bush White House, *and* that it was consistent with an altered Republican and conservative understanding of a large network of health centers in Leninist terms, rather than "Trojan-horse" terms. Even if this argument is correct, however, it is unclear, given the new post-ACA landscape, what the partisan and policy understandings will be that shape future conflict over the health centers program.

Health Centers amid Obama's Health Care Reform

It might be better to be lucky than good, but the health centers movement has been both, especially of late. While the current and last few Congresses are the most ideologically polarized in almost a century, the health centers movement and trade association have displayed an impressive ability to bring members of Congress together to increase health centers funding. In 2008 Bush signed into law the highly popular Health Care Safety Net Act (Pub. L. 110–355), which both provided substantial new funding and reauthorized the program for an additional four years. Also in 2008, for the first time ever, both major party presidential nominees sang the praises of community health centers. The program already had a great deal of momentum going into 2009 and 2010, as major new opportunities emerged with the combination of unified Democratic control of government and a massive economic recession.

The Obama administration has continued to push the program onward and upward, most importantly through the ACA.[53] The ACA authorized $11 billion in new funding over five years (FY 2011 to FY 2015) on top of the annual discretionary funding for the program, which is estimated to be about $2.6 billion per year. Thus, for this five-year period, the federal government is providing health centers with more than $22 billion (Senate Budget Committee 2010; CBO 2010). Perhaps even more important, the ACA included a number of important features that improved the program's financial standing (see Rosenbaum, this volume). Over the past decade, the program doubled its patient coverage, from about ten million to twenty million. The current plan is to double its coverage again, to forty million, by 2015.[54] The health centers program has reached a critical new stage: it is larger, financially more sure-footed, and more popular than ever before. It is also now shouldering increasingly weighty expectations and public and political scrutiny.

America's health safety net was fraying substantially *before* the current economic recession.[55] In the first year of the recession, total visits to health centers increased by 14 percent; among the uninsured, visits increased by 21 percent. There has also been an explosion in Medicaid enrollments; in 2009 the program experienced its single largest one-year increase since the program began in the 1960s, with almost four million new enrollees (NACHC 2009b; Iglehart 2011, 8). Meanwhile, over the past decade, charity care provided by all physicians declined by 10 percent (Cunningham and May 2006).

If the ACA goes according to plan, by the end of the decade an estimated thirty-two million Americans will join the ranks of the insured. Given the limited number of primary care providers, experts predict that, as in Massachusetts after its move to near-universal coverage, health centers could be overwhelmed by new patients (Ku 2009). Conversely, twenty-three million Americans are likely to remain uninsured or underinsured, eight million of whom will likely be undocumented immigrants. They will continue to seek treatment in ERs and health centers (Thomas 2010). And health centers can expect less support from the states. As of FY 2011, state funding has dropped 42 percent since FY 2008 (NACHC 2010a, 2). The expansion in the number of centers, their size, and their service provision has (and will) put enormous pressure on their chief limitation: their workforce. Many centers are being pushed to their limits, and this is true even before we reckon with the move from twenty million to forty million patients, which would require fifteen thousand new health professionals (see Rosenbaum, this volume).[56]

But another problem facing the program may well be political. The program has survived and thrived due to luck, hardworking advocates, an impressive federated lobby, and some very motivated supporters in Congress. However, many involved with the program think it has survived and thrived in part *because* it has remained a low-salience, uncontroversial, small program doing redistributive politics in the guise of distributive politics. Health centers can no longer remain an open secret. The ACA, increased funding, and the anemic condition of other safety-net providers have made the already central health centers absolutely critical to US primary care. Can the program emerge from the shadows and still remain shielded from increasingly embittered congressional politics? Moreover, can it do so once roughly ten million of its patients are Hispanic, many of them undocumented immigrants? Will states continue to fund relatively generous Medicaid reimbursement schemes for centers that have gone from "ghetto medicine" to "barrio medicine"? Will the "gentleman's agreement" that allows health centers to treat undocumented immigrants hold?

Now that national health reform has begun, Republicans have begun to revive arguments against health centers that have not been voiced for more than two decades. For instance, Sen. Tom Coburn (R-OK) attacked the program for providing unfair competition for private practices and decried the program as a "government-centered" rather than a "patient-centered" solution (Favole 2010). More recently, presidential aspirant Gov. Haley Barbour (R-MS) has moved further, along a parallel track, in castigating an updated version of the archetypal Cadillac-driving welfare queen (in his version, BMW-driving individuals receive Medicaid treatments and claim they cannot afford a co-payment) (Goldstein and Balz 2011). In 2011 House Republicans departed from several years of kid-glove treatment for health centers by proposing $1.3 billion in budget cuts for health centers (along with $174 million in cuts for the National Health Service Corps). In one estimate, almost three million Americans would lose their regular primary care provider in 2011 if these proposed cuts were enacted (Senate Appropriations Committee 2011, 8). While this effort failed, the fact that it was even attempted suggests that there may be some fraying in the health centers' bipartisan political safety net. As their visibility, costs, and links to the increasingly criticized Medicaid program become more visible, there are good reasons for their advocates to wonder.

I have sought in this chapter to contextualize some lessons that interested parties think they may have learned about health politics as they have engaged over the last four decades with this remarkable, "strange" program. I have made what is only a highly suggestive argument: the fate of federally funded health centers has been caught up in larger battles over national health reform and party competition. The political forces shaping the world's largest primary care network will no doubt change in a post-ACA world. However, for good or ill, the development of the health centers program will surely provide both constraints and opportunities for political contestants as they continue to battle over the place of the state in the provision of primary care.

Notes

1. Data on centers and facilities include the US states and territories. The figure of twenty million includes one million patients served by "look-alikes." These are centers that fulfill all the requirements of federally funded centers but do not rely on federal grants; however, they qualify for the reimbursement relationships that benefit federally qualified health centers (FQHCs).

2. Additional citations and discussions of archival, interview, and other data used in this chapter can be found on the author's Web site (http://www-personal.umich.edu /~rmickey/). This research is based in part on interviews the author conducted in 2007 and 2008 with Lee Schorr, Joyce Lashof, Dan Hawkins, and participants at a policy and issues forum of the National Association of Community Health Centers (NACHC).

3. In the early part of the century, this meant southern and eastern European immigrants; in the 1960s, it meant blacks and (in the urban West and Southwest) Hispanics (Davis 1921; Rosen 1971).

4. This grew out of the Sheppard–Towner Act of 1921 and ended by 1929, in part due to the AMA's opposition.

5. From the late 1930s until 1947, the Farm Security Administration established and operated more than one thousand health cooperatives across rural America. These federally subsidized prepaid health plans emphasized preventive care and served some one-half million people (Grey 1999).

6. Local public health departments were usually underfunded, captured by local medical establishments, or patronage operations for political machines; they rarely attacked barriers to access and were not sites of policy innovation. Schools of public health—potential sources of new models of primary care delivery—were minor players on the policy landscape. In 1958, seven years before the first health centers began operation, the United States had only eleven accredited schools of public health and fewer than 1,200 students enrolled (Richmond and Fein 2005, 17–18, 95).

7. In one estimate, this share (among all physicians) declined from 80 to 28 percent from 1931 to 1963 (Richmond 1969, 86; Sardell 1988, 44; Stevens 1999).

8. Johnson's analysis that the passage of the Civil Rights Act had "lost the South" for the Democratic Party only amplified this need.

9. Since the 1950s the National Medical Association, the membership association of black doctors, had stepped up their calls to end several racially exclusionary practices of medical facilities in the South and North, and had demanded inclusion into county and state medical societies and the AMA (membership in which was often required to secure hospital staff privileges) (Langer 1965, 282–283, 328; Smith 1999).

10. The National Medical Association had encouraged black doctors to join with liberal white physicians—Jack Geiger among them—to protect civil rights workers in the Deep South. The organization developed out of this experience, the Medical Committee for Human Rights, quickly established thirty branches across America's cities; these protested longstanding patterns of racial discrimination in health care, and agitated for better health care delivery for ethnic and racial minorities (McBride 1991, 154–155; 1993, 322–323; Dittmer 2009).

11. Geiger, Gibson, and OEO staff especially sought to attack racial disparities in health access, care, and outcomes for blacks and Hispanics (Geiger 1993, 946–947).

12. OEO's director, former Peace Corps director Sargent Shriver, was initially quite skeptical about the health centers project; the support of Dr. Julius Richmond, founder of Head Start, was critical in convincing Shriver to approve the centers as a demonstration project (Schorr 1988, 130–131; Lefkowitz interview with OEO staffer Sandy Kravitz, in Lefkowitz 2007, 9).

13. Section 207 of the EOA of 1964 (Administrative History Papers 1974, 333).

14. Author's interview with Lee Schorr. By that time, other major OEO programs, including VISTA, Head Start, and Job Corps, had begun medical projects. The Community Action Program established its own Office of Comprehensive Health Services in late 1966.

15. Black GPs near health centers sometimes voiced their opposition. Dr. Paul B. Cornely, the most prominent black figure in American public health, complained that black inner-city doctors were ignored in the planning of the health centers. Still, black inner-city physicians remained more supportive of health centers and other

safety-net institutions than local (white) medical societies (*New York Times*, Nov. 14, 1968; Richard 1969).

16. Kennedy served on the Senate health subcommittee of the Committee on Labor and Public Welfare, which had jurisdiction over health centers.

17. EOA, as amended, Section 211–2 (Administrative History Papers 1974, 335; Sardell 1988, 66).

18. The Comprehensive Health Planning and Public Health Services Act of 1966 (Pub. L. No. 89–749) was amended by the Partnership for Health Amendments of 1967 (Pub. L. No. 90–174). These became known as 314(e) projects.

19. President Johnson rarely mentioned the program in public and never discussed it in detail in public (fewer than a dozen times, compared to about eighty mentions [and much longer discussions] of Head Start).

20. The AMA did not require its state affiliates to begin desegregating themselves until 1968.

21. Generalists at the HEW, as well as OMB staff, rejected Rumsfeld's "power play" on behalf of the OEO. Also, OMB officials doubted the capacity of heath centers to become financially self-sufficient (Starr 1982, 396; Brown 1983, 214–216, 490–491; Reynolds 1999, 10).

22. Many public health reformers and policy analysts had called for block grants since the Truman administration, and Wilbur Cohen and other important voices during the Johnson administration also backed block grants, such as the 1966 Partnership for Health program.

23. In a July 8, 1970, press conference, OEO director Donald Rumsfeld stated, "the single most exciting thing going on in the country, from a research standpoint or development standpoint on the supply side [of medical care], is the neighborhood health center concept."

24. Medicare began to do so in 1977, but only for rural health centers (Sardell 1988, 131).

25. The Health Maintenance Act of 1973 (Pub. L. 93–222); Brown 1983.

26. Ford claimed that the problems of access for the underserved could be met simply by "health care financing programs—such as Medicare and Medicaid" (Ford 1975).

27. In 1979 NACHC had a budget of $54,000, compared to $11 million for the American Hospital Association.

28. The 1977 Health Services Extension Act (Pub. L. 95–83) had extended the 1975 authorization for another year.

29. According to one participant on the Hill, it was "difficult to get people in the room for the hearing and the markup" (Sardell 1988, 141).

30. Through "positive programming," the HEW staffers used formulas and other indices to determine those areas in greatest need; it then helped them develop proposals (Sardell 1988, 114).

31. Sen. Ted Kennedy (D-MA) claimed that only 158 of 574 centers provided comprehensive services (Senate Report 95–860 [1978], 27; Sardell 1988, 126).

32. Similarly, the NACHC complained that smaller grant awards for new and existing centers, coupled with inflation, had forced centers to cut some of their medical services and now rarely could fund supplementary services (Senate Committee on Human Resources, Hearings, 110–114; Sardell 1988, 147).

33. David Winston, author of the chapter, was an influential Republican health policy analyst and minority staff director of the Senate Committee on Labor and Human Resources (Winston 1981, 248–249, 269, 274–275, 286, 291).

34. The reduction was from about $325 million in FY 1981 to $248 million in FY 1982 (Sardell 1988, 177).

35. *Washington Post*, Nov. 4, 1981. Of the eighty medically underserved areas losing their designations, seventy won back their designations on appeal (Sardell 1988, 187). In 1982 two Public Health Service agencies, the Health Services Administration and the Health Resources Administration, were combined into what remains the Health Resources and Services Administration (HRSA). The new Bureau of Health Care Delivery and Assistance within HRSA would administer community health centers, migrant health centers, and the National Health Service Corps. Metrics for designating medically underserved areas and health professional shortage areas continue to be hotly debated.

36. This legislation (Pub. L. 99–280 [1986]) was drafted jointly by Kennedy and Hatch (who was now on board with the program) (Reynolds 1999, 29–30).

37. Pub. L. 101–508, The Omnibus Budget Reconciliation Act of 1990 (Reynolds 1999; Lefkowitz 2007, 21; Rosenbaum, Jones, and Shin 2010, 4); Pub. L. 101–239 (1989, for Medicare), and Pub. L. 101–508 (1990, for Medicaid).

38. The black National Medical Association, concerned about the failure of Carter's health insurance proposal to tackle access problems, opposed it—a major step for an organization that had backed every NHI proposal since 1945 (McBride 1993, 325–326).

39. Clinton secured SCHIP in exchange for substantial cuts in domestic discretionary spending as part of the Balanced Budget Act of 1997.

40. OMB associate director for health and personnel Dan Mendelson argued along these lines (*Washington Post*, Aug. 26, 1999).

41. House Republicans had also included an expansion of health centers in their counterproposal to the Clinton plan in 1993 (Rich 1993).

42. In 1998 Hatch helped lead the Senate's effort to increase funding for FY 1999 by $100 million. By the late 1990s he saw health centers as necessary to "fill in the cracks" as other safety-net programs were cut. However, Hatch had not embraced a cynical "fig leaf" strategy. He opposed a large expansion of the program, and doubted whether "three billion dollars would be sufficient to cover expensive services outside the CHC's scope and to cover the infrastructure costs in areas which did not currently have CHCs" (Pub. L. 105–277 [1998]; Reynolds 1999, 107, 93, 127).

43. For an articulation of the fear of the health centers as "fig leaf," see Taylor 1999.

44. The date was Sept. 29, 2004.

45. Republican party platforms have lauded health centers since 1992. See *The American Presidency Project*, http://www.presidency.ucsb.edu/platforms.php.

46. The health centers initiative also found expression in the 2000 Republican Party platform. There was no mention of health centers in Democratic Party platforms from 1980 through 2004.

47. Orrin Hatch first used the phrase while defending his support for another War on Poverty program, Job Corps: "I'm a compassionate conservative. I'm not some kind of ultra-right-wing maniac" (*New York Times*, Mar. 13, 1981).

48. Rove's was a "campaigning and governing philosophy that puts a set of core policies *in the service of politics to an unusually direct degree*. Some elements of this approach are tonal and symbolic, while others . . . are more concrete" (emphasis added; *New York Times*, Nov. 5, 2004).

49. Of course, the increasingly heated debates over immigration policy since 2006 have made this effort even more difficult.

50. Another target of health-centers-as-bankshot politics may be Hispanics, who now comprise more than one-third of all health center patients nationally. In a small number of states, they comprise a large majority of the patient pool. While many of these users are undocumented, it could be argued that Rove and other Republican strategists viewed their treatment in health centers, along with national immigration reform, as attractive to Hispanic voters.

51. Another departure from traditional Republican prerogatives regarding federalism was the infamous Act for the Relief of the Parents of Theresa Marie Schiavo (Pub. L. 109–3).

52. It is possible that a vast increase in health centers would lower uncompensated care rates, relieve pressure on local safety nets, and thereby marginally decrease local insurance premiums.

53. Additionally, the Economic American Recovery and Reinvestment Act of 2009 (Pub. L. 111–5) (the "stimulus package") provided a one-time $2 billion increase to the HHS to finance health centers.

54. NACHC estimates that the number of patients served would increase by more than 25 percent in a single year (from 2014 to 2015, from 31.6 to 40.0 million). This seems highly optimistic (NACHC 2010b).

55. On the role of adults with Medicaid in driving the rapid increase in the rate of emergency department visits, see Tang et al. 2010.

56. Author's telephone interview with Dan Hawkins, NACHC, Mar. 2008. The American College of Physicians estimates that the current shortfall in primary care providers is forty thousand (Howell 2010; Neergaard 2010).

References

Administrative History Papers. 1974. "Administrative History of the OEO during the Johnson Administration, 1963–1969." Austin, TX: Lyndon B. Johnson Library.

Agency for Healthcare Research and Quality (AHRQ). 2006. "US Medical Expenditure Panel Survey." Rockville, MD: AHRQ. meps.ahrq.gov/mepsweb.

Barnes, F. 2003. "A 'Big Government Conservatism.'" *Wall Street Journal*, Aug. 15.

Bartlett, B. 2006. *Impostor: How George W. Bush Bankrupted America and Betrayed the Reagan Legacy*. New York: Doubleday.

———. 2007. "'Starve the Beast:' Origins and Development of a Budgetary Metaphor." *The Independent Review* 12:15–26.

Boyce, J. 1969. "Negro Doctors Label US Health Care a 'Conspiracy.'" *Chicago Tribune*, Feb. 18.

Brandt, A. M., and M. Gardner. 2000. "Antagonism and Accommodation: Interpreting the Relationship between Public Health and Medicine in the United States during the 20th Century." *American Journal of Public Health* 90:707–715.

Brown, L. D. 1983. *Politics and Health Care Organization: HMOs as Federal Policy*. Washington, DC: Brookings Institution Press.

Bush, G. W. 2000a. "Lowering Costs is Key." *USA Today*, Apr. 13: 16A.

———. 2000b. "2000 Republican Presidential Nomination Acceptance Speech." Philadelphia. Aug. 3.

Butler, S., and P. Germanis. 1983. "Achieving Social Security Reform: A 'Leninist' Strategy." *Cato Journal* 3:547–556.

Clymer, A. 2000. "Bush and Texas Have Not Set High Priority on Health Care." *New York Times*, Apr. 11.

Colgrove, J. 2007. "Reform and Its Discontents: Public Health in New York City during the Great Society." *Journal of Policy History* 19:3–28.

Conason, J. 2003. "Where's the Compassion?" *The Nation*, Sept. 15.

Congressional Budget Office (CBO). 2010. "Revised Estimate for H.R. 3590 (The Patient Protection and Affordable Care Act (PL 111–48)." Washington, DC: US Congress. May 11.

Conlan, T. J. 1998. *From New Federalism to Devolution: Twenty-Five Years of Intergovernmental Reform.* Washington, DC: Brookings Institution Press.

Conlan, T., and J. Dinan. 2007. "Federalism, the Bush Administration, and the Transformation of American Conservatism." *Publius* 37:279–303.

CQ Almanac. 1995. "Bill for Labor, Health and Human Services Requires Trade-Offs." Washington, DC: Congressional Quarterly.

Cunningham, P. J., and J. H. May. 2006. "A Growing Hole in the Safety Net: Physician Charity Care Declines Again." Tracking Report No. 13. Mar. Washington, DC: Center for Studying Health Systems Change.

Davis, K. 1981. "Reagan Administration Health Policy." *Journal of Public Health Policy* 2:312–332.

Davis, K., and C. Schoen. 1978. *Health and the War on Poverty: A Ten-Year Appraisal.* Washington, DC: Brookings Institution.

Davis, M. M. 1921. *Immigrant Health and the Community.* New York: Harper and Brothers.

———. 1927. "Goal-Posts and Yardsticks in Health Center Work." *American Journal of Public Health* 17:433–440.

Derickson, A. 2002. "'Health for Three-Thirds of the Nation': Public Health Advocacy of Universal Access to Medical Care in the United States." *American Journal of Public Health* 92:180–191.

Derthick, M., and S. M. Teles. 2003. "Riding the Third Rail: Social Security Reform," in *The Reagan Presidency.* ed. W. E. Brownlee and H. D. Graham, 182–208. Lawrence: University Press of Kansas.

Dilulio, J., and R. Suskind. 2002. "John Dilulio's Letter." *Esquire,* Oct. 2.

Dittmer, J. 2009. *The Good Doctors: The Medical Committee for Human Rights and the Struggle for Social Justice in Health Care.* London: Bloomsbury Press.

Dubose, L. 1999. "Running on Empty: The Truth about George W. Bush's 'Compassionate Conservativism.'" *The Nation,* Apr. 26.

———. 2000. "Read My Chips." *Austin Chronicle,* Sept. 1.

Duffy, J. 1990. *The Sanitarians: A History of American Public Health.* Urbana: University of Illinois Press.

Favole, J. A. 2010. "Funds Double for Health Clinics." *Wall Street Journal,* Mar. 25.

Flanagan, R. M. 2001. "Lyndon Johnson, Community Action, and the Management of the Administrative State." *Presidential Studies Quarterly* 31:585–608.

Ford, G. R. 1974. "Presidential Message." Public Papers of the President, 1974. Dec. 23.

———. 1975. "Veto of a Public Health Services Bill." Public Papers of the President, 1975. July 26.

Geiger, H. J. 1984. "Community Health Centers: Health Care as an Instrument of Social Change." In *Reforming Medicine: Lessons of the Last Quarter Century.* ed. V. Sidel and R. Sidel. New York: Pantheon.

———. 1993. "Community-Oriented Primary Care: The Legacy of Sidney Kark." *American Journal of Public Health* 83:946–947.

———. 2002. "Community-Oriented Primary Care: A Path to Community Development." *American Journal of Public Health* 92:1713–1716.

———. 2005. "The First Community Health Centers: A Model of Enduring Value." *Journal of Ambulatory Care Management* 28:313–320.

General Accounting Office (GAO). 1973. "Implementation of a Policy of Self-Support by Neighborhood Health Centers." *Report to the Subcommittee on Health*. Committee on Labor and Public Welfare: US Senate. May 2.

Gingrich, N. 2003. "Conservatives Should Vote 'Yes' on Medicare." *Wall Street Journal*, Nov. 20.

Glenn, B., and S. M. Teles. 2009. *Conservatism and American Political Development*. New York: Oxford University Press.

Goldstein, A., and D. Balz. 2011. "Governors Differ on Extent of Flexibility for Medicaid." *Washington Post*, Feb. 28.

Green, J. 2007. "The Rove Presidency." *Atlantic Monthly* September, 52–72.

Grey, M. R. 1999. *New Deal Medicine: The Rural Health Programs of the Farm Security Administration*. Baltimore: Johns Hopkins University Press.

Health, Education, and Welfare (HEW), Department of. 1967. "Delivery of Health Services for the Poor." Washington, DC: Government Printing Office.

Henig, J. 2009. "Education Policy from 1980 to Present: The Politics of Privatization." In *Conservatism and American Political Development*, ed. B. J. Glenn and S. M. Teles, 291–323. New York: Oxford University Press.

Hillman, B., and E. Charney. 1972. "A Neighborhood Health Center: What the Patients Know and Think of Its Operation." *Medical Care* 10:336–344.

Hiscock, I. V. 1935. "The Development of Neighborhood Health Services in the United States." *Milbank Memorial Fund Quarterly* 13:30–51.

Hoffman, B. 2003. "Health Care and Social Movements in the United States." *American Journal of Public Health* 93:75–85.

———. 2006. "Emergency Rooms: The Reluctant Safety Net." In *History and Health Policy in the United States: Putting the Past Back In*, ed. R. A. Stevens, C. E. Rosenberg, and L. R. Burns. New Brunswick, NJ: Rutgers University Press.

Hollister, R. M. 1974. "Neighborhood Health Centers as Demonstrations." In *Neighborhood Health Centers*, ed. R. M. Hollister, B. M. Kramer, and S. S. Bellin. Lexington, MA: Lexington Books.

Hollister, R. M., B. M. Kramer, and S. S. Bellin. 1974. "Neighborhood Health Centers as a Social Movement." In *Neighborhood Health Centers*, ed. R. M. Hollister, B. M. Kramer, and S. S. Bellin. Lexington, MA: Lexington Books.

Howell, J. D. 2010. "Reflections on the Past and Future of Primary Care." *Health Affairs* 29:760–765.

Iglehart, J. K. 1978. "The Carter Administration's Health Budget: Charting New Priorities with Limited Dollars." *Milbank Memorial Fund Quarterly* 56:51–77.

———. 2010. "Health Centers Fill Critical Gap, Enjoy Support." *Health Affairs* 29:343–345.

———. 2011. "After Midterm Elections, Changes Are in Store." *Health Affairs* 30:1–8.

Jacobs, L. R. 2007. "The Medicare Approach: Political Choices and American Institutions." *Journal of Health Politics, Policy, and Law* 32:159–186.

Ku, L., E. Jones, B. Finnegan, and S. Rosenbaum. 2009. "How Is the Primary Care Safety Net Faring in Massachusetts? Community Health Centers in the Midst of Health Reform." Issue Brief No. 7878. Washington, DC: Kaiser Commission on Medicaid and the Uninsured.

Ku, L., P. Richard, A. Dor, E. Tan, P. Shin, S. Rosenbaum. 2010. "Strengthening Primary Care to Bend the Cost Curve: The Expansion of Community Health Centers Through Health Reform." Policy Research Brief No. 19. June 30. Washington, DC: Geiger Gibson/RCHN Community Health Foundation Research Collaborative, George Washington University School of Public Health and Health Services.

Langer, E. 1965. "AMA (II): Doctors' Organization Faces Growing Outside Criticism, Wide Range of Problems." *Science* 149:282–328.

Lashof, J. C. 1968. "Medical Care in the Urban Center." *Annals of Internal Medicine* 68:242–245.

Leal, D. L., M. A. Barreto, J. Lee, and R. O. de la Garza. 2005. "The Latino Vote in the 2004 Election." *Political Science* Jan., 41–49.

Lefkowitz, B. 2007. *Community Health Centers: A Movement and the People Who Made It Happen.* New Brunswick, NJ: Rutgers University Press.

Marcus, I. 1981. *Dollars for Reform: The OEO Neighborhood Health Centers.* Lexington, MA: Lexington Books.

McBride, D. 1991. *From TB to AIDS: Epidemics among Urban Blacks Since 1900.* Albany: SUNY Press.

———. 1993. "From Community Health Care to Crisis Medicine." *Journal of Health Politics, Policy, and Law* 18:322–323.

Mullan, F. 1976. *White Coat, Clenched Fist: The Political Education of an American Physician.* New York: Macmillan.

Nathan, R. P. 1975. *The Plot That Failed: Nixon and the Administrative Presidency.* New York: Wiley.

National Association of Community Health Centers (NACHC) and the Robert Graham Center. 2009a. "Primary Care Access: An Essential Building Block of Health Care Reform." Washington, DC: NACHC.

———. 2009b. "Recession Brings More Patients to Community Health Centers." Fact Sheet No. 0209. September. Washington, DC: NACHC.

National Association of Community Health Centers (NACHC). 2010a. "Entering the Era of Reform: The Future of State Funding for Health Centers." State Policy Report No. 33, Oct. Washington, DC: NACHC.

———. 2010b. "Expanding Health Centers Under Health Care Reform: Doubling Patient Capacity and Bringing Down Costs." June. Washington, DC: NACHC.

Neergaard, L. 2010. "Health Overhaul Likely to Strain Doctor Shortage." *Associated Press,* Mar. 29.

Nixon, R. 1971. "Special Message to the Congress Proposing a National Health Strategy." Speech Addressing Congress. February 18. Public Papers of the President, 1971. The American Presidency Project. http://www.presidency.ucsb.edu/ws/index.php?pid=3311&st=&st1=#axzz1Zqe0Qi00.

Oliver, T. R. 1999. "The Dilemmas of Incrementalism: Logical and Political Constraints in the Design of Health Insurance Reforms." *Journal of Policy Analysis and Management* 18:652–683.

Peterson, M. A. 2000. "The Fate of 'Big Government' in the United States: Not over, But Undermined?" *Governance* 13:256–257.

Pierson, P., and T. Skocpol. 2007. "American Politics in the Long Run." In *The Transformation of American Politics: Activist Government and the Rise of Conservatism,* ed. P. Pierson and T. Skocpol. Princeton, NJ: Princeton University Press.

Politzer, R. M. 2005. "The United States Health Centers Initiative." *Journal of Public Health Policy* 26:418–429.

Rasco, C., and L. Tyson. 1996. "Memorandum to the President." *Chris Jennings Papers.* Domestic Policy Council Papers. Little Rock, AR: William Jefferson Clinton Presidential Library. Aug. 16, Folder 1 (Box 11), 8–9.

Reynolds, D.A.V. 1999. "An Analysis of the Political and Economic Viability of Community Health Centers: Implications for Their Future." Ph.D. dissertation, University of Michigan.

Rich, S. 1993. "House Republicans Propose Alternative Health Care Plan." *Washington Post,* Sept. 16.

Richard, M. P. 1969. "The Negro Physician: Babbitt or Revolutionary?" *Journal of Health and Social Behavior* 10:265–274.

Richmond, J. B. 1969. *Currents in American Medicine: A Developmental View of Medical Care and Education.* Cambridge, MA: Harvard University Press.

Richmond, J. B., and R. Fein. 2005. *The Health Care Mess: How We Got Into It and What It Will Take to Get Out.* Cambridge, MA: Harvard University Press.

Rosen, G. 1971. "The First Neighborhood Center Movement—Its Rise and Fall." *American Journal of Public Health* 61:1620–1637.

Rosenbaum, S., E. Jones, and P. Shin. 2010. "Community Health Centers: Opportunities and Challenges of Health Reform." Issue Paper No. 8098. Aug. Washington, DC: Kaiser Commission on Medicaid and the Uninsured.

Rudalevige, A. 2008. "'The Decider': Issue Management and the Bush White House." In *The George W. Bush Legacy,* ed. C. Campbell, B. A. Rockman, and A. Rudalevige. Washington, DC: Congressional Quarterly Press.

Sardell, A. B. 1988. *The US Experiment in Social Medicine: The Community Health Center Program, 1965–1986.* Pittsburgh: University of Pittsburgh Press.

Schorr, L. B. 1988. *Within Our Reach: Breaking the Cycle of Poverty.* With D. Schorr. New York: Doubleday.

Schorr, L. B., and J. English. 1974. "Background, Context and Significant Issues in Neighborhood Health Centers." In *Neighborhood Health Centers,* ed. R. M. Hollister, B. M. Kramer, and S. S. Bellin, 289–296. Lexington, MA: Lexington Books.

Senate Appropriations Committee. 2011. "Chairman Inouye Releases Analysis of House CR Proposal." Washington, DC: Press Release. Feb. 15.

Senate Budget Committee. 2010. Chairman's Mark: FY 2011 Senate Budget Resolution. Washington, DC. Apr. 21.

Senate Human Resources Committee. 1978. "Health Services Extension Act of 1978: Hearings before the Subcommittee on Health and Scientific Research." 95th Congress, 2nd sess., pp. 110–114.

Shalala, D. 1999. "Memo to the President, Dec. 26, 1999. History of the Department of HHS." Memos for the President. Little Rock, AR: William Jefferson Clinton Presidential Library. Box 31 (Folder 6).

Sinclair, B. 2008. "Living (and Dying?) by the Sword: George W. Bush as Legislative Leader." In *The George W. Bush Legacy,* ed. C. Campbell, B. A. Rockman, and A. Rudalevige, Washington, DC: Congressional Quarterly Press.

Smith, D. B. 1999. *Health Care Divided: Race and Healing a Nation.* Ann Arbor: University of Michigan Press.

Solomon, J., A. MacGillis, and S. Cohen. 2007. "How Rove Directed Federal Assets for GOP Gains." *Washington Post,* Aug.19.

Starr, P. 1982. *The Social Transformation of American Medicine: The Rise of a Sovereign Profession and the Making of a Vast Industry.* New York: Basic Books.

Stern, B. J. 1946. *Medical Services by Government: Local, State, and Federal.* New York: Commonwealth Fund.

Stevens, R. 1999. *In Sickness and in Wealth: American Hospitals in the Twentieth Century.* Baltimore: Johns Hopkins University Press.

Tang, N., J. Stein, R. Y. Hsia, J. H. Maselli, and R. Gonzales. 2010. "Trends and Characteristics of US Emergency Department Visits, 1997–2007." *Journal of the American Medical Association* 304:664–670.

Tanner, M. D. 2007. *Leviathan on the Right: How Big-Government Conservatism Brought Down the Republican Revolution.* Washington, DC: Cato Institute.

Taylor, D. H. 1999. "Do Targeted Efforts for the Rural Underserved Help Kill Comprehensive Reform?" *Journal of Rural Health* 15:55–60.

Teles, S. M., and M. Derthick. 2009. "Social Security from 1980 to Present: From Third Rail to Presidential Commitment—and Back?" In *Conservatism and American Political Development.* ed. B. J. Glenn and S. M. Teles, 261–290. New York: Oxford University Press.

Thomas, M. 2010. "After Reform, 23 Million to Remain Uninsured." *Chicago Sun-Times,* Apr. 20.

Tilson, H. H. 1973. "Stability of Physician Employment in Neighborhood Health Centers." *Medical Care* 11:384–400.

Torrens, P. R. 1971. "Administrative Problems of Neighborhood Health Centers." *Medical Care* 9:487–497.

White House. 1994. "Presidential Briefing Book. Access for Underserved and Vulnerable Populations." Papers of the White House Health Care Interdepartmental Working Group. Little Rock, AR: William Jefferson Clinton Presidential Library. Folder 3 (Box 644).

———. 2004. "Making Health Care More Affordable." Office of the Press Secretary, Sept. 2. Washington, DC.

———. 2006. "Reforming Health Care for the 21st Century," National Economic Council, Feb. Washington, DC. http://georgewbush-whitehouse.archives.gov/stateoftheunion/2006/healthcare/healthcare_booklet.pdf.

Wilensky, S., and D. H. Roby. 2005. "Health Centers and Health Insurance: Complements, Not Alternatives." *Journal of Ambulatory Care Management* 28:348–356.

Wills, G. 2006. "A Country Ruled by Faith." *New York Review of Books* 53:8–12.

Winston, D. A. 1981. "The Department of Health and Human Services." In *Mandate for Leadership: Policy Management in a Conservative Administration*, ed. C. L. Heatherly. Washington, DC: The Heritage Foundation.

Zelizer, J. 2007. "Seizing Power: Conservatives and Congress since the 1970s." In *The Transformation of American Politics*, ed. P. Pierson and T. Skocpol. Princeton, NJ: Princeton University Press.

Zwick. D. I. 1972. "Some Accomplishments and Findings of Neighborhood Health Centers." *Milbank Memorial Fund Quarterly* 50:392, 404.

Reinventing a Classic

Community Health Centers and the Newly Insured

On March 23, 2010, forty-five years after the first community health centers opened their doors in Mound Bayou, Mississippi, and Boston's Columbia Point housing projects, President Obama signed into law arguably the most sweeping overhaul of the nation's health insurance system ever attempted. Unlike Medicare and Medicaid, the Patient Protection and Affordable Care Act (ACA) does not merely fill the chasms created by voluntary health insurance.[1] Instead, it tackles the fundamental problems that arise in a system that gives healthy individuals the freedom to opt out, bars coverage for the sick, and allows private insurers to select the healthiest customers and then walk away when the tide turns.

The ACA addresses these problems by creating a five-pillar approach to health reform. First, as of January 1, 2014, the law eliminates health insurers' ability to choose only the healthiest risks by barring various types of discriminatory practices including, among others, rescissions of coverage, discrimination based on health status, and application of preexisting condition exclusions.[2] Second, by requiring virtually all individuals who can afford to do so to obtain coverage, the law creates the national pool of healthy lives essential to any viable, stable approach to universal coverage.[3] Third, to ensure that coverage is affordable, the legislation creates a system of refundable tax credits and cost-sharing subsidies.[4] Fourth, the legislation creates a more robust individual and small-group market for health insurance coverage through the establishment of state health insurance exchanges.[5] Finally, the law restructures Medicaid to ensure coverage of the poorest individuals.[6]

But even as the ACA establishes a new foundational base for health insurance, it pretty much leaves untouched the organization and practice of health care. Important pilot efforts are authorized that aim to use Medicare and (at state option) Medicaid to incentivize greater quality and efficiency among health care providers.[7] But these pilots do not alter providers' freedoms to select the patients they wish to treat, practice in what they perceive to be desirable locations, reject patients considered too difficult to manage, or specialize in accordance with the practice area of their own choosing. Nothing in the law compels physicians—the gateway into the health care system—to locate in poor communities, to accept Medicaid beneficiaries or uninsured people, to learn to speak multiple languages, or to become skilled in caring for patients whose health burdens extend far beyond a relatively simple set of presenting clinical symptoms. By contrast, adaptation of health care to medically underserved communities and populations is the hallmark of the health center program.[8]

The ACA makes a number of major investments in community health centers. A primary purpose of these investments is to address the chronic shortage of health care professionals to serve the low-income and medically underserved populations who are the principal beneficiaries of health reform. An additional purpose is to prepare for the surge in health care use that can be expected to flow from a major expansion of insurance (Kessler 2009) to thirty-two million persons, including the sixteen million mostly adult poor people who will gain Medicaid eligibility.[9] The aim of these reforms is to more than double the size of the program by 2019, growing health centers from the twenty million patients served in 2009 (NACHC 2009) into a health care gateway for some fifty million medically underserved children and adults by 2019 (Rosenbaum, Jones, and Shin 2010). Most of these patients will be insured, but more than one in five is projected to remain without health insurance as a result of gaps in coverage, the lack of affordable options, or legal status (ibid.). This is to be expected, of course, given the mission of health centers.

How health centers respond to this updated mission and the opportunities and challenges that lie ahead are the focus of this chapter. The chapter begins with an overview of the health centers program and its key characteristics. It then describes the major elements of the law that will help shape their ability to achieve this expanded gateway mission. It also discusses broader currents moving through the health care system as a whole—including the pressures toward clinical and financial integration—that ultimately will bear directly on health centers' success in opening a window onto the entire health care system for their patients.

Overview

Health Centers' Origins and Affiliations

Chapter 2 reviews the history of community health centers in depth; briefly, they were established in 1965 by the Office of Economic Opportunity as a War on Poverty demonstration program and with roots in the civil rights movement (Davis and Schoen 1978; Lefkowitz 2007; Adashi, Geiger, and Fine 2010). The program was transformed in 1975 from federal demonstration status to a formal component of the Public Health Service Act (PHSA).[10] Today community health centers represent an important national investment whose goal is to anchor accessible and affordable health care in communities and populations identified as medically underserved by a combination of health risk characteristics and a shortage of primary health care services (HRSA 2010b).[11]

The program's mission is evident from the core statutory requirements that define it: first, location in, or service to, a medically underserved population; second, an obligation to make care affordable through the use of prospectively adjusted charges tied to income; third, a duty to provide (either directly or through referrals) comprehensive care that transcends that found in a traditional clinical practice and that traverses clinical care, public health, and social interventions (table 3.1); and finally, governance by a board the majority of whose members are patients of the health center.[12]

While these requirements are fixed in statute, it is important to note that health centers come about in many ways. An independent community organization might sponsor a health center. A health center can also be initially sponsored by another health care entity (such as a hospital system) that itself does not meet the requirements of the law; indeed, many of the earliest health centers were sponsored by hospitals and were later spun off as independent corporations capable of satisfying all PHSA requirements including community board governance. Health centers are permitted to—indeed, they are encouraged to—enter into a wide range of affiliations; without affiliations (with other medical care practices, managed care organizations, hospitals, nursing facilities, laboratories, and other types of health care entities), it is not possible for health centers to meet their broad health care obligations, which, as table 3.1 shows, do not stop at primary care (Rosenbaum et al. 2011).

Nor is economic viability possible without affiliation. As discussed at greater length in the following section, health centers rely principally on Medicaid for their funding. As Medicaid has moved steadily toward the use of managed care arrangements, failure to enter into formal agreements with managed care plans would effectively cut health centers off from their patients and their principal source of revenue while placing them in violation of the requirement that health centers participate in all health insurance programs used by their patients.[13]

In sum, by statute and by mission, health centers must affiliate.[14] While health centers are community-based entities subject to unique board governance requirements, they also are corporate health care enterprises designed to take maximum advantage of the types of resources available in poor communities, including any available source of public and private health insurance. Furthermore, as health care providers with broad clinical care obligations, health centers are expected to display the degree of relationship to other parts

Table 3.1   **Primary and Supplemental Services at Health Centers**

Primary Health Services	Supplemental Health Services
Medical diagnostic and treatment services	Inpatient and outpatient hospital services
Diagnostic laboratory and radiologic services	Home health services
Preventive health services for children and adults including preventive pediatric care, prenatal and postpartum care, immunizations, and voluntary family planning services	Extended-care facility services
Emergency medical services	Rehabilitative services
Transportation services	Mental health services
Preventive dental services	Dental services other than those provided as primary health services
Services, including those of outreach workers, that promote and facilitate optimal use of primary health services and services referred to above and, if a substantial number of individuals in the population served by the center are of limited English-speaking ability, the services of outreach workers and other personnel fluent in the language or languages spoken by such individuals	Vision services, including routine eye and vision examinations and provision of eyeglasses, as appropriate and feasible
	Allied health services
	Pharmaceutical services, including the provision of prescription drugs
	Therapeutic radiologic services
	Public health services (including nutrition education and social services)
	Ambulatory surgical services
	Health education services

Source: 42 USC §254b

of their community health systems that are integral to the successful delivery of health care. Although health centers' ability to secure services for their patients invariably suffers the types of constraints that can be expected to affect the performance of providers whose services are aimed at medically disenfranchised patients, federal law nonetheless establishes a health center's duty to act essentially as "committed sponsor" to its patients (Duff and Hollingshead 1968).[15] The working clinical, teaching, and managed care collaborations that health centers have developed in numerous communities over the years are all evidence of the high degree of community integration they have achieved, and the federal law establishing health centers anticipates such integration (Rosenbaum et al., 2011).

Health Center Penetration, Patients, and Services

One reason health centers have enduring strength lies in the data produced by the program; unlike state health care block grants, the program produces extensive (and for the most part publicly available) information about what it does, which in turn elucidates health centers' contributions at the national, state, and community levels.

Twelve hundred community and migrant health center grantees operating sites in more than eight thousand locations served some twenty million patients in 2009 (Adashi, Geiger, and Fine 2010). The health centers statute actually encompasses several grantee categories (one grantee can in fact hold awards under multiple categories), but all grantee types share the program's basic characteristics of affordability, comprehensiveness, location in or service to medically underserved areas and populations, and community governance. At the same time, each grantee category has its own history, traditions, and mission. What might be thought of as the traditional model grew out of the original pilot demonstrations and has an obligation to serve all residents within its defined service area. Migrant health centers, whose origins actually predate the 1965 pilot program (Lefkowitz 2007), are designed to meet the unique health care needs of migrant and seasonal farmworkers; in 2002, 125 of the nation's 843 health center grantees received migrant health grants (Rosenbaum and Shin 2005); in 2009, health centers served more than 940,000 migrant and seasonal farmworker patients (NACHC 2009). In addition, the health center family includes grantees whose mission is aimed at providing health care for homeless individuals and families as well as residents of public housing. As with migrant health centers, many of these providers also may hold general-purpose health center grants. In 2009 health centers served one million homeless patients (NACHC 2009).

Health centers are found in all states, but certain states show higher numbers of grantees in relation to their low-income populations, with the greatest representation in the Northeast and the greatest deficits in the South and Southwest (Ku et al. 2011). At the same time, health centers are quite geographically dispersed, a testament to the high level of need (nearly 100 million persons live in urban and rural communities designated as medically underserved; Ku, Shin, and Rosenbaum 2009) and the program's popularity (regardless of political stripe, virtually all members of Congress desire health centers in their states and districts).

Health center patients reflect the centers' statutory mission and obligations: they are disproportionately poor, members of racial and ethnic minority groups, uninsured, and dependent on public health insurance. In 2008 racial minority patients made up 53 percent of all health center patients, and one-third of all patients were Hispanic/Latino. Compared to the US population, health center patients are nearly six times as likely to be poor, two and one-half times as likely to be uninsured, and nearly three times as likely to receive Medicaid (Rosenbaum, Jones, and Shin 2010). Uninsured patients (38 percent of all health center patients) and Medicaid patients (36 percent) account for almost 75 percent of health center caseloads (figure 3.1).

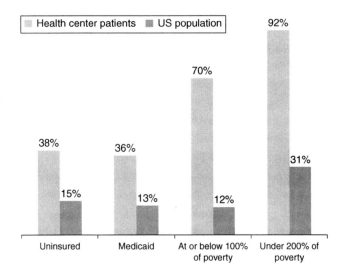

Figure 3.1 Health Centers Serve Disproportionately Poor, Uninsured, and Publicly Insured Patients, 2008

Source: Kaiser Commission on Medicaid and the Uninsured (2010); George Washington University Department of Health Policy analysis of 2008 Uniform Data System data and 2008 Current Population Survey

Although health centers can be found in all states, these national figures show considerable variation at the state level (Adashi, Geiger, and Fine 2010). In 2006 the proportion of uninsured health center patients ranged from 19 percent or lower to 40 percent or greater (NACHC 2008). Among Medicaid patients, the proportion served ranged from under 10 percent in seven states to more than 20 percent in twelve states and the District of Columbia (Rosenbaum, Jones, and Shin 2010). The proportion of Medicaid patients served by health centers is two and one-half times greater than their overall proportion in the population (NACHC 2009).

Although the health center program is commonly thought of as one skewed toward urban communities and populations, in fact the opposite is true. Compared to the general population, health center patients are more likely to live in rural areas (44 percent of health center patients, compared with 21 percent of the population; Rosenbaum, Jones, and Shin 2010). Health center patients are also more likely to be younger and female, although the number of Medicare beneficiaries served by health centers has risen significantly over the past decade. In 2008 children comprised 36 percent of all health center patients while nearly 60 percent of patients were female (ibid.).

Health center patients exhibit a greater burden of poor health. Compared with patients receiving care from private physicians, health center patients are nearly three times more likely to seek care for serious and chronic conditions (figure 3.2).

Consistent with their penetration into poor and medically underserved communities, health centers have the potential to influence the accessibility, quality, and outcome of health care, not only for individual patients but also at the community level. The earliest health center studies show measurable community-wide impact on infant mortality and the immunization status of children (Davis and Schoen 1978), and research has found an association between the presence of health centers and reductions in health disparities (Falik et al. 2006; NACHC 2007; Gold et al. 2009; Probst, Laditka, and Laditka 2009). Of particular note has been health centers' performance in the area of preventive health care; research suggests that low-income, Medicaid, and uninsured patients served by health centers are more likely than low-income patients served in other clinical settings to receive preventive services (Dor et al. 2008). But, consistent with the high number of Medicaid and uninsured patients they serve, health centers tend to experience more serious problems than physicians in office-based practice in securing specialty referrals for their uninsured and publicly insured patients (figure 3.3). At the same time,

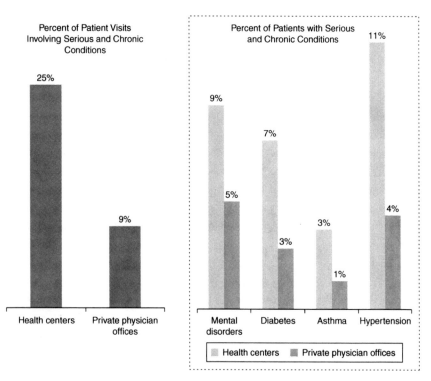

Figure 3.2   Health Center Patients and Visits Are Chronic Illness–Related, Compared with Office-Based Physicians

Note: Estimates based on comparable diagnoses of diabetes, hypertension, asthma, heart disease, and mental illness as a proportion of total medical visits. *Source*: Burt, McCaig, and Rechtsteiner 2007; health center data from 2007 Uniform Data System, Health Resources and Services Administration.

Source: Kaiser Commission on Medicaid and the Uninsured 2010; private physician data from 2006 National Ambulatory Medical Care Survey (Centers for Disease Control, National Center for Health Statistics, 2008); 2006 Uniform Data System, Health Resources and Services Administration.

consistent with the higher prevalence of serious conditions, health centers outperform private physicians in referral rates for their privately insured patients (Rosenbaum, Jones, and Shin 2010).

Part of health centers' ability to effectively reach low-income populations is the extent to which their care and services have been adapted to their patients through enabling services such as outreach, translation, and transportation. In addition, health centers employ a wide range of clinical staff including physicians, nurse practitioners and physician assistants, dentists, and behavioral health specialists. Because health centers are organized as staff-model clinics, they are able to achieve practice efficiencies and greater levels

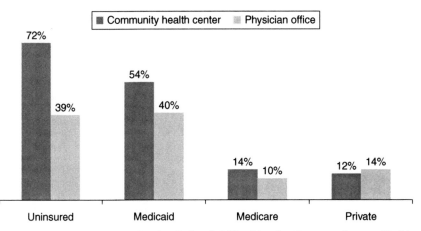

Figure 3.3 Patients Experiencing Referral Difficulties, by Coverage Source: Health Centers and Physician Practices, 2006

Source: Kaiser Commission on Medicaid and the Uninsured; CDC/NCHS, 2006 National Ambulatory Medical Care Survey by Esther Hing and David A. Woodwell, "Differences in Physician Visits at Community Health Centers and Physician Offices: United States, 2008"

of integration (Dor et al. 2008; Dor et al. 2009; Ku et al. 2009; Ku, Rosenbaum, and Shin 2009; Rosenbaum et al. 2009).

Health Center Staffing and Revenues

Health centers contribute significantly to the presence of clinical staff in medically underserved communities. In 2008 health centers employed more than fifty-one thousand medical, dental, and mental health/substance abuse staff. Health centers make extensive use of National Health Service Corps (NHSC) personnel; between 2003 and 2008, health centers employed approximately 5,350 full-time equivalent NHSC-supported clinicians, making them the nation's single largest NHSC placement site (HRSA 2010a). Beyond clinical staff, health centers represent a significant source of community employment; one analysis found a 4:1 return on the health center investment in the form of direct economic benefits into poor communities and indirect benefits as a result of job creation (Shin, Finnegan, and Rosenbaum 2008; Shin et al. 2010).

Federally funded health centers derive their revenues from multiple payers, including public and private health insurance and federal, state, and local grants and contracts (figure 3.4). In the early days, federal grant funding comprised health centers' overwhelming source of funding. By 2008 PHSA grants accounted for only 18.3 percent of all health center revenues. Medicaid revenues, by contrast, accounted for 37 percent, two and one-half times their

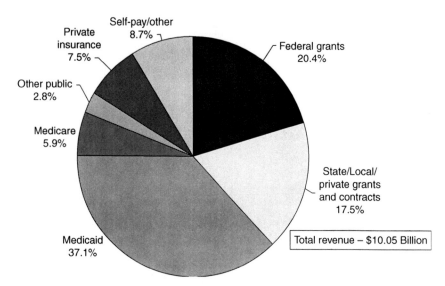

Figure 3.4   Sources of Health Center Revenue, 2008

Source: Kaiser Commission on Medicaid and the Uninsured 2010; GWU Department of Health Policy analysis of 2008 Uniform Data System data

relative importance in 1985. The rise in Medicaid revenues as the central source of health center funding can be attributed to the significant expansions in Medicaid eligibility that have occurred since the 1980s as well as the enactment of special coverage and payment rules for health centers in 1990.[16]

The effect of public health insurance expansions on the size and scope of community health centers is best evidenced by the following statistics: between 1990 and 2004, Medicaid revenues grew by 250 percent while the number of uninsured patients increased by 141 percent, even though, in real-dollar terms, discretionary grant funding for health centers remained essentially flat (Rosenbaum and Shin 2006). To be sure, federal grant funding plays a crucial role because it serves as the foundation of the health center model. From a purely financial perspective, however, Medicaid has built the modern health center and served as the program's growth engine. For this reason, it is the ACA's Medicaid expansions (as well as, to a lesser extent, the coverage that will become available through state health insurance exchanges) that will propel health centers forward.

Under Medicare and Medicaid amendments, community health centers are known as federally qualified health centers (FQHC). Federal qualification makes health centers eligible for Medicaid and Medicare coverage and federal grants, and entitles them to special cost-related payment rules and federal grants. (Entities that meet all federally funded health center requirements but do not receive a federal grant are called look-alike centers.) The goal of the FQHC amendments was to protect federal and state grant funds meant for care of the uninsured from cross-subsidizing the cost of treating publicly insured patients. These provisions have had a major impact on health center financing. The payment protections extend to health centers participating in managed care arrangements, with state Medicaid programs and Medicare both responsible for reconciling revenues received from managed care entities against the reasonable cost of care for the population.[17]

The FQHC payment methodology creates several noteworthy incentives. Health centers are paid on a per-encounter basis, which incentivizes volume. At the same time, payments for each encounter are bundled into an all-inclusive rate reflecting all available clinical and ancillary services. The payment methodology thus captures the broad array of services furnished by health centers (including clinical overhead costs) and recognizes the higher volume of encounters that might arise from a sicker patient population while at least potentially encouraging efficiencies within any single encounter or class of encounters as a result of payment bundling.

Additional, if indirect, sources of financial support for health centers come from two important federal legal provisions. First, FQHCs receive their malpractice coverage under the Federal Tort Claims Act, thereby alleviating the need to purchase professional and institutional liability insurance on the open market.[18] Second, FQHCs are qualified to participate in the Section 340B prescription drug program, which entitles them to deeply discounted rates for outpatient prescription drugs.[19]

The Affordable Care Act and Health Center Investments

The Affordable Care Act elevates the status and profile of health centers, both through direct investment and indirectly as a result of its structure, which rests a reformed private insurance system on a much-expanded Medicaid base. Because health centers play such a pivotal role in Medicaid and in care of lower-income populations more generally, the ACA essentially commits an advance investment in health centers to pave the way for the surge in health care use that can be expected among the lower-income population as a result of newly acquired insurance coverage.

The ACA Prelude

Prior to passage of the ACA, Congress made important investments in health centers, appropriating additional funds as part of the 2008 reauthorization of the program and the 2009 American Reinvestment and Recovery Act (ARRA, the stimulus law) to enable growth and modernization. The Health Care Safety Net Act of 2008 reauthorized the program for four years and appropriated funds aimed at growing the program by 50 percent over this period.[20] The act also reauthorized and increased funding for the NHSC.

The stimulus law appropriated an additional $2 billion for investment in health center expansion. ARRA included funding to further increase health center capacity and provided direct funding through a combination of Medicaid and grants to enable the adoption of health information technology (HIT). About 99 percent of health center physicians are predicted to be eligible for Medicaid HIT adoption incentive payments, which invest in HIT infrastructure for providers that serve a disproportionate share of Medicaid patients. By 2010 the ARRA investment led to the establishment of 126 new health center access points and three million additional patients served, with more funds reaching communities with the highest unemployment rates (Finnegan et al. 2009).

Elements of the ACA

The ACA builds on this series of investments in multiple ways while also positioning health centers to send even deeper roots into the health care landscape. The ACA reforms include both expansion of health insurance for low-income populations served by health centers and direct investment in health center capacity and increased access.

Expanded Health Center Capacity

The ACA provides mandatory funding (not subject to discretionary appropriations) to expand health centers and the National Health Service Corps, providing $11 billion for health center expansion and $1.5 billion for NHSC growth over the FY 2011–2015 time period. In addition, health reform permanently authorizes both programs.

Of the $11 billion allocated to health centers, $9.5 billion is allocated to the expansion of health center operational capacity, with the remaining funding allocated to helping health centers meet their capital needs, such as renovating existing sites and upgrading HIT systems (table 3.2).

In combination, the health center and NHSC expansion funding is expected to add sufficient service capacity to reach an additional thirty to forty million patients by 2015, with a projected patient capacity of between thirty-six and fifty million more patients by 2019 (Rosenbaum, Jones, and Shin 2010). Because the ACA is projected to leave some twenty-four million individuals without health insurance, and because health centers have service to the uninsured as a core part of their mission, the number of uninsured health center patients is anticipated to remain at a significantly elevated 22 percent by 2019, down from 38 percent in 2009 (Ku et al. 2010).

Medicaid and Medicare

By far the most important growth generator under the ACA for health centers is the expansion of Medicaid to all children and adults with family incomes below 133 percent of the federal poverty level. When fully phased in, the Medicaid expansion is projected to reach some sixteen million persons and can be expected to have a major impact on the insurance status of health center patients. One estimate shows that the proportion of patients served by health centers who are enrolled in Medicaid can be expected to rise from 35 percent in 2008 to 43 percent by 2019 (Ku et al. 2010). Although FQHC services are not part of a modified Medicaid "benchmark benefit" package to which newly eligible beneficiaries will be entitled, they remain a covered benefit for the traditional Medicaid insureds. The "benchmark" package, like the "essential benefit" package for individuals who will receive coverage through health insurance exchanges, includes coverage for many of the services that health centers provide, such as ambulatory medical care, prescribed drugs, maternity care, comprehensive pediatric care, and laboratory and diagnostic tests—all of which are basic health center service features. At the same time, however, other services required of all health centers, such as preventive dental services, enabling services, and transportation, are not covered by the

Table 3.2   **Increases in Health Center Program and National Health Service Corps Funding (FY 2011–FY 2015)**

Health Centers	National Health Service Corps
Total five-year funding increase: $11 billion	Total five-year funding increase: $1.5 billion
Capital needs: $1.5 billion	
Operating funds:	Operating funds:
FY 2011: $1.0 billion	FY 2011: $290 million
FY 2012: $1.2 billion	FY 2012: $295 million
FY 2013: $1.5 billion	FY 2013: $300 million
FY 2014: $2.2 billion	FY 2014: $305 million
FY 2015: $3.6 billion	FY 2015: $310 million

Source: Kaiser Commission on Medicaid and the Uninsured; calculations by George Washington University Department of Health Policy

Medicaid benchmark and are only optional benefits for traditional Medicaid (see table 3.1). Medicaid payment policy addresses this issue by providing a bundled payment to FQHCs that is intended to compensate for this full range of services for any Medicaid patient, either current or newly eligible.[21]

Recognizing FQHCs' burgeoning Medicare beneficiary population, the ACA also improves Medicare's payment rates, reducing the impact of the artificially low payment structure that was imposed on health centers in 1992 by the first Bush administration.

Private Health Insurance through State Health Insurance Exchanges

The creation of health insurance exchanges, with their ability to offer subsidized private health insurance coverage to individuals regardless of health status, represents another key growth generator for health centers. Most uninsured health center patients who do not qualify for Medicaid will likely qualify for subsidies in the exchanges unless they are undocumented immigrants. The availability of this new coverage and the associated drop in uninsured health center patients will have a major impact on health center operations. One estimate shows that by 2019, more than 9 percent of health center patients will be covered by exchange plans (Ku et al. 2010). Approximately 30 percent of all health center patients have family incomes that exceed the federal poverty level; this figure may rise as health centers grow and reach greater numbers of communities that, while underserved, are not deeply impoverished.

Figure 3.5 shows the projected health insurance composition of health center patients over a ten-year period ending in 2019. The proportion of patients who are uninsured is expected to decline significantly, but uninsured

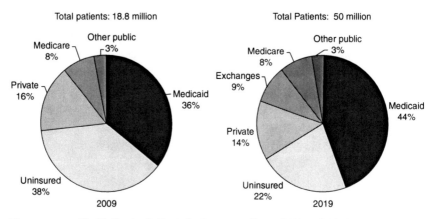

Figure 3.5   Health Center Patients by Insurance Type, 2009 and 2019

Source: Ku et al. 2010

patients will remain at the core of the health center system, and, as is the case today, health center grants can be expected to cover only that portion of the care these patients need that is primary in nature.

For health plans to qualify to sell through the new exchanges, they will be required to contract with essential community providers such as health centers.[22] In the case of health centers, qualified health plans also will be required to pay providers at the Medicaid FQHC payment rate, a reform prompted by evidence of major revenue shortfalls (50–60 percent) experienced by health centers in treating privately insured patients (Shin et al. 2008).[23] Furthermore, because the system of subsidies for lower-income persons enrolled in exchange plans includes cost-sharing assistance to individuals below 250 percent of the federal poverty level, health centers will benefit financially from being shielded, at least partially, from the cost of uncovered deductibles and coinsurance.

Medical Residency Training Programs

An additional important investment that contemplates a significant role for health centers is establishment of "teaching health centers" to finance community-based residency training and to link community-based health care providers such as health centers more closely to the medical and osteopathic professions' residency and training programs.

Investments in Health System Change

The ACA deals with the imperative to address terrible financial costs that health care exacts on the US economy, chiefly through a series of demonstration and pilot efforts. Their purpose is to put Medicare and (at the option of each state) Medicaid to work on new payment models that, taken together, do two things. First the law encourages health care providers to become more efficient in managing complex patients—particularly those with extensive physical and mental health conditions—through the use of a medical-home approach to patient care.[24] The medical-home model has been a feature of the health policy landscape for some forty years (AAP 2010) but has ascended in importance in the past decade.[25] Embracing the concept aims to boost the role of primary health care providers as active managers of the full range of patient needs, especially in the case of patients with chronic illnesses and conditions. Because the law's concept of a medical home turns on broad coordination activities and expanded primary care access, the move to emphasize medical homes in primary health care financing inevitably dovetails with the essential attributes of a community health center.[26] Indeed, in November 2010 the

Centers for Medicare and Medicaid Services (CMS) announced a partnership with five hundred community health centers to launch a medical-home demonstration for up to 195,000 Medicare beneficiaries who are health center patients (CMS 2010).

A second health care financing reform model—and one that by November 2010 had worked the health care industry into a frenzy of buzzwords, conferences, and business positioning in the market—is the accountable-care organization (ACO).[27] Defining ACOs through a range of functionality attributes and institutional characteristics, the ACA essentially offers financial incentives through Medicare (and again, at state option, through Medicaid) as a means of promoting more integrated health care practice. The law seeks to achieve this result by encouraging the creation of vertically integrated health care arrangements or joint ventures of individual professionals and smaller groups that agree to operate in a shared governance fashion and to assume responsibility for comprehensive patient care through the collective use of professional and financial resources. Collective accountability for costs, quality, and information about performance and outcome are essential elements of an ACO. The inducement is the ability to profit if overall costs remain below projected expenditures for a patient population. For ACOs to work, the providers that form the new enterprises must be able to adapt to practice styles that encourage efficiencies and that are geared to holding down costs while improving quality.

As with medical homes, health centers would appear to be logical—and indeed essential—partners in ACO formation and operation in medically underserved communities. This logic rests on their location, their scope of services, their integrated operations, their emphasis on management of patients with multiple chronic conditions, and their legal and mission-driven obligation to achieve clinical integration, at least at the primary care level.

Health Reform's Great Transformation

Health reform promises to transform health centers from an important but modest program for underserved communities into a permanent part of the health care landscape, a national enterprise capable of serving one in seven Americans, fully integrated into the community health systems in which health centers operate. The ACA achieves this health care gateway goal through a series of direct investments, but most notably through an expansion of subsidized health coverage for low-income individuals and families, particularly Medicaid. Some might think that insurance coverage expansion will obviate the need for health centers by opening access to "mainstream" health care providers. The experience of Massachusetts's health centers in the wake of that state's landmark reform suggests just the opposite, in fact. As a result of issues related to capacity, place, and population characteristics, medically underserved communities remain medically underserved despite coverage expansions. In this respect, the integration of health centers into broader care arrangements remains essential if these integrated care arrangements are to reach populations most in need of improved health care access.

Throughout their history, health centers have shown a nimbleness and resilience that helps explain their success. Part of their nimbleness comes from the fact that health centers must adapt to their communities in order to fulfill their obligations. Part of their resilience comes from the fact that, given their mission and the financing and populations they serve, health centers have had to build relatively complex systems of care with limited resources. Yet even with their history of nimbleness and resilience, health centers will face considerable challenges under health reform. These challenges can be categorized into two major groups: the need to double their capacity within a decade; and the need to not merely undergo the clinical and financial evolution that increasingly will be demanded of broader community health systems but also to lead the way for the populations they serve. Simply put, the nation's ability to financially sustain universal health insurance depends on the degree to which the health care system can work smarter and within realistic resource constraints. Indeed, the very first people to lose coverage if the achievements of 2010 fail will be the very patients and communities that health centers are committed to serve. Considering this, the successful evolution of health centers will need to address four major tasks.

Strengthening Adult Medicine Programs While Preserving Their Strength in Maternal, Child, and Women's Health

Health centers historically have served a population that skews toward young women and children. Appropriate clinical care for these populations presents a major challenge to be sure, but health centers have been able to achieve important results in maternal and child health over the years. Now health centers face a major demand for growth in their adult medicine capabilities, including managing the needs of older men and women who are indigent and who may have gone years without appropriate care. (Nearly 40 percent of uninsured adults received virtually no health care in the preceding two years [KCMU 2010].) In addition, health centers can be expected to face increasing health care demands among low-income Medicare beneficiaries, who consume a disproportionate amount of Medicare and Medicaid funding and whose appropriate management is crucial not only to population health but also to long-term cost containment.

Strengthening health centers' adult medicine performance—in particular the ability to further improve their management of patients with multiple, chronic physical and mental health conditions—while holding fast to their performance in the area of maternal, child, and primary reproductive health for women of childbearing age will constitute a major test of skills. Meeting the test will involve not only new staff recruitment and the continuing adoption of health information and clinical quality improvement systems but also the forging of new community affiliations around chronic disease management and the negotiation of payment arrangements that test payment bundling and shared savings.

Payment Reforms That Do Not Jeopardize Care for the Uninsured

As health centers move to strengthen their chronic disease management capabilities, they will continually confront the need to develop new payment systems in which health centers are a part of an integrated enterprise that receives aggregated payment covering most if not all aspects of clinical and related treatment. This more fully integrated system is very different from the current FQHC payment system, which is encounter-based and thus rewards volume, and which captures into bundled payments for any particular condition the costs that health centers incur for the full range of services they provide to all patients.

The new payment arrangements, with different amounts for particular types of patients and conditions, will be far more targeted in what services they will recognize, and these payment systems can further be expected to reward efficiency rather than volume. Both of these expectations hold implications for health centers, which have utilized the broad revenue-generating aspects of the FQHC payment structure to propel growth and an increasing depth of care.

Despite the ACA's considerable capital and operational investments, the per capita payments that health centers receive under their federal grants will continue to recognize only the cost of on-site care, not those costs associated with supplemental and specialized treatments. At the same time, health centers can be expected to play an increasingly important role in caring for the uninsured, as discussed previously. While ACA projections suggest that 6 percent of the population will be uninsured by 2019, separate projections for health centers show that the rate of uninsured patients at health centers will be nearly four times as great. To be sure, this is to be expected, given their history, mission, and federal obligations, but in a world in which no payer wants to incur costs for treatments and services other than what it needs for its particular patients, the reality of uncompensated care at health centers looms as a major impediment to their broader integration.

The answer lies in the formulation of updated policy regarding how to compensate health centers for the uninsured populations they treat and manage as well as the services they furnish that enable care and improve health for all patients but that are not recognized as covered or payable under traditional concepts of health insurance, including the essential benefit package established under the ACA in the individual and small-group markets. The ACA's interim policy position is to preserve the Medicare and Medicaid FQHC payment methodology (which ensures compensation of reasonable costs of FQHC services on a per-encounter basis) and to extend this methodology to qualified health plans operating inside exchanges, but to leave FQHCs to normal market forces outside of exchanges. How long this interim policy will last is anyone's guess. However, state Medicaid programs have placed increasing pressure on the CMS to waive application of the FQHC coverage and payment requirements as part of broader demonstrations conducted under Section 1115 of the Social Security Act.[28] The ultimate answer may lie in an express all-payer uncompensated care add-on, a separate supplemental payment (similar to Medicare and Medicaid DSH), an increase in discretionary appropriation, an additional federal stop-loss payment, or some other approach. Regardless, a decision will clearly be needed about how to allow health centers to lead in the evolution to population-based payment structures, in which revenues and rewards often flow through broader market-based enterprises while protecting uninsured patients and services at a health center and community-specific level.

Attention to Affiliation

By law, health centers can and must affiliate and become an integral part of the health care systems in which they operate. Nonetheless, important legal considerations arise for health centers that seek to affiliate. Some of these considerations are matters for all health care providers, such as fraud and antitrust concerns and tax law implications for nonprofit entities. But other legal issues are unique to health centers. These include the challenge of coordinating the legal aspects of affiliations and joint ventures with PHSA grant requirements, Federal Tort Claims Act legal considerations (which cover certain but by no means all health center operations in a broadened affiliation arrangement), and considerations related to other aspects of health centers' unique structure. One matter that is in all likelihood a nonissue is governance structure. Like all nonprofit entities, health centers have certain obligations related to governance. It so happens that in the case of health centers, fiduciary power lies with a board whose majority is composed of patients rather than other members of the communities in which they practice. The fact that governance is patient-majority should be no more a barrier to affiliation than the legal questions that arise when any nonprofit corporation affiliates with other entities.

Finding Good Partners with a Commitment to Community Health

Clearly, health centers must find partners that recognize their potential for high quality and efficient care. But health centers need partners that also recognize their mission. Two major sets of partners come to mind. The first is public hospital and health care systems that, like health centers, share their mission and obligations and that have the breadth of supplemental services and specialty arrangements that health center patients need. The second is nonprofit hospitals and health systems that, under Internal Revenue Code reforms contained in the ACA, must document their community benefit activities in the area of community-wide health planning and uncompensated care (Burt, McCaig, and Rechtsteiner 2007). Affiliations with health centers that specify a range of referral and support services flowing from the hospital to health centers and that include public health agencies and health programs in the community could constitute a specific form of community benefit in furtherance of both strategic community-wide service activities and as evidence of commitment to uncompensated care. These affiliations could in turn form the basis for community-oriented ACOs.

The list of challenges clearly could be lengthened, but these are the major issues and opportunities that will confront health centers in the coming years. The good news is, first, that there is no set of health care providers that has demonstrated a greater ability to rise to new challenges, and second, that health centers come to the table with real resources and remarkably bipartisan goodwill. In the coming years, much of the ACA's success in medically underserved communities and populations rests with health centers. It is no exaggeration to note that health centers' ability to meet these challenges will help determine the extent to which the seminal insurance achievements of the ACA are sustainable.

Notes

1. Pub. L. 111–148, as amended by the Health Care and Education Reconciliation Act, Pub. L. 111–152.
2. Public Health Service Act (PHSA), §§2701–2794 as amended by Patient Protection and Affordable Care Act (PPACA) §§1001 and 1201.

3. Internal Revenue Code §5000A as added by PPACA §1501.
4. PPACA §1401.
5. PPACA §1311.
6. Social Security Act (SSA) §1902(a) as amended by PPACA §2001.
7. See, e.g., PPACA §3021 (Center for Medicare and Medicaid Innovation), §3022 (Medicare Shared Savings Program (Accountable Care Organizations), §3023 (national pilot on payment bundling), §3502 (establishing community health teams to support the patient-centered medical home), §2703 (state Medicaid option to provide health homes for enrollees with chronic conditions, and §2706 (pediatric accountable care organizations).
8. 42 U.S.C. §254b.
9. The report found long waits for primary care and elevated emergency department use rates as a result of a limited supply of physicians coupled with maldistribution of available health care resources.
10. PHSA §330, codified at 42 U.S.C. §254b.
11. An area or population is designated as medically underserved, according to 1976 regulations issued by the Department of Health and Human Services, if its score on an "index of medical underservice" (IMU) shows high need. HRSA notes that the "IMU involves four variables—ratio of primary medical care physicians per 1,000 population, infant mortality rate, percentage of the population with incomes below the poverty level, and percentage of the population age 65 or over." Thus, while there are more than 6,200 areas as of 2010 holding designations as primary care health professions shortage areas (HPSAs), the medical underservice area designation (MUA) denotes not only a shortage of providers but one or more patient populations whose overall health status is compromised. All MUAs are treated as HPSAs, which determine placement of National Health Service Corps professionals. See generally HRSA's discussion at http://bhpr.hrsa.gov/shortage/ (accessed Nov. 21, 2010).
12. PHSA §330(a), (b) and (k)(3)(H) (2009).
13. PHSA §330(k)(3)(E).
14. PHSA §330(k)(3)(B).
15. The term "committed sponsor" is used by Duff and Hollingshead to denote clinicians who exhibit the highest duty of loyalty to their patients to secure what they judge to be medically necessary health care.
16. Pub. L. 101–508, The Omnibus Budget Reconciliation Act of 1990.
17. SSA §§1923(aa)(1)(A)
18. 28 U.S.C. §1346(b).
19. PHSA §340B.
20. Pub. L. 110–355.
21. PPACA §2001. Section 1937 (b)(4) specifically provides for the provision of FQHC services and prospective payment system (PPS) reimbursement to FQHCs as provided under §1902(bb) even in the benchmark or benchmark-equivalent packages provided for in Section 1937(b); thus, it would appear that FQHC payment rules apply to newly eligible beneficiaries.
22. PPACA §1311(c)(1)(C).
23. PPACA §1302.
24. For reasons that relate to the politics of semantics in health professionalism, medical homes in Medicaid are known as "health homes." PPACA § 2607.
25. The center reports that the first discussions of medical homes began in 1967 with the issuance of the *Standards for Child Health Care*.

26. PPACA §3502.
27. PPACA §3302.
28. 2 U.S.C. §1315. The 2010 approval of California's Medicaid waiver, for example, included waiver of the FQHC payment methodology. See CMS waiver approval letter referencing special terms and conditions. http://www.chhs.ca.gov/Documents/Waiver.pdf (accessed Feb. 9, 2011).

References

Adashi, E. Y., H. J. Geiger, and M. D. Fine. 2010. "Health Care Reform and Primary Care: The Growing Importance of the Community Health Center." *New England Journal of Medicine* 362:2047–2050.

American Academy of Pediatrics (AAP). 2010. "National Center for Medical Homes Implementation Overview." National Center for Medical Home Implementation. http://www.medicalhomeinfo.org/about/ (accessed Nov. 21, 2010).

Burt C. W., L. F. McCaig, and E. A. Rechtsteiner. 2007. "Ambulatory Medical Care Utilization Estimates for 2005." Advance data from *Vital and Health Statistics* 388. Hyattsville, MD: National Center for Health Statistics.

Centers for Medicare and Medicaid Services (CMS). 2010. "CMS Introduces New Center for Medicare and Medicaid Innovation, Initiatives to Better Coordinate Health Care." *CMS Media Releases: Press Releases.* Washington DC: US Department of Health and Human Services. http://www.cms.gov/apps/media/press/release.asp?Counter=3871&intNumPerPage=10&checkDate=&checkKey=&srchType=1&numDays=3500&srchOpt=0&srchData=&keywordType=All&chkNewsType=1%2C+2%2C+3%2C+4%2C+5&intPage=&showAll=&pYear=&year=&desc=&cboOrder=date (accessed Nov. 21, 2010).

Davis, K., and C. Schoen. 1978. *Health and the War on Poverty.* Washington DC: Brookings Institution Press.

Dor, A., Y. Pylypchuck, P. Sin, and S. Rosenbaum. 2008. "Uninsured and Medicaid Patients' Access to Preventive Care: Comparison of Health Centers and Other Primary Care Providers," Brief No. 4. Geiger Gibson/RCHN Community Health Foundation Research Collaborative. Washington DC: George Washington University School of Public Health and Health Services. http://www.gwumc.edu/sphhs/departments/healthpolicy/dhp_publications/index.cfm?mdl=pubSearch&evt=view&PublicationID=A5EFC6C5–5056–9D20–3DBB2F5E5B966398 (accessed Nov, 21, 2010).

Dor, A., P. Richard, E. Tan, S. Rosenbaum, P. Shin, and L. Repasch. 2009. "Community Health Centers in Indiana: State Investments and Returns," Brief No. 12. Geiger Gibson/RCHN Community Health Foundation Research Collaborative. Washington, DC: George Washington University School of Public Health and Health Services.

Duff, R. S., and A. Hollingshead. 1968. *Sickness and Society.* New York: Harper and Row.

Falik, M., J. Needleman, R. Herbert, B. Wells, R. Politzer, and M. B. Benedict. 2006. "Comparative Effectiveness of Health Centers as a Regular Source of Care." *Journal of Ambulatory Care Management* 29, no. 1: 24–35.

Finnegan, B., L. Ku, P. Shin, and S. Rosenbaum. 2009. "Boosting Health Information Technology in Medicaid: The Potential Effect of the American Recovery and Reinvestment Act." Brief No. 9. Geiger Gibson/RCHN Community Health Foundation Research Collaborative. Washington DC: George Washington University School of Public Health and Health Services.

Gold, R., J. DeVoe, A. Shah, and S. Chauvie. 2009. "Insurance Continuity and Receipt of Diabetes Preventive Care in a Network of Federally Qualified Health Centers." *Medical Care* 47:431–439.

Health Resources and Services Administration (HRSA). 2010a. "HRSA Data Warehouse." *United States Department of Health and Human Services.* http://datawarehouse .hrsa.gov/nhscdetail.aspx#anchor (accessed May 5, 2010).

———. 2010b. "Shortage Designation: Medically Underserved Areas and Populations." United States Department of Health and Human Services. http://bhpr.hrsa.gov/ shortage/muaguide.htm (accessed Nov. 21, 2010).

Kaiser Commission on Medicaid and the Uninsured (KCMU). 2010. "Community Health Centers: Opportunities and Challenges of Health Reform." Washington, DC: Kaiser Family Foundation. http://www.kff.org/uninsured/8098.cfm (accessed Feb. 5, 2011).

Kessler, M. 2009. "Despite High Coverage Rate, Mass. Residents Have Difficulty Finding Care" *BNA Health Policy Daily.* Washington, DC: Alliance of Community Health Plans. http://www.achp.org/newsroom/mmr/5710.html (accessed Nov. 19, 2010).

Ku, L., P. Richard, A. Dor, E. Tan, P. Shin, and S. Rosenbaum. 2009. "Using Primary Care to Bend the Curve: Estimating the Impact of a Health Center Expansion on Health Care Costs," Brief No. 14. Geiger Gibson/RCHN Community Health Foundation Research Collaborative. Washington DC: George Washington University School of Public Health and Health Services.

———. 2010. "Strengthening Primary Care to Bend the Cost Curve: The Expansion of Community Health Centers through Health Reform." Brief No. 19. Geiger Gibson/ RCHN Community Health Foundation Research Collaborative. Washington DC: George Washington University School of Public Health and Health Services.

Ku, L., S. Rosenbaum, and P. Shin. 2009. "Using Primary Care to Bend the Cost Curve: The Potential Impact of Health Center Expansion in Senate Reforms," Brief No. 16. Geiger Gibson/RCHN Community Health Foundation Research Collaborative. Washington DC: George Washington University School of Public Health and Health Services.

Ku, L., P. Shin, B. Bruen, and K. Hayes. 2011. "The States' Next Challenge: Securing Primary Care for Expanded Medicaid Populations." *New England Journal of Medicine* 364:493–495.

Ku, L., P. Shin, and S. Rosenbaum. 2009. "Estimating the Effects of Health Reform on Health Centers' Capacity to Expand to New Medically Underserved Communities and Populations." Geiger Gibson/RCHN Community Health Foundation Research Collaborative Policy Research Brief No. 11. Washington, DC: George Washington University School of Public Health and Health Services. http://www.gwumc.edu/sphhs/ departments/healthpolicy/dhp_publications/pub_uploads/dhpPublication_9889E996– 5056–9D20–3D1F89027D3F9406.pdf (accessed October 11, 2011).

Lefkowitz, B. 2007. *Community Health Centers: A Movement and the People Who Made It Happen.* New Brunswick: Rutgers University Press.

National Association of Community Health Centers (NACHC). 2007. *Access Granted: The Primary Care Payoff.* Washington DC: The Robert Graham Center, and Bethesda, MD: Capital Link.

———. 2008. "Health Centers and Uninsured: Improving Health and Access to Care." http://www.nachc.com/client/documents/Uninsured_Fact_Sheet_FINAL912.pdf.

———. 2009. "United States at a Glance." Washington DC. http://www.nachc.com/ client/documents/United%20States%20FSv2.pdf (accessed Nov. 21, 2010).

Probst, J. C., J. N. Laditka, and S. B. Laditka. 2009. "Association between Community Health Center and Rural Health Clinic Presence and County-Level Hospitalization Rates for Ambulatory Care Sensitive Conditions: An Analysis across Eight US States." *BMC Health Services Research* 9:134.

Rosenbaum, S., E. Jones, and P. Shin. 2010. *Community Health Centers: Opportunities and Challenges of Health Reform.* Kaiser Commission on Medicaid and the Uninsured. Washington, DC: Kaiser Family Foundation. http://www.kff.org/uninsured/8098.cfm (accessed Nov.21, 2010).

Rosenbaum, S., and P. Shin. 2005. "Migrant and Seasonal Farmworkers: Health Insurance Coverage and Access to Care." Kaiser Commission on Medicaid and the Uninsured. Washington DC: Kaiser Family Foundation. http://www.kff.org/uninsured/7314.cfm (accessed November 21, 2010).

———. 2006. "Health Centers Reauthorization: An Overview of Achievements and Challenges." Kaiser Commission on Medicaid and the Uninsured. http://www.kff.org/uninsured/upload/7471.pdf (accessed Feb. 5, 2011).

Rosenbaum, S., P. Shin, B. Finnegan, and R. Whittington. 2009. "Primary and Preventive Healthcare: A Critical Path to Healthcare Reform for Florida: The Role of Florida's FQHCs." Geiger Gibson Program in Community Health Policy. Washington DC: George Washington University Department of Health Policy.

Rosenbaum, S., M. Zakheim, J. Leifer, M. Golde, J. Schulte, and R. Margulies. 2011. "Assessing and Addressing Legal Barriers to Clinical Integration among Community Health Centers," July. Washington, DC: The Commonwealth Fund.

Shin, P., B. Bruen, E. Jones., L. Ku, and S. Rosenbaum. 2010. "The Economic Stimulus: Gauging the Early Effects of ARRA Funding on Health Centers and Medically Underserved Populations and Communities," Brief No. 17. Geiger Gibson/RCHN Community Health Foundation Research Collaborative. Washington DC: George Washington University School of Public Health and Health Services.

Shin, P., B. Finnegan, and S. Rosenbaum. 2008. "How Does Investment in Health Centers Affect the Economy?" Brief No. 1. Geiger Gibson/RCHN Community Health Foundation Research Collaborative. Washington DC: George Washington University School of Public Health and Health Services. http://www.gwumc.edu/sphhs/departments/healthpolicy/dhp_publications/pub_uploads/dhpPublication_A5C8D79 4–5056–9D20–3DD5D5A9CD2DAFD1.pdf (accessed Nov. 21, 2010).

Shin, P., B. Finnegan, J. Sharac, and S. Rosenbaum. 2008. "Health Centers: An Overview and Analysis of Their Experiences with Private Health Insurance." Kaiser Commission on Medicaid and the Uninsured. Washington DC: Kaiser Family Foundation.

Applying Lessons from Social Psychology to Repair the Health Care Safety Net for Undocumented Immigrants

"Our history tells us that immigration in the American story has always been controversial—associated always with both benefits and costs. . . . For native populations, European immigration meant death by disease, warfare, and social disorganization, a virtual genocide in which their populations fell by 90 percent by 1600. . . . When these death-bringing European immigrants became Americans by birth, their own response to further immigration was mixed. Industrious immigrants were indispensable in expanding colonial populations, and they were welcomed in the abstract and upon arrival. However, the quality of immigrants . . . was [and remains] a constant issue of concern."

—Otis L. Graham (2001)

"[Immigrants'] search for a better life is one of the most basic desires of human beings. Many undocumented workers have walked mile after mile, through the heat of the day and the cold of night. Some have risked their lives in dangerous desert border crossings, or entrusted their lives to the brutal rings of heartless human smugglers. Workers who seek only to earn a living end up in the shadows of American life—fearful, often abused and exploited."

—President George W. Bush (January 7, 2004)

This chapter offers a new tool to advance the discussion about how the law should respond to the presence of undocumented immigrants in America.

The Common Group Identity Model, formulated by social psychologists, explains the process of social categorization by which human beings naturally organize themselves into in-groups and out-groups and thus develop social perceptions to reinforce intergroup conflict. However, where group identities can be realigned, conflict can be reduced. This realignment, called "recategorization," introduces members of two previously separate groups of people to the recognition of their membership in an altogether different, single, inclusive, superordinate group. The result is that members of the two groups change their attitudes and behavior as they become involved in shared causes defined by the new in-group. Social psychologists have empirically shown it is possible to create new in-groups and improve intergroup relations by the deliberate exercise of recategorization (Dovidio et al. 2005). This chapter proposes that immigration policymakers consciously employ the lessons learned from the Common Group Identity Model to reform immigration law. My thesis is that the problems arising from social categorization—prejudice, stereotyping, discrimination, hatred, conflict, and violence—can be reversed by the process of what social psychologists call recategorization; therefore, state lawmakers may strengthen the health care safety net by applying recategorization theory to shape immigration law and policy.

I apply the Common Group Identity Model to the question of whether public funds should be spent to extend the health care safety net to undocumented immigrants. This is a question that the US Congress as well as a number of state and local legislative bodies have recently addressed by enacting a wave of statutes that limit the access undocumented immigrants have to publicly funded benefits. The generally restrictive trend in these laws that deny most health care benefits to the estimated twelve million noncitizens living in America has created what one commentator has described as a public health "nightmare" (Costich 2001). To date, most legal analysts have focused on the civil and human rights issues or the national safety concerns that these laws raise or address. I believe social psychologists might better explain the reasons underlying public benefit restrictions than lawyers. Moreover, social psychologists might also offer lawmakers the understanding they need to write a better law.

Undocumented immigrants are known to experience both high fertility rates and a higher incidence of communicable diseases. Noncitizens are frequently employed in jobs such as food service and preparation, domestic household employment, and agriculture where they will come into close contact with the larger population of citizens (Passel and Cohn 2009). Oddly, the current legal policy regime responds to these obvious public health concerns by legislatively restricting access by undocumented immigrants to all publicly supported services except emergency and basic public health care. Notwith-standing the threat these laws may present to the community's overall health and safety, the intent of these statutes is to discourage noncitizens from overburdening public resources. On its face, such a policy saves public benefit money. But closer inspection reveals these laws also increase the threat of disease spreading throughout the entire population. Psychologists offer insights that could help explain what motivates this policy and generate ideas to improve the immigration laws that implement it.

I argue here that American immigration policy would benefit from the Common Group Identity Model in two ways. First, by embracing the understanding that social psychologists have about the fundamental nature of the human tendency toward social categorization, the conversation about inclusivity and exclusivity among citizen and noncitizen groups might discard many of the polarizing presumptions and rhetoric about the current group interaction that has characterized the discussion about immigration reform. Second, by employ-ing the theory's wisdom about recategorization, at least with respect to the dis-tribution of health care benefits, scarce resources might be allocated in a way that relies much more on functionality, shared purposes, and a realignment of currently competing interests than upon differences between citizens and noncitizens turn on their mode of arrival in this country, their length of stay in America, or fears associated with their immutable characteristics. In the end, I hope that by situating Common Group Identity Model to shed light on the policies that underlie the law pertaining to noncitizens' access to health bene-fits we might develop a fresh perspective that will introduce new solutions to the ongoing conversation about reforming immigration law.[1]

The Public Policy Problem: Undocumented Immigrant Access to Publicly Funded Health Care

This chapter focuses specifically on one aspect of immigration policy: the question of how to regulate undocumented immigrants' access to the American health care system. I choose this focus for three reasons. First, we know empir-ically that virtually no one immigrates to the United States solely or even primarily to participate in our health care system (Goldman, Smith, and Sood 2006). Of all the benefits and services excluded by immigration control statutes—education, public assistance, employment—access to American health care is the least likely to lure immigrants to our American shores. While the world may look with envy upon the excellently trained practitioners, spectacularly well-equipped facilities, and stunningly advanced medical technology and procedures available in the United States, the world also knows that before passage of the Patient Protection and Affordable Care Act of 2010 (ACA), nearly fifty million American citizens did not have access to the wonders of American medicine until they needed it emergently. Moreover, the fact that some remain dedicated even after passage of health reform, to fighting the ACA's near universalization of access to health care, is lost on few outside the United States of America.

Thus, with some notable exceptions, the prospect of leaping over citizens to gain access to American medical services would be an irrational reason to come to this country. In fact, the evidence shows that the primary reason most foreigners immigrate to the United States is to obtain employment, not health or other public benefits. This evidence squarely confronts the soundness of a public policy that assumes withholding public benefits from undocumented immigrants will decrease the incentive for people to come across our borders illegally. A discussion about restrictions on health care benefits forces a deeper look at this reasoning and urges more plausible explanations.

Second, the conversation about disparate access to health care that is already proceeding has not meaningfully included foreign-born patients. We have considerable data to demonstrate that patterns of access and quality are unequal (Smedley, Stith, and Nelson 2003), but most of the evidence fails to identify the incidence of disparities that impacts immigrants generally and is virtually silent about undocumented immigrants specifically. Moreover, while the statistical evidence of disparities is abundant, we know much less about the causes of and reasons for disparities. This chapter seeks to enlarge the conversation about disparate access to health care to address the circumstances unique to undocumented immigrants.

Finally, by considering the current trend toward enactments that deny health care access to undocumented immigrants, we may learn more about our underlying motivations for distributing access as we do throughout American society. I suggest here that even to the extent that they are accurate, continuing to rely upon the existing "stories" that commonly explain the shortcomings of immigration policy generally, and public benefit provisions specifically, is unlikely to yield new solutions. The explanations that turn on proving a resurgence of nativism (Barkan 2003) or that highlight the impact of class divisions on immigration policy (Hatton and Williamson 2005) may shed light as far as they go. However, they seldom take serious note of the competing interest in managing scarce medical resources that necessarily also animates immigration policy. For example, in 1994 the Urban Institute conducted a systematic assessment of the economic impact of undocumented immigrants in the United States, focusing on the seven states in which approximately 86 percent of all undocumented immigrants live. This study concluded that the costs imposed by undocumented immigrants include: criminal incarceration ($471 million), education ($3.1 billion), and Medicaid and emergency medical care ($200 million to $300 million). The Institute for Taxation and Economic Policy reported in 2010 that these costs were offset by the economic contributions that undocumented immigrants make including sales, property, and state income tax revenues totaling $11.2 billion (Immigration Policy Center 2011). Moreover, these existing explanations do not necessarily point to a set of possible solutions or invite opposing sides of the debate to explore positions of consensus. At the very least, the discussion of social psychology presented in this chapter will offer a new vocabulary and toolbox to consider when looking at ways to set policy pertaining to undocumented immigrants. With these three goals in view, I turn now to outlining the major federal and state law provisions that control noncitizens' access to American health care.

The Current Law

Much has been written about the shifting balance of authority between the federal and states' governmental efforts to regulate immigration over the past quarter century. Whether and on what terms to distribute health care benefits to undocumented immigrants presents an especially disorganized picture of one aspect of immigration policy. It is instructive, for our purposes, to highlight the ways in which old paradigms have failed to yield any satisfactory approaches to immigration policy overall. The right to control immigration is constitutionally delegated to the federal government and is inherent, the Supreme Court has said, in the nation's sovereignty.[2] Yet Congress has within the past twenty-five years alternately exercised its authority to prohibit states from providing public benefits to immigrants; retracted its prohibition; and, finally, thrown it open to the states to determine whether to extend or withhold public benefits from undocumented immigrants. The states have responded in conflicting ways, sometimes even passing contradictory enactments within the same state. When states have gone too far, the federal courts have stepped in to reverse their actions. To set the stage for applying the social psychology analysis that follows, it is useful to briefly summarize the recent federal and state enactments that currently control access to health care by undocumented immigrants.

Federal Rules That Define Access for Undocumented Immigrants

The list of major federal enactments that control undocumented immigrants' access to health care begins with a statute not directed specifically at immigrants at all. Enacted in 1965 as Title XIX of the Social Security Act, the Medicaid Act created joint partnerships between the federal government and each state government to fund a safety net that made medical care available to the "categorically needy."[3] Generally, undocumented immigrants have been prohibited from enrolling in Medicaid since the program began. Even most legal immigrants are ineligible to receive Medicaid for the first five years that they live in the United States. However, because states have considerable discretion to define their Medicaid programs, it has been said that Medicaid is really a loose collection of fifty different health care programs for the poor, disabled, and chronically ill. Depending upon individual state laws, noncitizens may be eligible to receive health care through Medicaid because of their low-income levels, with 21.3 percent of noncitizens living in poverty compared to 11.8 percent of the general population (US Census Bureau 2001).

The second relevant federal statute is the Emergency Medical Treatment and Active Labor Act (EMTALA), passed in 1986 to grant access to emergency health care to all in an emergency medical condition. The statute is colloquially known as the "Anti-Dumping Act" because it requires health care providers to provide emergency medical services to all patients, notwithstanding their ability to pay for those services and without any reference to their immigration status. Thus, EMTALA guarantees that undocumented immigrants will receive free emergency medical care, even if no other health care services are publicly provided by either the federal government or the state in which they reside. Despite EMTALA, research shows that noncitizens are significantly less likely to use emergency rooms to obtain health care than citizens do (Goldman, Smith, and Sood 2006).

Thirdly, the Personal Responsibility and Work Opportunity Act of 1996 (PRWOA) established the terms and conditions upon which undocumented immigrants may receive public benefits in the United States.[4] The PRWOA divides immigrants into those who are "qualified aliens" eligible to obtain state funded benefits and all other aliens who are not qualified to receive benefits. Those qualified include legally admitted permanent residents under the Immigration and Naturalization Act, asylees, refugees, or those granted conditional entry under the act. Also, qualified aliens include certain Cuban and Haitian entrants as well as victims of violent battering and their children. Access to publicly funded health care is included among the benefits PRWOA regulates, along with other essential services such as housing, education, food stamps, and disability benefits. However, Congress did leave considerable discretion with state governments that wished to modify the PRWOA's federal restriction of public benefits to include only qualified aliens. The statute creates exceptions to allow all immigrants to receive emergency medical services, immunizations, testing and treatment services for communicable diseases, and any other assistance necessary to protect life or safety.[5] Moreover, the federal law allowed that after August 22, 1996, any state legislature that wished to extend public benefits to unqualified immigrants could do so by affirmative enactment. Finally, the PRWOA also permitted states to further restrict the public benefits available even to qualified aliens, within certain time limits set by the federal law. In short, the PRWOA set a broad federal agenda aimed at limiting access to public benefits by all immigrants and then invited states to exercise their discretion to either expand or further limit those benefits within their respective borders.

All fifty state legislatures have accepted the federal invitation (Matthew 2010). In 2006 alone, state legislatures enacted eighty-four immigration measures, and they doubled that number in 2007. That year, twenty-three states passed ninety-two laws to address immigrants' eligibility to receive publicly funded health care services (Preston 2007).

Since passage of the PRWOA, Congress has been working to reign in its harsh provisions, rolling back some of its most far-reaching restrictions. In 1997 the Balanced Budget Act (BBA) limited the group of immigrants affected by PRWOA to those arriving after August 1996. The BBA also allocated $25 million per year to each of twelve states with the highest number of undocumented aliens, to cover the cost of emergency care provided under EMTALA to these patients.[6] In 2003 the Medicare Modernization Act included a provision that allocated $1 billion over a three-year period to reimburse hospitals for the cost of providing safety-net care to undocumented immigrants.[7] Court challenges to the PRWOA have also resulted in narrowing the statute's prohibitory reach. For example, in *Lewis v. Thompson*, the Second Circuit ruled that PRWOA's denial of prenatal care to immigrant mothers not qualified to receive public benefits under its terms had a rational basis and thus did not violate the Constitution, but applying the act to deny automatic Medicaid coverage for the children of undocumented aliens born in this country violated the equal protection rights of these new Americans.[8]

The effect of these federal rules is to grant undocumented immigrants emergency medical assistance (so long as that assistance is not related to an organ transplant procedure and the patient meets the relevant state's eligibility requirements), emergency disaster relief, and public health assistance for communicable diseases including immunizations, testing, and treatment of symptoms (even if the symptoms turn out not to be caused by a communicable disease). The federal government's patchwork of legislation that regulates the availability of these health benefits evinces an ambivalent series of line-drawing exercises, dividing qualified from unqualified immigrants, distinguishing emergency from chronic or public health care, and separating children from their parents once they have exited the womb of an undocumented alien. This congressional approach leaves broad discretion to the states with little guidance. The result has been a conflicting and erratic flurry of immigration legislation passed at the state level.

Access to Health Care under State Immigration Laws

By 2009 twenty-eight states had enacted legislation to restrict access to publicly funded health benefits by noncitizens (Clark 2008). Examining the laws passed most recently by the nine states that enacted these statutes during the last five years provides a current and comprehensive survey of the variety of legislative approaches that operate across the country to limit health care access by noncitizens.

Arizona enacted its statute restricting immigrant access to public benefits in 2004 pursuant to passage of a state initiative called the Arizona Taxpayer and Citizen Protection Act. This voter initiative, also known as Proposition 200, was approved by 56 percent of Arizona voters and a remarkable 47 percent of Latino voters. It included the requirement that all state agencies verify the immigration status of those applying to avail themselves of public benefits including medical services, and it required the agencies to report the information to federal immigration authorities. Not only does the law make the failure to report violation of federal immigration statutes a Class 2 misdemeanor but it also creates a private cause of action for Arizona citizens wishing to sue any agent or agency for failure to comply with the verification and reporting requirements under the statute.

In 2006 Georgia, Virginia, and Colorado all enacted statutes to restrict access to health care and other public benefits by noncitizens; Idaho and Oklahoma followed in 2007. The South Carolina and Mississippi legislatures enacted statutes in 2008 and Utah promulgated its law in 2009. Virginia and Mississippi each took unique approaches to protecting their publicly funded resources. Virginia's legislature opted to specifically outline the narrow range of medical services that undocumented immigrants have access to in that state while Mississippi's law is void of any specific directives and instead announces this statement of legislative findings and purpose: "The Legislature finds that when illegal immigrants have been sheltered and harbored in this state and encouraged to reside in this state through the benefit of work without verifying immigration status, these practices impede and obstruct the enforcement of federal immigration law, undermine the security of our borders, and impermissibly restrict the privileges and immunities of the citizens of Mississippi. The Legislature further finds that illegal immigration is encouraged when public agencies within this state provide public benefits without verifying immigration status."[9]

Colorado's statute is virtually identical to the language used in the Georgia, Oklahoma, South Carolina, and Utah laws. Colorado was one of the first states to act after PRWOA to reinstate Supplemental Security Income and Medicaid eligibility for legal immigrants excluded under the federal statute. Yet Colorado's experience is instructive more because of what happened after the state's enactment than for the language of the provision itself. The stated legislative objective, as articulated in Colorado's House Bill 1023, was that "all persons eighteen years of age or older shall provide proof that they are lawfully present in the United States prior to receipt of certain public benefits." Although Colorado taxpayer monies may be spent under the law to provide undocumented immigrants with access to a K–12 education or services of a soup kitchen, the core prohibition under the law restricts access to health care.

The law requires medical providers to verify the lawful presence of any applicant for medical care before treatment, excluding services for medical emergencies, prenatal care, immunizations, and treatment of communicable diseases. As a consequence, hospitals, clinics, and treatment centers that serve the indigent have turned away patients in nonemergency conditions until their health deteriorated enough to warrant treatment under the law's exception for medical emergencies. On the other hand, there is evidence that private donations are being used in place of public funds to provide some medical services to undocumented immigrants, thereby reducing the state's cost of providing publicly funded care. Nevertheless, the question of whether tougher immigration laws actually save Colorado taxpayer dollars is unsettled.

The 2006 Colorado law reached far beyond the central limitation on health care benefits. It addressed many other aspects of the state government's relationship to undocumented immigration, including providing for tougher measures to penalize and control smuggling or human trafficking, greater authority for law enforcement to verify and report arrestees' immigration status, penalties against employers who hire undocumented labor, and prohibitions against unlawful voting. For example, its employment provision requires employers to verify employees' work status or risk fines or loss of economic development awards. Deliberately voting in an election without authorization of one's immigration status is penalized as a Class 5 felony under the law. Colorado's law heavily penalizes use of counterfeit identification documents and creates a full-time investigative position to find those using falsified immigration documents. Colorado's immigration law instructs the state's attorney general to seek reimbursement from the federal government for the cost of incarcerating, educating, and providing health care to illegal immigrants and requires police officers to report the suspected illegal status of any arrestees.

Colorado's governor declared the law to be "the toughest law in the country dealing with illegal immigration" and explained its purpose as "a major breakthrough in the fight to control the costs of illegal immigration," urging other states to follow Colorado's lead.[10] Since 2006, using Colorado's HB 1023 as a template, eight other states have enacted similar restrictions on undocumented immigrants' access to public services. These other states also vied for bragging rights to claim the "toughest immigration law" (Matthew 2010).

Idaho's benefit restriction law uses a different tactic altogether. Like the other statutes, Idaho's law requires verification that an applicant for certain public benefits is lawfully present in the United States before receiving benefits. The last sentence of the statute contains a telling disclaimer: "The intent of the legislature is not to regulate immigration but to control public expenditures for certain public benefits not inconsistent with federal law."[11]

This language provides a dramatic contrast to the Mississippi pronouncement that "declare[d] that it is a compelling public interest of this state to discourage illegal immigration by requiring all agencies within this state to fully cooperate with federal immigration authorities."[12] Distinguish the Idaho disclaimer from the language of California's first attempt to limit access to public benefits afforded to undocumented immigrants in the ballot initiative passed overwhelmingly by California voters in 1994. Proposition 187, as it was popularly called, contained ten sections that together required public service agencies to verify the citizenship status of those they served, notify federal Immigration and Naturalization Service (INS) officials of anyone suspected of being in the United States illegally, and deny benefits or services to those suspected of being undocumented immigrants. Section 6 excluded undocumented immigrants from receiving nonemergency health care while other sections penalized falsification of immigration documents; provided for cooperation between local, state and federal INS officials; and restricted access to other public benefits such as education and welfare assistance. According to its preamble, Proposition 187 was intended to address "economic hardship" resulting from the cost of providing public services to "illegal aliens." However, the preamble also referenced a desire to address suffering, injury, and damage caused by "the criminal conduct of illegal aliens in this state."[13] This connection between economic hardship, criminal conduct, and providing public benefits has led many to see Proposition 187 as an "anti-immigrant" measure aimed at stopping the flow of immigration to California (Cooper 2004). The initiative was quickly declared unconstitutional and its implementation permanently enjoined.[14] However, the proposition's objectives roused support even among Hispanic voters.[15]

Professor Brietta Clark has thoughtfully challenged the dominant narratives that the Mississippi statute and California's voter initiative embrace to create an "us/them" dichotomy and label immigrants as "outsiders" or "others in ways that fuel misunderstanding, fear, and mistrust" (Clark 2008). She points to the use of stereotypes and threatening caricatures that paint a vivid picture of the "illegal immigrant whom we should fear, punish, and exclude." Thus, exclusionary statutes are explained as ways to deter immigrants from making the choice to come to the United States. Alternatively, the us/them dichotomy explains that immigrants threaten the availability of medical resources or that exclusionary rules are limited to the undeserving who are "illegals" just as any other criminals but distinguishable from "legal aliens." This discourse depends upon exciting the imagination to reinforce the picture of immigrants as outsiders who are criminals, welfare abusers, thieves, and threats to the safety and security enjoyed by insiders.[16] Clark points out that the us/them narrative is reinforced by highlighting the foreignness or strangeness of immigrants and the urgent need to protect everything familiar from their reach.

However, the irony that Clark reveals is the similarity between the us/them language of those who seek to exclude undocumented immigrants on one hand, and the language used by those who advocate granting full access to immigrants as a matter of equity, justice, and common sense on the other hand. Clark concludes, "By engaging restrictionists on their terms and under the existing health care paradigm, pro-access advocates can unwittingly reinforce the 'Us–Them' dichotomy that pervades health policy decision-making" (Clark 2008, 273).

Clark recognizes that the solution is not just to change the narratives that describe health care but to go deeper to change the fundamental notions of how citizens and noncitizens are connected, creating partnerships, coalitions, and collaborations that will result in "reforming the health care system in ways that may or may not be immigrant-specific, but that will ultimately benefit immigrants as well" (ibid., 274). It is here that the Common Group Identity Model can add structure and direction to operationalize the call for changes in the immigrant health care narrative that Clark has raised.

The Common Group Identity Model

Social psychologists begin from the shared and established premise that "social categorization is a fundamental aspect of human functioning and perception" (Dovidio et al. 2005). This recognizes the normalness and value neutrality of the human tendency to separate into "multiple groups or categories" to give "structure to an otherwise bewildering world" (Krueger and DiDonato 2008). Importantly, this understanding removes the initial stigma attached to the simple fact that humans sort themselves into groups that include some and exclude others. Group membership among humans is not problematic in and of itself. Indeed, social categorization—the ability to sort ourselves into smaller, meaningful categories to allow interdependent cooperation and minimize risks and costs—is a "universal facet of human perception essential for efficient functioning" (Tajfel and Turner 1979). Yet it is unassailable that social group categorization comes at a cost.

Groups divide and segregate not only for cooperative good but also to exaggerate the differences between groups, thus nurturing stereotypes and prejudice. In-group members favor one another in sharing resources, providing social support, and distributing rights and responsibilities within a larger community or society. Beyond the basic levels of inclusionary behavior, in-group members may also define societal boundaries by stigmatizing those outside the group—the out-group members—or even establishing institutional criteria, such as quotas for inclusion, to define members of the in-group and out-group categories (Abrams, Hogg, and Marques 2005).

Here is how the us/them dichotomy plays out. Insiders argue that immigrants are lazy or criminals, yet the empirical evidence is plainly contradictory. Of the estimated 11.9 million undocumented immigrants in the United States, an estimated 7.2 million are working. America's in-group members ignore the fact that undocumented immigrants are largely taxpayers, contributing more in taxes withheld from their wages than we will ever spend on providing them social services. Insiders have excluded immigrants, by law, based solely upon their race or country of origin. To date, legal scholars such as Clark have been able to identify the irony, irrationality, or perhaps even travesty of the exclusionary tendencies of American immigration policies, but they have had no systemic paradigm for changing the way the us/them dichotomy controls the law.

The remarkable contribution that the Common Group Identity Model offers is evidence that negative attitudes, conduct, and even the law that grows out of patterns of inclusion and exclusion can be modified. For example, one group of social psychologists showed through two studies that it is possible to manipulate perceptions of national and international identity that lead to neg-ative attitudes toward immigrants and immigration by using persuasive com-munications in the form of four editorial articles written to target in-group and out-group attitudes (Esses et al. 2005). The editorial articles were "designed to induce a common, inclusive national identity"—in other words, to encourage recategorization of in-group and out-group members among the study partici-pants. These researchers found they could promote a common national in-group identity among Canadian students by presenting fictitious editorials that described the common ethnic roots among Canadians who shared a his-tory and tradition of immigration to Canada, and by emphasizing the national pride that "ethnics" in Canada could commonly share. The editorials, written to "induce a common, inclusive national identity" produced more positive attitudes toward immigrants. However, the first study did not produce any change in the participants' attitudes toward immigration. In the second study, editorials emphasizing a common international identity did prove to have a significant impact on turning previously negative attitudes held by Canadian students toward immigration into "significantly more favorable attitudes toward immigration following the persuasive communication that emphasized a common international identity" (ibid., 331). These researchers conclude that the support their studies provide for the Common Group Identity Model trans-lates into effective immigration policy for nations seeking to "foster acceptance of immigration and immigrants" (ibid., 334). However, even with the explana-tory power of the Common Group Identity Model and its potential influence on social behavior, the salient question that remains is what, if anything, should the law do in response.

From Theory to Practice

Behavioral realists suggest a three-step process to determine what legal responses to social psychology information might be taken. This analytical framework is useful to understand what influence the social psychology stud-ies discussed here might have on immigration law and policy. My discussion thus far has addressed only the first two steps of the behavioral realist's proce-dure. Citing the Common Group Identity Model, I have identified advances in behavioral science that I suggest provide a more accurate model of human cog-nition and behavior toward the scarce public benefit resources that undocu-mented immigrants may avail themselves of in the health care context. This is step one. Next, I have suggested that the recategorization remedy reflects a more commonsense approach to ordering behavior and decision-making between citizens and noncitizens than the us/them dichotomy that underlies our current immigration law regime. My proposal addresses step two. The third question posed by behavioral realists asks lawmakers to account for the disparity between the new model suggested by social psychology insights presented here and the latent exclusivity theories that drive public benefit laws. The Common Group Identity Model offers the possibility of revising immigration law—and, consequently, in-group and out-group behavior—by creating new law that changes collective behavior and interests (Kang and Lane 2010).

To change public benefit restrictions, lawmakers and their constituents must have the opportunity to examine the increasing importance of superordinate membership beyond the in- and out-group memberships that form to divide citizens from noncitizens. For example, reframing the immigration debate may explain to American laborers that their superordinate group is composed of "low-paid workers" who seek to achieve fair wages, improved working conditions, and reasonable health and retirement benefits. If so, American workers may come to accept that joining forces with noncitizens will more effectively prevent their goals from being undermined than by excluding noncitizen laborers whose interests are in fact consistent with their own. Similarly, citizens in a locality may be convinced that all families are currently excluded from the assurance that basic health care benefits will be afforded them even in the event of catastrophic illness, without the threat of bankruptcy. Therefore citizens might perceive the superordinate group to be those who seek to cooperate to create a sustainable health care delivery system that eliminates the premium paid by the insured to cover acute emergency care for the uninsured, thereby driving up the cost of health care for all.

We have seen superordinate groups form where two insider and outsider groups had previously existed. To create exceptions to exclusionary health care laws as they pertain to undocumented immigrants who have been battered, women's rights advocates and immigration rights advocates worked together to form a superordinate group of immigrants fleeing domestic violence. This is an example of recategorization. To replicate its success, first, policymakers must minimize the differences between in-group and out-group members so that these differences may be replaced. Second, the object becomes to disperse information about the shared objectives, needs, and priorities that both groups have in common so that these will be retained, even if for self-interested reasons.

The objective of this chapter will have been served if it inspires new dialogue among lawmakers interested in examining ways that existing public benefit rules might be reframed to construct cooperative and interdependent allocations of publicly funded resources. The Graham and Bush quotes that open this chapter betray the circularity of those who were once immigrants who arrived in America as outsiders and later became insiders. These former "aliens" are precariously reliant on a new group of outsiders who came to work in America, motivated by the same dreams that today, rather than threaten the existence and livelihoods of earlier immigrants, may be much better understood as a search for shared outcomes and futures. The Common Group Identity Model offers a way to progress beyond the law of inclusion and exclusion by redefining the "national interest" to construct the superordinate group to which both citizens and noncitizens belong.

Notes

1. This chapter is based on an earlier publication (Matthew 2010).
2. *Nishimura Ekiu v. United States*, 142 U.S. 659 (1892) and *Plyler v. Doe*, 457 U.S. 202 (1982). Both decisions construed Article I, §8, cl. 4 of the US Constitution, which grants the federal government "the power to establish a uniform Rule of Naturalization, and to regulate Commerce with foreign Nations."
3. 42 U.S.C. §§1396–1396v (1994).
4. Pub. L. No. 104–193, 110 Stat. 2198–2260 (1996), codified at 8 U.S.C. §1641.
5. 8 U.S.C. §1621(b).
6. Balanced Budget Act of 1997, Pub. L. No. 105–33, §4723(a), 111 Stat. 251, 515 (Sec. 4723) (providing payments for four consecutive years from 1998 to 2001).
7. The Medicare Modernization, Improvement, and Prescription Drug Act of 2003, Pub. L. No. 108–173, §1011(a)(1) codified at 42 U.S.C. §1395dd (2003). Also, Weeks (2006) explains that hospitals had only three sources of funds for reimbursement of costs for caring for undocumented immigrants before the MMA appropriation. These were short-term Medicaid coverage, disproportionate share hospital reimbursements, and the BBA payments available to twelve states with the highest numbers of undocumented immigrants.
8. 252 F.3d 567 (2nd Cir. 2001).
9. Press Release, "Owen Signs Immigration Legislation Considered Strongest in U.S.: Governor Approves Ten Bills Passed During Recent Special Session," July 31, 2006. http://www.verificationsinc.com/pdf/co-e-verify-press-release.PDF.
10. Ibid.
11. Idaho Code §67–7901, added by S.L. 2007, ch. 311, §1, eff. July 1, 2007.
12. The preamble language as well as the text of Proposition 187 in its entirety may be found in the appendix of Lolita K. Buckner Inniss, "California's Proposition 187—Does It Mean What It Says? Does It Say What It Means? A Textual and Constitutional Analysis," *Georgetown Immigration Law Journal* 10, no. 577 (Summer 1996).
13. Mississippi Code §71–11–1 Laws 2008, Ch. 312 §1, eff. July 1, 2008.
14. *League of United Latin American Citizens v. Wilson*, 1998 WL 14325 (C.D. Cal) ("Sections 1, 4, 5, 6, 7, 8 and 9 of Proposition 187 are declared to be in violation of the Supremacy Clause, preempted by federal law, and of no force or effect"). See also *Plyler v. Doe*, 457 U.S. 202 (1982), in which the US Supreme Court had already declared unconstitutional bans on access to public benefits based upon immigration status.

15. According to exit polls, 31 percent of Hispanic voters supported Proposition 187 along with 64 percent of nonwhite Hispanics, 57 percent of Asians, and 56 percent of African Americans (Preston 2007).
16. The fact is irrelevant that the deterrence discourse is contradicted by studies showing that immigrants underutilize health care services rather than greedily and fraudulently steal these benefits from those who are entitled (Clark 2008).

References

Abrams, D., M. A. Hogg, and J. M. Marques. 2005. "A Social Psychological Framework for Understanding Social Inclusion and Exclusion." In *The Social Psychology of Inclusion and Exclusion*, ed. D. Abrams, M. A. Hogg, and J. M. Marques. New York: Psychology Press.

Barkan, E. R. 2003."Return of the Nativists?" *Social Science History* 27, no. 2: 229–283.

Clark, B. R. 2008. "The Immigrant Health Care Narrative and What It Tells Us about the US Health Care System." *Annals of Health Law* 17, no. 2: 229–243.

Cooper, E. 2004. "Embedded Immigrant Exceptionalism: An Examination of California's Proposition 187, the 1996 Welfare Reforms and the Anti-Immigrant Sentiment Expressed Therein." *Georgetown Immigration Law Journal* 18:345–367.

Costich, J. F. 2001. "Legislating a Public Health Nightmare: The Anti-Immigrant Provisions of the 'Contract with America' Congress." *Kentucky Law Journal* 90:1043–1470.

Dovidio, J. F., S. L. Gaertner, G. Hodson, M. A. Houlette, and K. M. Johnson. 2005. "Social Inclusion and Exclusion: Recategorization and the Perception of Intergroup Boundaries." In *The Social Psychology of Inclusion and Exclusion*, ed. D. Abrams, M. A. Hogg, and J. M. Marques. New York: Psychology Press.

Esses, V. M., J. F. Dovidio, A. H. Semenya, and L. M. Jackson. 2005. "Attitudes Toward Immigrants and Immigration: The Role of National and International Identity," In *The Social Psychology of Inclusion and Exclusion*, ed. D. Abrams, M. A. Hogg, and J. M. Marques. New York: Psychology Press.

Graham, O. L., and R. Daniels. 2001. "The Unfinished Reform: Regulating Immigration in the National Interest." In *Debating American Immigration, 1882–Present*. Lanham, MD: Rowman & Littlefield.

Goldman, D. P., J. P. Smith, and N. Sood. 2006. "Immigrants and the Cost of Medical Care." *Health Affairs* 25, no. 6: 1700–1711.

Hatton, T. J., and J. G. Williamson. 2005. "A Dual Policy Paradox: Why Have Trade and Immigration Policies Always Differed in Labour-Scarce Economies?" Center for Economic Policy Research, Discussion Paper Series No. 5443. Boston: National Bureau of Economic Research.

Immigration Policy Center. 2011. "Unauthorized Immigrants Pay Taxes, Too: Estimates of the State and Local Taxes Paid by Unauthorized Immigrant Households." Washington, DC: American Immigration Council. http://immigrationpolicy.org/just-facts/unauthorized-immigrants-pay-taxes-too.

Kang, J., and K. Lane. 2010. "Seeing through Colorblindness: Implicit Bias and the Law." *UCLA Law Review* 58:465–520.

Krueger, J. I., and T. E. DiDonato. 2008. "Social Categorization and the Perception of Groups and Group Differences." *Social and Personality Psychology Compass* 2, no. 2: 733–750.

Matthew, D. B. 2010. "The Social Psychology of Limiting Health Care Benefits for Undocumented Immigrants." *Houston Journal of Health Law and Policy* 10:201–226.

Passel, J. S., and D. Cohn. 2009. "A Portrait of Unauthorized Immigrants in the United States." Washington, DC: Pew Research Center: Pew Hispanic Center. http://pewhispanic.org/files/reports/107.pdf.

Preston, J. 2007. "Surge in Immigration Laws around US" *New York Times*, Aug. 6.

Smedley, B. D., A. Y. Stith, and A. R. Nelson, eds. 2003. *Unequal Treatment—Confronting Racial and Ethnic Disparities in Healthcare*. Washington DC: The National Academies Press.

Tajfel, H., and J. C. Turner. 1979. "An Integrative Theory of Intergroup Conflict." In *The Social Psychology of Intergroup Relations*, ed. W. G. Austin and S. Worchel. Florence, KY: Brooks/Cole.

US Census Bureau. 2001. "Profile of the Foreign Born in the United States: 2000." Current Population Reports. Washington, DC: Economics and Statistics Administration.

Weeks, E. 2006. "After the Catastrophe: Disaster Relief for Hospitals." *North Carolina Law Review* 85:223–275.

Community Health Center and Academic Medical Partnerships to Expand and Improve Primary Care

A lengthy debate over how to build a more effective and affordable health care system culminated in the enactment of the Patient Protection and Affordable Care Act of 2010 (ACA). The legislation is neither the beginning nor the end of efforts to improve health care and health outcomes in the United States. Many more steps, both large and small, will be needed to establish a stable, high-performing health care system.

Among its many provisions, the ACA sets in motion an unprecedented expansion of health insurance coverage, projected to reach more than thirty million previously uninsured Americans. Over the next few years, a crucial test of health care reform will be whether the expansion of coverage is converted into a guarantee of cost-effective access to needed services. At the same time, expectations for better care will be raised for close to twenty million people who remain uninsured. Both the short-term and long-term success of health care reform will depend on the availability of high-quality primary care.

It seems clear that the capacity and cost-effectiveness of the nation's health care safety net, especially its community health centers (CHC), will be important determinants of how well the primary care needs of newly insured individuals and still-uninsured individuals are met as national health care reform proceeds (Adashi, Geiger, and Fine 2010). As chapter 3 of this volume explains, the ACA and the American Recovery and Reinvestment Act of 2009 (ARRA) include a number of incremental steps to strengthen CHCs, including funds to acquire new health information technology, support construction and expansion of centers, and support new clinical positions through the National Health Service Corps (NHSC).

While these are all necessary steps, an additional innovation could produce a catalytic effect and yield broad, lasting health system improvement. We propose an expansion of partnerships between the nation's CHCs and the nation's academic medical centers. The innovation we propose—the Community Health Center and Academic Medical Partnership (CHAMP)—would build upon current collaboration in the areas of patient care, health professions education, and community health services research (Morris et al. 2008; Brutger 2010).

This chapter explains how CHAMP would expand graduate medical education and ambulatory-training opportunities for primary care residents in CHCs designated as "teaching health centers." Such a partnership would improve the quality of primary care training and at the same time help CHCs meet the increasing demand for their services (Rieselbach, Crouse, and Frohna 2010). This initiative would help provide more affordable care and better outcomes for many of the people who will acquire health insurance as of 2014 and who are likely to be cared for by CHCs.

A major expansion of these collaborative relationships is now possible. Enactment of the ACA, with its support for primary care and teaching health centers, provides the initial basis for CHAMP to further establish CHCs as a key component of a reformed, cost-effective health care system. Primary care residents would receive their final year of training in these centers, followed by the incentive of NHSC debt repayment for subsequent practice in an underserved area. Residents trained in this setting would immediately increase the clinical capacity of CHCs and ultimately expand the primary care physician workforce.

We believe that this new visible commitment of our academic institutions to community health improvement may well inspire a new generation of medical students to consider primary care as a career choice. This partnership should be an integral part of a strategy to provide the number of well-trained and highly motivated clinicians needed to ensure a strong future for primary care across the US health care system. It would also respond to the recent call by a consortium of academic medical centers for leadership and cooperation with other sectors to address the social determinants of health and reduce disparities across population groups (Blue Ridge Academic Health Group 2010).

This chapter develops the case for CHAMP first by outlining the problems in health care delivery this proposal would address and then by describing a variety of past and present initiatives intended to strengthen the link between primary care training and safety net providers. After specifying the key features of CHAMP, we discuss how this proposal meshes with various provisions in the ACA that encourage such initiatives and identify areas in which further steps in policy and implementation will be required for broad development of this form of community–academic partnership.

Confronting Key Problems in American Health Care Delivery

An expanded partnership of CHCs and academic medicine is both well-targeted and timely. It addresses the confluence of three significant problems: inadequate access to affordable care, a depleted primary care workforce, and suboptimal primary care training.

The Continuing Problem of Access to Primary Care

Even under the most optimistic scenarios for health care reform under the ACA, millions of Americans will remain without adequate insurance coverage. Millions more will gain coverage through state Medicaid programs, which provide comprehensive benefits but often cannot provide reliable access to private primary care medical practices. Many of these individuals, therefore, will likely be dependent on current programs offering health services in underserved areas, most prominently the CHC program.

As Robert Mickey documents in chapter 2 of this volume, the network of federally qualified CHCs has grown substantially since its inception in the 1960s, gaining bipartisan political support and a solid reputation for quality, affordable care (Sardell 1986; Lefkowitz 2007; Iglehart 2010). The US Health Resources and Services Administration (HRSA) now helps fund about twelve hundred centers with some eight thousand rural and urban sites located in every state and US territory. They are the primary source of care for more than twenty million people, more than 5 percent of the US population, and in some states they serve more than 10 percent of the population (Adashi, Geiger, and Fine 2010).

These centers have established themselves as a vital part of the nation's safety net and are increasingly an option for mainstream medical care. The National Association of Community Health Centers (NACHC) has set its sights on CHCs growing to serve thirty million people by 2015 and fifty-one million by 2020 (Robert Graham Center 2007). Federal policymakers appear to recognize the need for such growth, but it will not be realized unless health centers are able to overcome the present challenges in recruiting primary care physicians (Rosenblatt et al. 2006; Morris et al. 2008).

The experience in Massachusetts after the state enacted a major expansion of health insurance coverage in 2006 suggests that the demand for services in CHCs will likely increase, not abate, as implementation of the ACA proceeds. When Massachusetts extended coverage to several hundred thousand individuals, many of them faced the challenge of finding a primary care practice that would accept new patients (Steinbrook 2008a). Although CHCs in Massachusetts saw a reduction in the proportion of patients who were uninsured, the total number of patients seeking care at those centers increased by 12 percent from 2005 to 2007. Newly insured individuals, particularly those with coverage through Medicaid or the Children's Health Insurance Program, accounted for most of the increased demand for services (Ku et al. 2009).

The Worsening Shortage of Primary Care Physicians

A second key problem is the worsening shortage of primary care physicians. Primary care is regarded by many experts as "the essential foundation for an effective, efficient, and equitable health care system" (Grumbach and Mold 2009, 2589). High-quality primary care serves as the first point of entry for patients into the health care system, as well as a source of continuing care for chronic conditions and coordination with a comprehensive range of secondary, tertiary, and complementary health services (Starfield 1992; Shi and Singh 2008).

A substantial body of evidence demonstrates that countries with a stronger orientation toward primary care have better health outcomes, higher satisfaction with health services, and relatively lower health care costs (Starfield 1994; Starfield, Shi, and Macinko 2005). The US health system fares poorly in international comparisons, largely due to the weakness of its primary care infrastructure (Ginsburg et al. 2008; Commonwealth Fund 2010). Within the United States, states with higher ratios of primary care physicians and more available primary care have better health outcomes, fewer hospitalizations for conditions treatable with primary care, and fewer pronounced health disparities across population groups (Parchman and Culler 1994; Shi et al. 1999; Shi and Starfield 2000, 2001; Shi et al. 2002; Starfield, Shi, and Macinko 2005).

Yet American primary care is in need of a lifeline (Bodenheimer, Grumbach, and Berenson 2009). The financial, structural, and human resources devoted to primary care in the United States are depleted and threatened further by a number of trends. About one-third of US physicians are currently in primary care—already a small proportion by international standards—and this is expected to decrease as large numbers of older primary care physicians retire in the next few years.

Medical students, who typically incur a large debt to finance their education, increasingly elect to pursue residency training in specialties they perceive as having a greater economic return on their investment, better working conditions, and more prestige (Lee 2008; Steinbrook 2008b; COGME 2010).

For more than a decade, the proportion of medical school graduates choosing to pursue residencies in primary care has declined (Bodenheimer, Grumbach, and Berenson 2009). Even within traditional primary care fields such as internal medicine and pediatrics, residents are choosing to pursue subspecialty training or hospital-based practice (Salsberg et al. 2008; NEHI-Macy 2010). New physicians are filling 15 percent fewer family medicine residency positions compared with a decade ago, and fewer than half of all family medicine residents are US medical school graduates (National Resident Matching Program 2008).

An important source of funding for graduate medical education (GME) is Medicare, which pays teaching hospitals to help support the costs associated with residency programs such as salaries and benefits for trainees and instructors, office space, and administrative expenses. The Balanced Budget Act of 1997 and subsequent budget reconciliation acts in 1999 and 2000 modified the basis for GME payments and placed a cap on the total number of residency slots eligible for Medicare support at each teaching institution, but not the type of residency positions (Oliver, Grover, and Lee 2001; MedPAC 2009). Teaching hospitals have not had any reason, therefore, to counter the demand for greater specialty training and less primary care training.

A long-run strategy to revitalize primary care must address three current weaknesses in the system: financial compensation, practice conditions, and workforce development (Bodenheimer, Grumbach, and Berenson 2009). These three barriers interrelate in complex ways, but the bottom line is that fewer primary care physicians are entering the workforce at a time when more are needed.

Suboptimal Training in Primary Care

The problems associated with traditional primary care training have been developing for decades. During the 1970s and 1980s, the growth of health maintenance organizations (HMO) put them in competition for patients with teaching hospitals. HMOs typically reduced hospital admissions and reduced the average length of stay for patients who were hospitalized, and this trend was dramatically accelerated when Medicare adopted a new prospective payment system for hospital services in 1983.

The combined effect of these changes has left many teaching hospitals with patient populations inadequate for primary care clinical instruction; they consist mainly of people with uncommon illnesses whose treatment needs differ substantially from patients routinely encountered in ambulatory settings. In addition, most training is not well aligned with the goals of delivery system reform (COGME 2010; Hackbarth and Boccuti 2011). The Medicare Payment Advisory Commission (MedPAC) argued in its 2009 report to Congress:

> Of particular concern is the relative lack of formal training and experience in multidisciplinary teamwork, cost awareness in clinical decision making, comprehensive health information technology, and patient care in ambulatory settings. Residency experience in nonhospital and community-based settings is important because most of the medical conditions that practicing physicians confront should be managed in nonhospital settings. However, inherent financial incentives and Medicare regulations strongly encourage teaching hospitals to confine their residents' learning experiences to within the hospital.
>
> (MedPAC 2009, xiii)

These problems persist even though primary care residency programs have begun to increase training in community settings. Internal medicine requires that a minimum of one-third of training time take place in ambulatory settings (ACGME 2008a) and family medicine and pediatrics require an even higher proportion of ambulatory care training (ACGME 2008b).

But this is far from a satisfactory experience for young primary care physicians because many academic medical centers have a difficult time establishing well-organized, well-supervised, and well-supported ambulatory-training sites that reflect the full scope of community health needs (Keirns and Bosk 2008). Residency programs commonly fulfill ambulatory-training requirements by rotating residents through hospital-based outpatient departments, clinics, and physician offices (MedPAC 2009, 29). Many residents reach the end of their training with little practical knowledge of how to deliver high-quality primary care—where they and other members of a health care team are responsible for comprehensive, continuous, coordinated care of most acute and chronic conditions for their patients (Starfield 2008). Many have little experience, as well, with the information and processes associated with quality improvement and demands for more accountable care. In short, they are unprepared for the gradual but still revolutionary shift in demands on the medical profession, a shift that "requires reconsidering the very definition of a 'good doctor'" (Swensen et al. 2010). As Swensen and colleagues summarize: "In the past, a stereotypical good doctor was independent and always available, had encyclopedic knowledge, and was a master of rescue care. Today, a good doctor must have a solid fund of knowledge and sound decision-making skills but also must be emotionally intelligent, a team player, able to obtain information from colleagues and technological sources, embrace quality improvement as well as public reporting, and reliably deliver evidence-based care, using scientifically informed guidelines in a personal, compassionate, patient-centered manner."

New Initiatives to Strengthen the Health Care Safety Net

The ACA and other recent initiatives offer a historic opportunity to modernize and complete a badly needed expansion of the nation's network of CHCs (Adashi, Geiger, and Fine 2010; Iglehart 2010). In 2009 more than 40 percent of medically underserved areas lacked a CHC site (Bascetta 2009). With leadership from the president and bipartisan support, annual appropriations to the CHC program doubled to $2.1 billion in the last years of the Bush administration.

The 2009 ARRA economic stimulus package adopted at the outset of the Obama administration authorized an additional one-time $2 billion appropriation for construction, equipment, health information technology, and new services in CHCs. In addition, the ARRA provided $300 million to add positions in the National Health Service Corps, "the indispensable CHC partner" that recruits health care professionals for placement in underserved communities, as well as $48 million for primary care training programs for physicians, physician assistants, and dentists (Adashi, Geiger, and Fine 2010).

The ACA goes well beyond these efforts; it authorizes $12.5 billion to expand CHCs and the National Health Service Corps over a five-year period from 2011 through 2015. Overall, these initiatives envision adding fifteen thousand primary care providers, enabling CHCs to serve as the usual source of care for forty million Americans (Adashi, Geiger, and Fine 2010). Given the significant new resources and new expectations for CHCs, the crucial question is how to develop—in relatively short order—a commensurate supply of primary care physicians to provide patient care and provide leadership to the clinical and management teams of CHCs.

One Step Further: Expanded Primary Care Training in CHCs

The basic proposition that academic medical centers should bear more responsibility for community health is not new. In 1983 Lewis and Sheps turned a critical eye on their colleagues and programs in academic medical centers:

> Certainly the road taken by our medical schools and hospitals since the Flexner report has brought brilliant and important successes in research, education and practice. Now, after a period of great growth in size, research productivity, and prestige, the centers somehow appear not to be good enough. It is as though something happened to them on the way to the future. More is demanded of them. But not more of the

same. Something different is expected—a much more direct relationship with community needs and social policy and the assumption by the centers of a set of direct responsibilities for the nature, effectiveness, and cost of the delivery of medical care itself.

(Lewis and Sheps 1983)

Nor is the idea of extending academic medical training into the community novel. In 1986 Rieselbach and Jackson proposed a link between primary care training and care for low-income patients. They suggested a program through which teaching hospitals would provide ambulatory-training sites in community-based clinics on the grounds that primary care residents would receive better training and become more aware of the needs of underserved populations. This proposal also included recommendations that each teaching hospital reserve at least 60 percent of its residency positions for primary care physician training and that the National Health Service Corps allow qualified members to satisfy their corps commitments by serving as faculty (Rieselbach and Jackson 1986).

These ideas were incorporated into legislation, the Ambulatory Training Act, proposed by Sen. Edward Kennedy in 1986 but never enacted. The bill would have redirected Medicare GME funding used to support residency training for some international medical graduates into community-based primary care residency programs. Included in this proposal was a provision to establish full reimbursement for the Medicare share of GME in the ambulatory setting and to temporarily increase reimbursement for direct GME costs. Residency positions in which the resident devoted greater than 25 percent of time to education in the ambulatory setting would receive extra support.

Further support for a link between GME and community health care centers resulted from a 1989 report by the Institute of Medicine (IOM) on "strategies to overcome barriers to financing graduate medical education for primary care practitioners in ambulatory settings." The study was based primarily on a workshop held in Washington, DC, attended by leaders in the primary care specialties of general internal medicine, general pediatrics, and family medicine as well as experts in medical education financing, hospital and academic administration, policy analysis, and the insurance industry.

The IOM study committee concluded that the most efficient ways to improve GME support in primary care settings would also increase the number of medical graduates choosing careers in primary care. The committee also concluded that a lack of primary care GME support would threaten the availability of care for underserved populations; therefore, the committee's solutions focused on care for these populations within the context of primary care GME (IOM 1989).

The report included recommendations for a variety of organizations and programs. Many were directed to Medicare; these included adoption of a resource-based relative-value scale method of payment for physicians then being considered by Congress and subsequently enacted in the 1989 Omnibus Budget Reconciliation Act; adjustment to the Medicare payment for the direct costs of GME that would create an incentive to establish residencies in primary care and to place those residents in primary care ambulatory settings; and adjustment to Medicare payments for indirect medical education to account for the time spent by primary care residents in all primary care ambulatory settings. Other recommendations included suggestions that states, through their Medicaid programs and other means, increase their financial support of GME, particularly in the primary care specialties (IOM 1989).

Current Efforts in Community-Based Primary Care Training

Over the ensuing two decades of private and public sector health care reforms, the problems of an inadequate supply of primary care providers and access to affordable care worsened, yet efforts to solve these problems on a systematic basis failed to advance. As a result, partnerships between academic health centers and local CHCs have developed on an ad hoc basis without an overarching policy framework or an assured source of financial support.

The Association of Academic Health Centers (AAHC) recently surveyed its member institutions regarding their partnerships with CHCs (Brutger 2010). Thirty-nine academic health centers, or 40 percent of the AAHC membership, responded to the survey. Of those responding, 89 percent currently have established partnerships with federally qualified health centers, rural health centers, other community clinics, and homeless health centers. The survey does not provide a complete picture of such partnerships due to the low participation rate and lack of details regarding the extent of collaborative activities. The AAHC does identify limited funding and restrictive regulatory policies as potential barriers to forming relationships and improving upon existing ones.

To date, perhaps the strongest effort to address the CHC primary care workforce crisis through partnerships with academic training programs is the Education Health Center Initiative. It is a collaboration of the Northwest Regional Primary Care Association, University of Washington Family Medicine Residency Network (also covering Alaska, Montana, and Idaho), University of Washington Department of Family Medicine, and Community Health Association of Mountain/Plains States (NRPCA 2010). It was established with the aim of evaluating residency training in health centers and "creating a model for training primary care physicians in the health care safety net" (Morris et al. 2008).

One of the key partners in the Education Health Center Initiative, the University of Washington Department of Family Medicine, has also created programs designed to expand the family medicine workforce in underserved areas. These programs include the Underserved Pathway, which allows students to focus on specific underserved populations throughout the educational process; the Rural/Underserved Opportunities Program, which is a four-week immersion experience in community medicine during which students live and work in underserved areas; and the Targeted Rural/Underserved Track, which seeks to connect underserved communities with the University of Washington and its affiliated residency programs.[1] All of these programs inform the development of models for other community–academic partnerships.

The premise of current and proposed community–academic partnerships is that they will provide medical residents with the necessary skills, cultural experience, and motivation to continue working in underserved areas after they complete their formal training. The well-established partnerships spearheaded by the University of Washington offer empirical evidence of the importance of community-based training in building a primary care workforce for underserved areas. Morris and colleagues surveyed two groups of family medicine residency graduates from Washington, Alaska, Montana, and Idaho. One group consisted of family physicians who completed their residencies between 1986 and 1999 while the other group completed their residencies between 2000 and 2002. Both groups were questioned about the locations of their residency training, their current job locations, job satisfaction, and scope of work. The results indicated that graduates of CHC-based residency programs were almost three times as likely as graduates of non-CHC residency programs to work in underserved areas after graduation. Furthermore, CHC-trained graduates indicated a level of job scope and satisfaction similar to non-CHC trained graduates (Morris et al. 2008).

Key Features of CHAMP

While there is sufficient experience to justify an expansion of existing primary care training in CHCs, the challenge of creating such partnerships can only be met by establishing a new framework for policy and institutional development. This does not require a major new federal program, however. Important innovations often stem from a recombination of existing technologies or processes rather than the invention of entirely new ones (Oliver and Paul-Shaheen 1997; Oliver 2004). Such is the case with CHAMP, our proposed program for community health center and academic medicine partnerships. It builds upon programs and organizational relationships that have been in place for many years in some communities, and have been emerging in many others, as well as new or expanded initiatives in the ACA.

The key building blocks for CHAMP are primary care residency programs, the CHC program, Medicare funding of graduate medical education, and the National Health Service Corps. CHAMP also accommodates, indeed accelerates, the most positive elements of the current revolution in primary care practice.

The CHAMP program would incorporate the following set of features:

1. A CHC would be eligible to become a CHAMP center by affiliating with an accredited family medicine, pediatrics, or internal medicine residency program, much like the ACA calls for new "teaching health centers." In addition, CHCs would need to implement the Tier 2 requirements for a patient-centered medical home established by the National Committee for Quality Assurance. This model would support the core functions of primary care, use electronic medical records, and emphasize prevention and chronic disease management (PCPCC 2007). Finally, a CHAMP health center would need a community governing board committed to supporting both the educational and service missions—in particular, meeting standards for accreditation of the affiliated residency program (Rieselbach, Crouse, and Frohna 2010).

2. A CHAMP center would be the site for selected third-year primary care residents to receive their final year of clinical training. Residents in their first and second years could be assigned to a CHAMP center for brief continuity clinics while devoting the majority of their time to inpatient training. This schedule could be modified for family medicine residents to meet their unique training requirements. Under faculty supervision, residents would care for a panel of patients while learning how to work within clinical and management teams in a medical home model. Compared with most current arrangements, this extended period of ambulatory care training would provide senior residents with a much better opportunity to practice continuous and coordinated care, and to understand the community and social context of their patients' conditions and treatments. The key advantage for the CHC would be the opportunity to greatly expand its clinical staff and volume of services.

3. We believe that large numbers of primary care residents would choose CHAMP centers for their training. This generation has grown up with

the concept and practice of community service during elementary and secondary school, and annually submits tens of thousands of applications to join Teach for America, AmeriCorps, and other volunteer programs. The combination of delivering urgently needed care in the community and gaining experience in the practice environment of the future, the patient-centered medical home, would be very attractive to many young physicians.

The reduction in potential career earnings facing physicians entering primary care would merit adding a significant financial incentive: Primary care residents participating in CHAMP would be encouraged to apply for positions in an expanded National Health Service Corps and would be given the highest priority for an appointment. The loan repayment offered by the Corps provides sixty thousand dollars in exchange for two years of service, with an option to extend the service until all qualifying loans are repaid. Along with the opportunity for loan repayment, CHAMP participants would be given preference to preselect the NHSC site for their service in the Corps, including the opportunity to remain part of the clinical and management team in the CHAMP center where they trained. This would improve recruitment and retention of staff in many CHCs.

4. We believe that faculty positions in CHAMP would also make it easier for CHCs to attract established primary care physicians, who could draw full-time or part-time academic salaries and be more heavily engaged in teaching than is normally possible in academic clinical settings (Morris et al. 2008). Primary care faculty would also be able to more easily participate in practice-based research networks focused on real-world tests of clinical effectiveness, prevention strategies, reduction of health disparities, and other means of population health improvement.

5. A critical component of CHAMP is financial support for establishing and maintaining graduate medical education in CHCs. More than 42 percent of CHCs already serve as training sites for some form of primary care education and training, but most do not receive any financial support to help cover the costs of training (NACHC 2008). Adding senior primary care residents to CHC medical staffs under CHAMP should substantially increase the volume of services and reimbursement for patients with health insurance coverage. Larger and longer-term funding sources for teaching health centers will be needed, however, to support residents and faculty as well as indirect education expenses.

Critical Issues for CHAMP Development and Implementation

Despite new support in the ACA related for teaching health centers, several challenges remain for systemwide development of CHAMP. A primary challenge, as noted earlier, is securing resources to establish and sustain a growing network of participating CHCs. The Teaching Health Center program authorized by the ACA recently announced a modest initial phase of funding through HRSA. Section 5508 of the ACA provides for payments to qualified teaching health centers with approved residency programs to help cover direct and indirect costs associated with operating those training programs, analogous to the direct and indirect GME payments made by Medicare to hospital-based residency programs. Funding of up to $230 million for such payments is available for the five-year period from FY 2011 to FY 2015. Despite this unprecedented authority and funding under the ACA, the resources are sufficient to support only a small number of prototype centers.

Development of a more automatic and budget-neutral funding source is crucial to the long-term growth and success of teaching health centers. A prominent option to provide stable funding for a much larger CHAMP program is to reallocate GME funds currently paid by Medicare to teaching hospitals. Overall, GME payments from Medicare exceed $9 billion annually to support training for about ninety thousand residents in over eleven hundred hospitals—an average of nearly $100,000 per qualifying medical resident (MedPAC 2009, 12; Hackbarth and Boccuti 2011). Direct GME payments help cover salaries and fringe benefits of residents and supervising faculty, office space, and other administrative costs related to operating a given residency program. The teaching hospital receives a fixed, per-resident payment and is then free to allocate those funds to its various residency programs as it sees fit. In addition, a teaching hospital receives an indirect medical education adjustment for episodes of patient care delivered either in inpatient or outpatient settings. These GME payments typically generate substantially more revenue than can be justified by the actual indirect costs associated with hospital-based training (MedPAC 2009, 13).

For those reasons, MedPAC and others have suggested reallocating some portion of GME payments to support residency programs in community, nonhospital settings (Rich et al. 2002; AAFP 2009; Mullan 2009; Hackbarth and Boccuti 2011). Expansion of primary care residency positions in CHCs under CHAMP would most likely require that teaching hospitals explicitly use some of their GME payments to support these CHC training sites and that the overall cap on residency positions eligible for Medicare support be raised or waived to accommodate these additional slots for primary care.

A second challenge in CHAMP development is generating mutual interest among CHCs and academic health centers in the difficult task of establishing fully accredited residency programs at community sites. Currently, many CHCs serve as sites for brief periods of training for medical students or residents. But long-term placement of primary care residents will require a variety of changes in CHCs, which may include expansion of clinical facilities, adoption of new clinical and management information systems, new governance arrangements, and acceptance of oversight from accrediting bodies.

The ACA support for teaching health centers goes directly to CHCs, not to teaching hospitals and existing residency programs. This design helps to ensure that CHCs will be full partners in the integration of residency training with their model of service delivery, but tensions are certain to arise over shared governance and funding. To secure accreditation, CHCs may need to establish separate nonprofit entities—presumably with greater representation of academic institutions—to develop and operate residency training in accordance with national standards. There are likely to be different standards for allopathic and osteopathic medical training as well as other health professions, which may create further tensions in selecting, funding, and administering training programs in CHCs.

A third challenge in CHAMP development is the needed size and scope of its critical partnership with the NHSC. New funding for the NHSC is now available, but that expansion is not commensurate with the expected demand for CHC growth.

Equally important to the long-run impact of community-based training on access to care is a modification in how the NHSC places participating health professionals. Currently, individuals electing to participate in the NHSC loan repayment program are assigned to communities and sites without any regard for where they received their prior training. To encourage new recruitment and especially retention of participants after their loan repayment obligations are fulfilled, the NHSC should allow residents who are trained in teaching health centers to "preselect" the site where they received their training, or another site they are familiar with. As they make the transition from their residency training to NHSC service, these individuals will already know the CHC management and much of the clinical team, will continue to work with the same patients and community members, and presumably will be far more likely to remain in practice in that community after their service commitment is fulfilled. This would help reduce the NHSC's longstanding problems with turnover and improve satisfaction among both CHC physicians and patients (Ginzberg 1994; Pathman et al. 2009).

Conclusion

A substantial expansion of primary care training in selected community health centers, as envisioned in the CHAMP strategy, would benefit the participating institutions and the communities they serve. If the pilot teaching health centers initiated under the ACA prove viable, increasing their numbers could greatly increase access to high-quality, affordable primary care for populations who will not be able to secure insurance coverage or whose communities currently face a shortage of primary care services.

CHAMP fits in well with the movement already under way within the CHC program to adopt higher standards of quality and effectiveness through chronic disease collaboratives and adoption of the patient-centered medical home model. It could serve as a cornerstone for innovations in health services delivery, including accountable care organizations, through Medicaid (Rieselbach and Kellerman 2011). It also could help provide a direct pipeline into an expanded and more prestigious NHSC program. Finally, it could provide a concrete point of action and source of enthusiasm within academic health centers whose leaders and students are looking for immediate ways to contribute to national health care reform efforts and their community (Mullan et al. 2010).

Note

1. University of Washington Department of Family Medicine Web site, http://depts .washington.edu/fammed/, accessed Oct. 5, 2010.

References

Accreditation Council for Graduate Medical Education (ACGME). 2008a. "Program Requirements for Residency Education in Internal Medicine." Chicago: ACGME. Accessed Dec. 28, 2008. www.acgme.org.
————. 2008b. "Program Requirements for Residency Education in Pediatrics." Chicago: ACGME. Accessed Dec. 28, 2008. www.acgme.org.
Adashi, E. Y., H. J. Geiger, and M. D. Fine. 2010. "Health Care Reform and Primary Care—The Growing Importance of the Community Health Center." *New England Journal of Medicine* 362:2047–2051.
American Academy of Family Physicians (AAFP). 2009. "Transforming Graduate Medical Education." Washington, DC: AAFP.
Bascetta, Cynthia. 2009. "Many Underserved Areas Lack a Health Center Site, and Data Are Needed on Service Provision at Sites: Statement of Cynthia Bascetta, Director, Health Care." April 30. Washington, DC: Health Resources and Services Administration. http://www.gao.gov/new.items/d09667t.pdf.
Blue Ridge Academic Health Group. 2010. "The Role of Academic Health Centers in Addressing the Social Determinants of Health." Report 14 (Jan.). Atlanta, GA: Emory University.
Bodenheimer, T., K. Grumbach, and R. A. Berenson. 2009. "A Lifeline for Primary Care." *New England Journal of Medicine* 360:2693–2696.

Brutger, R. 2010. "Academic Health Centers and Community Health Centers: The Landscape of Current Partnerships." Washington, DC: Association of Academic Health Centers. http://www.aahcdc.org/policy/reddot/AAHC_Community_Health_Centers_ The_Landscape.pdf.

Commonwealth Fund. 2010. *Mirror, Mirror on the Wall: How the Performance of the US Health Care System Compares Internationally.* New York: Commonwealth Fund.

Council on Graduate Medical Education (COGME). 2010. "Advancing Primary Care." Jan. Washington, DC.

Ginsburg, J. A., R. B. Doherty, J. F. Ralston, and N. Senkeeto. 2008. "Achieving a High-Performance Health Care System with Universal Access: What the United States Can Learn from Other Countries." *Annals of Internal Medicine* 148, no. 1: 55–75.

Ginzberg, E. 1994. "Improving Health Care for the Poor: Lessons from the 1980s." *Journal of the American Medical Association* 271:464–467.

Grumbach, K., and J. W. Mold. 2009. "A Health Care Cooperative Extension Service: Transforming Primary Care and Community Health." *Journal of the American Medical Association* 301, no. 24: 2589–2591.

Hackbarth G., and C. Boccuti. 2011. "Transforming Graduate Medical Education to Improve Health Care Value." *New England Journal of Medicine* 364:693–695.

Iglehart, J. K. 2010. "Health Centers Fill Critical Gap, Enjoy Support." *Health Affairs* 29, no. 3: 343–345.

Institute of Medicine (IOM). 1989. *Primary Care Physicians: Financing Their Graduate Medical Education in Ambulatory Settings.* Washington, DC: National Academies Press.

Keirns, C. C., and C. L. Bosk. 2008. "The Unintended Consequences of Training Residents in Dysfunctional Outpatient Settings." *Academic Medicine* 83:498–502.

Ku, L., E. Jones, B. Finnegan, P. Sin, and S. Rosenbaum. 2009. *How Is the Primary Care Safety Net Faring in Massachusetts? Community Health Centers in the Midst of Health Reform.* Washington, DC: Kaiser Family Foundation Commission on Medicaid and the Uninsured. Accessed Mar. 25, 2009. www.kff.org/healthreform/7878.cfm.

Lee, T. H. 2008. "The Future of Primary Care: The Need for Reinvention." *New England Journal of Medicine* 359:2085–2086.

Lefkowitz, B. 2007. *Community Health Centers: A Movement and the People Who Made It Happen.* New Brunswick, NJ: Rutgers University Press.

Lewis I. J., and C. G. Sheps. 1983. *The Sick Citadel: The American Academic Medical Center and the Public Interest.* Cambridge, MA: Oelgeschlager, Gunn, and Hain.

Medicare Payment Advisory Commission (MedPAC). 2009. "Report to the Congress: Improving Incentives in the Medicare Program." June. Washington, DC.

Morris C. G., B. Johnson, S. Kim, and F. Chen. 2008. "Training Family Physicians in Community Health Centers: A Health Workforce Solution." *Family Medicine* 40:271–276.

Mullan, F. 2009. "Workforce Issues in Health Care Reform: Assessing the Present and Preparing for the Future." Testimony before the Senate Finance Committee, Mar. 12. http://finance.senate.gov/hearings/hearing/?id=d82650ed-02b3-b69f-ad34–5d6c 8843a5de.

Mullan, F., C. Chen, S. Petterson, G. Kolsky, and M. Spagnola. 2010. "The Social Mission of Medical Education: Ranking the Schools." *Annals of Internal Medicine* 152:804–811.

National Association of Community Health Centers (NACHC). 2008. "Health Profession Training Opportunities at Community Health Centers." Bethesda, MD. Accessed Feb. 15, 2009. http://www.nachc.com/client/documents/HPT_Fact_Sheet_FINAL.pdf.

National Resident Matching Program. 2008. "Results and Data: 2008 Main Residency Match." March. Washington, DC. Accessed Dec. 28, 2008. www.nrmp.org.

New England Healthcare Institute and Josiah Jr. Foundation (NEHI-Macy). 2010. "Remaking Primary Care: A Framework for the Future." Jan. New York.

Northwest Regional Primary Care Association (NRPCA). 2010. "Education Health Center Initiative." Accessed Oct. 5. http://www.nwrpca.org/education-health-center-initiative.html.

Oliver, T. R. 2004. "Policy Entrepreneurship in the Social Transformation of American Medicine: The Rise of Managed Care and Managed Competition." *Journal of Health Politics, Policy and Law* 29 (Aug.–Oct.): 701–733.

Oliver T. R., A. Grover, and P. R. Lee. 2001. "Variations in Medicare Payments for Graduate Medical Education in California and Other States." June. Oakland: California HealthCare Foundation.

Oliver, T. R., and P. Paul-Shaheen. 1997. "Translating Ideas into Actions: Entrepreneurial Leadership in State Health Care Reforms. *Journal of Health Politics, Policy and Law* 22 (June): 721–788.

Parchman, M. L., and S. Culler. 1994. "Primary Care Physicians and Avoidable Hospitalizations." *Journal of Family Practice* 39:123–128.

Pathman, D. E., B. J. Crouse, L. F. Padilla, T. V. Horvath, and T. T. Nguyen. 2009. "American Recovery and Reinvestment Act and the Expansion and Streamlining of the National Health Service Corps: A Great Opportunity for Service-Minded Family Physicians." *Journal of the American Board of Family Medicine* 22, no. 5: 582–584.

Patient-Centered Primary Care Collaborative (PCPCC). 2007. "Joint Principles of the Patient Centered Medical Home." Feb. Washington, DC: PCPCC.

Rich, E. C., M. Liebow, M. Srinivasan, D. Parish, J. O. Wolliscroft, O. Fein, and R. Blaser. 2002. "Medicare Financing of Graduate Medical Education: Intractable Problems, Elusive Solutions." *Journal of General Internal Medicine* 17, no. 4: 283–292.

Rieselbach R. E., B. J. Crouse, and J. G. Frohna. 2010. "Teaching Primary Care in Community Health Centers: Addressing the Workforce Crisis for the Underserved." *Annals of Internal Medicine* 152:118–122.

Rieselbach, R. E., and A. L. Kellerman. 2011. "A Model Health Care Delivery System for Medicaid." *New England Journal of Medicine* 364:2476–2478. doi:10.1056/NEJMp 1104873.

Rieselbach R. E., and T. C. Jackson. 1986. "In Support of a Linkage between the Funding of Graduate Medical Education and Care of the Indigent." *New England Journal of Medicine* 314:32–35.

Robert Graham Center. 2007. "Access Denied: A Look at America's Medically Disenfranchised." Washington, DC: National Association of Community Health Centers. http://www.graham-center.org/online/graham/home/publications/monographs-books/2007/rgcmo-access-denied.html.

Rosenblatt, R. A., C. H. Andrilla, T. Curtin, and L. G. Hart. 2006. "Shortages of Medical Personnel at Community Health Centers: Implications for Planned Expansion." *Journal of the American Medical Association* 295:1042–1049.

Salsberg, E., P. H. Rockey, K. L. Rivers, S. E. Brotherton, and G. R. Jackson. 2008. "US Residency Training before and after the 1997 Balanced Budget Act." *Journal of the American Medical Association* 300:1174–1180.

Sardell, A. 1986. *The US Experiment in Social Medicine: The Community Health Center Program, 1965–1986.* Pittsburgh: University of Pittsburgh Press.

Shi, L., and D. A. Singh. 2008. "Outpatient and Primary Care Services." Chap. 7 in *Delivering Health Care in America: A Systems Approach*, 4th ed. Boston: Jones and Bartlett.

Shi, L., and B. Starfield. 2000. "Primary Care, Income Inequality, and Self-Related Health in the US: Mixed-Level Analysis." *International Journal of Health Services* 30:541–555.

———. 2001. "Primary Care Physician Supply, Income Inequality, and Racial Mortality in US Metropolitan Areas." *American Journal of Public Health* 91:1246–1250.

Shi, L., B. Starfield, B. Kennedy, and I. Kawachi. 1999. "Income Inequality, Primary Care, and Health Indicators." *Journal of Family Practice* 48, no. 4: 275–284.

Shi, L., B. Starfield, R. Politzer, and J. Regan. 2002. "Primary Care, Self-Rated Health Care, and Reductions in Social Disparities in Health." *Health Services Research* 37, no. 3: 529–550.

Starfield, B. 1992. *Primary Care: Concept, Evaluation, and Policy*. New York: Oxford University Press.

———. 1994. "Is Primary Care Essential?" *Lancet* 344:1129–1133.

———. 2008. "The Future of Primary Care: Refocusing the System." *New England Journal of Medicine* 359, no. 20: 2087, 2091.

Starfield, B., L. Shi, and J. Macinko. 2005. "Contribution of Primary Care to Health Systems and Health." *Milbank Quarterly* 83:457–502.

Steinbrook, R. 2008a. "Health Care Reform in Massachusetts—Expanding Coverage, Escalating Costs." *New England Journal of Medicine* 358:2757–2760.

———. 2008b. "Medical Student Debt—Is There a Limit?" *New England Journal of Medicine* 359:2629–2632.

Swensen, S. J., G. S. Meyer, E. C. Nelson, G. C. Hunt Jr., D. B. Pryor, J. I. Weissberg, G. S. Kaplan, J. Daley, G. R. Yates, M. R. Chassin, B. C. James, and D. M. Berwick. 2010. "Cottage Industry to Postindustrial Care—The Revolution in Health Care Delivery." *New England Journal of Medicine* 362:e12. doi:10.1056/NEJMp0911199.

Peter D. Jacobson, Valerie Myers,
Judith G. Calhoun, and Jodyn E. Platt

Chapter 6

Examining the Structure and Sustainability of Health Care Safety-Net Services

In a period of increasing patient demand and waning financial resources, the sustainability of health care safety-net organizations (SNO) is not guaranteed. This chapter focuses on primary care SNOs such as federally qualified health centers (FQHC) (also known as community health centers, or CHC) and community-based organizations such as free clinics. Their ability to remain financially viable while maintaining their mission of providing health care to uninsured and underinsured populations (the target populations), depends on developing innovative and efficient health care delivery designs and strategies.

Until now most SNOs have viewed themselves as mission-oriented; at best, attention to sound business practices has been a secondary consideration. But as financial pressures and growing unmet need threaten their survival, many SNOs have recognized the need to operate as small businesses with greater attention to efficiency (Jacobson et al. 2005). What they collectively lack, however, is the means to identify what those operational and organizational strategies should be and how they might be used. Despite their importance as providers of last resort for uninsured and underinsured populations, there is only limited empirical evidence about how SNOs are organized and how they deliver health care. Unlike the robust study of larger health care organizations, the thousands of clinics that comprise the health care safety net have not yet been studied thoroughly to determine which organizational structures would achieve the best outcomes and which practices would improve quality of care. One goal of this chapter is to stimulate rigorous health services research on SNOs.

The chapter will broadly examine the current organizational models that SNOs are using and will assess whether the organizational and operational structures are adequate to meet the primary care needs of the target populations. These needs include acute care, triage, referrals to specialists, chronic care management, and access to pharmaceuticals. The questions to be addressed include the following: Are FQHCs, free clinics, or hybrids (clinics that take insurance but are also committed to serving those without insurance) capable of acting as medical homes? To what extent are connections to larger health care systems necessary to sustain SNOs? How will SNOs adapt to changes in target population groups (such as undocumented immigrants and newly unemployed individuals)? What types of administrative support systems are needed to sustain health care SNOs? What is the role of SNOs, especially free clinics, after health reform? How will the Patient Protection and Affordable Care Act (the Affordable Care Act, or ACA) affect the models clinics use to provide primary care services?

After a summary of the background and context, we provide a synthesis of the current literature on models of care in SNOs. We then present results of a qualitative research project that examines organizational and operational efficiencies in Michigan's SNOs. We conclude with policy recommendations, focusing on alternative organizational strategies that could best serve the target populations and ensure a sustainable health care safety net along with innovative policies that states can adopt.

Background and Context

At the outset, we note that the ACA promises profound changes for uninsured populations and, hence, equally important challenges and opportunities for SNOs. For FQHCs, the ACA promises enhanced fiscal resources along with an anticipated increase in demand for services. For free clinics, it promises only increased demand without providing any fiscal help. Ironically, the ACA could exacerbate the central problems free clinics already confront: depleted resources and ever-increasing demand for services. Thus, one of the premises of this chapter is that successful implementation of the ACA, and particularly the effective use of new funding, will depend on improving operational efficiencies and developing effective organizational structures.

In 2000 the Institute of Medicine (IOM) provided an overview of the fraying health care safety net that was tellingly titled "America's Health Care Safety Net: Intact but Endangered" (IOM 2000). Ten years later, the ability of SNOs to meet the needs of the nation's uninsured and underinsured populations remains a major social problem in the United States. Administratively, safety-net clinics face budgetary constraints that impede their ability to operate efficiently and engage in strategic development and capacity building. Indeed, SNOs face a range of management challenges including: leadership training and staff development; recruiting and retaining qualified medical personnel; analyzing patient encounter data; acquiring resources; and using best clinical practices.

At the community level, gaining access to specialty care referrals for patients is a major challenge because of financial pressures confronting hospitals and private physicians. Compounding this problem, there are few mechanisms to assess continuity of care for referred patients. Fundraising is an increasingly challenging endeavor because of heightened competition for donor support from other nonprofit organizations.

A regional network is one way to provide the administrative support clinics need, but SNOs have been resistant to operating as a regional cooperative. Moreover, regional networks have not been able to take full advantage of their buying power to obtain group purchasing price efficiencies. Therefore, it is necessary to consider the organizational challenges that SNOs face individually as well as collectively.

Contributions of Free Clinics

Because other chapters in this volume address FQHCs in detail, here we provide more background about free clinics, which make a separate and yet unrecognized significant contribution toward serving uninsured persons. Free clinics rely on volunteer medical professionals and other forms of community support to serve uninsured patients. Nationwide, they are a critical entry point into the health care system for uninsured populations. Generally, they do not seek insurance reimbursement or seek payments from patients. FQHCs, in contrast, receive federal funds and accept insurance, especially from Medicaid, although they are expected to provide care for uninsured patients as well. Together these organizational types constitute the bulk of the health care safety net. Despite the infusion of federal money into FQHCs, free clinics will still be an indispensable health care venue for uninsured and underinsured patients in many metropolitan areas (Felt-Lisk, McHugh, and Howell 2002; MPCA and AHCC 2004; Salinsky 2004; Jacobson et al. 2005).[1]

With a mission of providing health care at no cost to uninsured and underinsured populations, free clinics are the only resource designed exclusively to serve uninsured populations. They represent a community-oriented, private sector response to a serious social problem: serving a large and growing patient population that has difficulty finding health care at other venues. Free clinics engage volunteer physicians and other medical professionals to evaluate, treat, and, where possible, refer patients for specialty and other health care needs. Free clinics are patient-centered organizations, existing solely to serve patient needs. Of necessity, they are sites of innovation in health care delivery and organization.

Without free clinics, many uninsured patients risk losing their connection to health care services for several reasons. First, local public health departments are substantially reducing their direct service capacity. Second, fiscal pressures prevent hospitals from expanding services to the uninsured population. Third, even though one might argue that FQHCs are likely to fill the void, especially with the influx of new money from the ACA, there are reasons to be concerned. In particular, FQHCs face their own financial and practical limitations (Felt-Lisk, McHugh, and Howell 2002; Rosenbaum, Shin, and Darnell 2004).[2] FQHCs are heavily dependent on Medicaid revenues, which are likely to be unstable over the next few years, and federal support, which may be limited by current budget deficits.

Challenges for All SNOs

A common problem among SNOs is that there are limited mechanisms for them to learn from one another. The IOM's landmark study emphasized this point. After examining claims that safety-net providers have been able to adapt to the changing environment, the report states that the committee was "continuously frustrated by its inability to find a single source where such information was collected and analyzed" (IOM 2000, 211). The IOM report then recommended efforts "to document and analyze the effects of changes in [safety net funding programs] on the safety net and the health of vulnerable populations" (ibid., 214).

Sharing information is particularly difficult within poor, urban areas because resources are limited, and just getting through the day is tantamount to success. Individual clinics have largely been isolated from one another, with limited sharing of information across clinics and no common organizational strategy. As discussed later, a regional network is one way to provide the administrative support clinics need.

At the clinic level, there are insufficient data regarding patient encounters, few technological resources for data analysis, and little ability to follow up with patients who are referred to other health care providers in the community (Wells and Weiner 2005). At the regional level, existing networks face limited capacity for real-time data feedback on patient-level benchmark measures, or for technical assistance in identifying and implementing administrative and clinical best practices.

SNOs need further information about which model of patient-centered care is most effective for linking the uninsured to the community's health care services. Free clinics and FQHCs generally follow one of three models: urgent care, primary care, or triage and referral. But other models, such as a health promotion and prevention strategy, may be more effective in improving patient outcomes and population health. The existing literature and the results of our recent study consider both current and potential models.

Literature Review: Models of Primary Care

The literature search for this review was performed with a keyword search in the PubMed and the Ovid Medline databases, examining articles published from 1998 to 2010. We identified models of primary care that might provide better quality of care than the traditional model and/or make primary care more accessible or affordable to the uninsured and underinsured population.

One problem with the literature is that we know very little in the aggregate about which care delivery models SNOs actually use (Darnell 2010). For instance, a recently completed survey of free clinics provides a wealth of information about services, patients, and the cost of care but no information about the model of care delivery.[3] Another major problem is that very few of these models have been tested empirically. As a result, much of what follows represents analytical possibilities as opposed to proven models.

For this review we focus on five major trends in the literature regarding organizational models for SNOs. First, we examine whether SNOs are natural settings to be patient-centered medical homes (PCMH), a high policy priority for primary care. Second, we consider workforce needs, which are compelling among SNOs. In particular, we explore the roles of diverse health professionals such as nurses, physician assistants, and volunteer medical and administrative staff in providing patient care that is efficient relative to quality and financial concerns. Third, we assess which primary care models might offer optimal long-term benefits, such as the reduction of emergency department (ED) visits. Fourth, we consider models that can improve chronic disease management and continuity of care while keeping costs manageable. Fifth, we look at alternative models that might complement and enhance the scope of care that SNOs can provide. For instance, strategies such as school-based health centers, retail clinics, telehealth/e-medicine, and local access-to-care programs are increasingly viable alternatives to a traditional primary care approach, particularly if they are able to leverage community resources and existing infrastructure, private–public partnerships, and technology.

Safety-Net Organizations as Patient-Centered Medical Homes

One of the major policy initiatives for primary care has been the concept of patient-centered medical homes. Many policymakers and researchers have promoted the PCMH concept as an answer to government agencies that seek political solutions to make quality health care affordable and accessible to all Americans (Rosenthal 2008). (For a summary and analysis of the PCMH principles from the American Academy of Family Physicians, see Strange, Nutting, and Miller 2010.) Yet it remains to be seen whether payers can be convinced of the value of medical homes and whether physicians can deliver what the medical home promises (Backer 2007).

As defined by the American College of Physicians, a PCMH is a physician-led, team-based model of care that provides continuous and coordinated care throughout a patient's lifetime to maximize health outcomes. The PCMH is responsible for providing all of a patient's health care needs or appropriately arranging care with other qualified professionals (Robeznieks 2007). In a PCMH, every patient has a personal physician who leads an integrated team of health care professionals that provides coordinated acute, chronic, preventive, and end-of-life care (Barr 2006; Robeznieks 2007; Rosenthal 2008). Patients also have enhanced access through extended hours and secure electronic communication options (Robeznieks 2007). Sound empirical evidence demonstrates that having a regular source of care and continuous care with the same physician over time, which PCMHs are designed to provide, leads to better health outcomes as well as lower costs (Starfield and Shi 2004; Backer 2007). Nevertheless, several potential roadblocks need to be addressed before we can realize the promise of medical homes (Schoenbaum 2007).

SNOs have shown mixed capabilities as PCMHs. A recent Commonwealth Fund report suggests that it may be premature for many clinics to meet major criteria constituting a PCMH (Reschovsky and O'Malley 2008; Cloeman and Phillips 2010). The report simultaneously documents many of the challenges that need to be overcome while stressing the advantages of a PCMH for the safety-net population. Regarding the challenges, the report notes that many of the surveyed SNOs lack adequate processes for scheduling, coordinating care, or implementing team-based care. In contrast, Friedberg and colleagues (2010) found that primary care practices that serve disproportionately vulnerable populations retained the structural capacity to serve as PCMHs. But as the authors note, their study is more applicable to FQHCs, was concentrated in Massachusetts, and differed from previous research findings.

Workforce

Like the public health system, SNOs face challenges in recruiting and retaining a well-trained workforce. Rieselbach, Crouse, and Frohna (2010) note that

CHCs are particularly at risk as the workforce struggles to meet demand because SNOs mostly offer primary care services. In all likelihood, the ACA will exacerbate the difficulties SNOs face in meeting the community's primary care needs. For free clinics, which rely on volunteer health providers, the key challenges are finding physician volunteers at a time of declining physician revenue, and finding nurses, who are in high demand in all medical care settings. A prominent theme in the literature is that nurse-managed clinics can help meet the demand at a reasonable cost. For CHCs, which are able to hire medical professionals, the challenge is to find enough practitioners willing to work in this environment to meet the anticipated demand resulting from the ACA. Fortunately, one of the significant achievements of the act is its focus on workforce issues, including debt repayment programs for public-health practitioners.

The literature suggests that nurse practitioners (NP) and physician assistants (PA) are ideally situated to staff nurse-managed clinics specifically and SNOs more generally. NPs and PAs have complementary skills and are trained to provide the full range of typical primary care. Nurses, especially NPs, are common providers in all the models presented in this chapter. Studies have shown that NPs provide primary care of the same quality as physicians in terms of patient satisfaction, future health services utilization, and patient outcomes (Robeznieks 2007; Rosenthal 2008). Nurse-managed clinics play a vital role in providing needed health services to vulnerable populations, and are further discussed in a subsequent section.

Students in health professional schools can be used effectively as SNO volunteers to address workforce shortages. Working in free clinics provides them with valuable service-learning experiences and the opportunity to develop empathy, social awareness, and social and cultural competence (Backer 2007). In this volume (chapter 5), Rieselbach, Crouse, and Frohna (2010) propose the establishment of primary care teaching health centers within CHCs. If implemented, students would receive their final year of training in CHCs. As an incentive to continue providing care in underserved areas, their proposal would include debt repayment through the National Health Service Corps. Although this proposal only includes medical students, nothing prevents its expansion to other health professional students, such as dental students. These trainees can complement lay volunteers in free clinics who are usually responsible for clerical and administrative tasks. Indeed, free clinics cannot function without significant help from lay volunteers who open more time for health professionals to spend with patients (Schoenbaum 2007).

Primary Care Models

As noted earlier, the literature on the organizational structure of SNOs is quite limited. Nonetheless, some studies indicate that urgent care models can reduce emergency room visits. Even though there is no nationally accepted definition, the Urgent Care Association of America defines urgent care as the delivery of ambulatory medical care outside of a hospital ED on a walk-in basis without a scheduled appointment.[4] Urgent care has a few distinguishing characteristics, such as an emphasis on walk-in or unscheduled patients, extended evening and weekend hours, and an array of services that exceeds those offered in a traditional primary care practice. Urgent care clinics apply a customer service approach to providing convenient care that is often not prevalent in doctors' offices and EDs, which are designed to accommodate the physicians' availability rather than the patients' (Weinick and Betancourt 2007). But unlike an ED, urgent care clinics are not open twenty-four hours and are rarely equipped to handle complex cases.

Limited information is available about the actual outcomes and cost savings resulting from the use of an urgent care center. Two studies that assess the impact of urgent care center use on the frequency of ED visits and primary care physicians' (PCP) visits (Merritt, Naamon, and Morris 2000; Kramer, Mitchell, and Epplen 2004) showed that using urgent care centers results in a statistically significant decrease in the frequency of ED visits and a significant increase in PCP use in the six months after a visit to an urgent care center.

The main concern about the care provided at urgent care centers is that it is episodic; there is no continuity of care (Weinick and Betancourt 2007). Urgent care aims to treat patients quickly by referring, recommending, and preparing them for further evaluation. The focus is on symptoms, and physicians do not routinely search past medical records. The motto is to "treat 'em and street 'em" (Guthmann 2002). More often than not, physicians are seeing a patient for the first time, yet very little time is available in which to gather a history, make a working diagnosis, and initiate a plan of therapy. Many patients present to an urgent care clinic after their illness has progressed and beyond the time when medical intervention is most effective (Wong 1996). Despite these concerns, the urgent care industry appears to be emerging as an important primary care model.

Chronic Care Models

While the literature on chronic care models is limited, the group-visit model shows some promise as a possible solution to the limits of current care structures on chronic illness management (Jaber, Braksmajer, and Trilling 2006). Group visits are subdivided into three different types.

One approach is the cooperative health care clinic, which begins with a few minutes of social time, followed by an educational segment lasting about half an hour (Pennachio 2003). Next, the physician and nurse take patients' vital signs, update their records, write prescription refills, sign forms, and give immunizations. A question-and-answer session follows. During the final hour, the physician sees some patients one-on-one. Visits last about two and a half hours and are limited to roughly twenty patients.

Drop-in group medical appointments work best as follow-up visits for established patients (Pennachio 2003). Patients with conditions that benefit from treatment in a group setting or in longer, supervised sessions, such as depression or anxiety, are well suited to drop-in models. Drop-in groups are typically held weekly and last about ninety minutes each, with a physician and a health behavior specialist leading the session. Like cooperative clinics, the groups can be disease-specific, but mixed groups are more common.

The Physicals Shared Medical Appointment model was designed mainly for primary care but is also now being used in many specialties for prenatal exams, well-baby checks, and school physicals (Pennachio 2003). This model typically triples the physician's efficiency by grouping patients by sex and age for physical examinations.

The literature suggests an increase in quality of care and patient satisfaction with group care. Group visits lead to a decrease in ED visits, visits to specialists, and hospitalization rates for patients with chronic illnesses (Jaber, Braksmajer, and Trilling 2006). Mixed results have been found for improving healthy behaviors, self-efficacy, physical function, depression, quality-of-life, and disease-specific outcomes (Jaber, Braksmajer, and Trilling 2006). Although results related to the cost of care have been mixed, a recent study showed that group visits decreased the cost of care and were feasible and acceptable to uninsured and inadequately insured patients with uncontrolled type 2 diabetes (Clancy et al. 2008). Group visits helped patients foster an improved sense of trust in their physician. Importantly, patients in groups reported receiving more coordinated, community-oriented, and culturally competent care (Clancy et al. 2003a, 2003b).

Other Models for SNOs

Safety-net organizations are often quite creative in the models they adopt and adapt to deliver services. Although not traditionally considered to be SNOs, some models should at least be mentioned as possibilities for serving uninsured populations. These models include nurse-managed clinics, school-based health centers, retail or convenient care clinics, e-medicine/telehealth, and local access-to-care programs, as examples.

Nurse-Managed Clinics

Nurse-managed clinics are primarily located in medically underserved areas within rural and urban communities. NPs, who serve as primary care providers, staff these centers and foster strong partnerships with the communities they serve. Providers in nurse-managed clinics view the health problems of their patients within the context of societal, environmental, and cultural influences and work to connect patients with information and resources that can positively affect their health (Pohl et al. 2007).

According to the literature, nurse-managed clinics have been successful in many ways. They consistently reach a variety of different demographics, particularly children and youth, which suggests that the centers are delivering vital services to underserved populations at an early age (Pohl et al. 2007). Nurse-managed clinics also serve a population that is strongly affected by health disparities. The preventive care that these centers emphasize, such as immunizations, screenings, and health education, is essential to combating these disparities. Finally, nurse-managed clinics have a strong reputation of "providing high-quality, cost-effective care and achieving high patient satisfaction rates in the communities they serve" (Mundinger et al. 2000).

School-Based Health Centers

School-based health centers began in the 1970s to improve access to health care for underprivileged children (Allison et al. 2007). School clinics are designed chiefly to provide primary care services for uninsured, underinsured, low-income, and minority children whose access to care is otherwise limited. The peer-reviewed literature provides strong evidence that school clinics improve access to care and provide better quality of care, especially for uninsured children, and are an effective way to cater to the health care needs of children and adolescents. School clinic users have a significantly higher number of primary care and dental visits, health maintenance visits, screening for high-risk behaviors, and immunizations as compared to nonusers (Kaplan et al. 1999; Allison et al. 2007). Several studies have shown a significant decrease in ED visits for children who receive care from a school clinic (Kaplan et al. 1999; Young, D'angela, and Davis 2001; Allison et al. 2007).

Convenient Care Clinics/Retail Clinics

Convenient care clinics (also called retail or minute clinics) can be controversial because of concerns regarding quality and continuity of care (Lin 2008, Woodburn, Smith, and Nelson 2007). But they continue to multiply at a rapid pace and clearly serve an important market niche (Schmidt, Kolar, and

Fairfield 2007). These clinics have proliferated in response to obstacles that hindered or prevented the delivery of primary health care services to millions of moderate- and low-income Americans. Convenient care clinics are retail-based medical clinics that offer a defined scope of diagnostic and treatment services for common medical ailments as well as preventive health services. They are conveniently located in places where people shop, and consumers can drop in without an appointment (Hansen-Turton et al. 2007). Because they charge for their services without regard to income or insurance (albeit at lower rates than otherwise available), they are not SNOs (Thygeson et al. 2008).

E-Medicine/Telehealth Model

In primary care, e-medicine is being used for online appointment scheduling, electronic prescription refills, general messaging capabilities, web visits with physicians, and to provide patients with online lab results (Kalb 2004; Stone 2007). The advantages of electronic medicine include significant cost and time savings for the patient because there is no time away from work and no cost of travel (Stone 2007). E-medicine also has the potential to provide improved access for people living in smaller rural communities (Bynum et al. 2003). At the same time, e-medicine introduces new questions for its providers about medical liability, cross-border licensure, reimbursement rates (Silverman 2003), possible breakdown in the doctor–patient relationship (Hjelm 2005), and the financial requirements necessary to install and maintain e-medicine systems.

Local Access-to-Care Programs

Many communities have begun to develop access-to-care programs that are locally organized and financed. These programs provide a structured set of health care benefits and services to uninsured working-age adults, though most offer only limited benefits or basic primary care services. Sometimes termed county health plans or "project access" programs, they have a formal enrollment process, eligibility determination, and enrollment fees that provide access to a network of providers who offer free or reduced-price health care services. The few studies that have been conducted show mixed results for their effectiveness vis-à-vis the target populations (Blewett, Ziegenfuss, and Davern 2008; Hall 2011).

Summary

Of the models presented earlier, the patient-centered medical-home model probably provides the best quality of primary health care and has won favor with physician organizations and lawmakers as the centerpiece for improving health care (Kruse 2007). Whether that model is achievable for SNOs remains an empirical question. More importantly, the literature suggests that each of the models considered has strengths and weaknesses for SNOs that should be studied empirically.

For instance, chronic diseases such as diabetes currently place the maximum burden on the health care system, and the group-visit model seems a viable means to maximize physician output and to effect behavioral changes in chronically ill patients. Urgent care clinics and convenient care clinics are more accessible and affordable from the point of view of the uninsured. But the major problem with both models is that there is no continuity of care; instead the care provided is episodic and patients cannot identify with a single provider. E-medicine has great potential, both by itself and in combination with any of the models presented. In all likelihood, the use of e-medicine will increase exponentially over time and the challenge will be to ensure that its use does not compromise quality of care. School-based health centers and nurse-based clinics play a vital role in improving health and well-being of children and in providing much-needed health care to uninsured youth. While promising, local access-to-care programs have yet to achieve sustained results in providing access to care for uninsured populations.

The Qualitative Interviews

Research Questions and Methods

In 2009 and 2010 we conducted qualitative interviews with representatives from twenty-nine SNOs in Michigan. The study purpose was to examine operational efficiencies and organizational structures that could improve the quality of health care for the target populations. We developed and tested an interview protocol and requested additional data if available. For purposes of this chapter, we describe responses to interview questions asked about the current primary care organizational model being used and whether the clinic had considered an alternative model.

The sample included fourteen FQHCs, eleven free clinics, and four hybrid clinics. Altogether, we interviewed ninety-six respondents, including clinic directors, medical directors, financial staff, and scheduling staff. The interviews ranged from one to two hours in length and were recorded for subsequent transcription. The data were coded and entered into NVivo software. During the coding process, interrater reliability was greater than 95 percent.

Results

Service Models

Our respondents cited multiple models for delivering their health care services. Table 6.1 lists the top five models cited by clinic type: primary care,
medical home, preventive, urgent care, and referral. Most common were
primary/preventive care (83 percent) and medical-home models (59 percent).
For free clinics, urgent care models figured prominently as well (27 percent).
In addition to the dominant model types, there were as many as fifteen other
types cited, ranging from health management organization (HMO) to dental to
behavioral health and pharmacy. Perhaps more aptly named bundles of services than models per se, the range and diversity of responses demonstrates the
fungibility and flexibility of nomenclature as well as practice. Our respondents
were much less concerned with how to label service provision than with being
able to provide services at all. Put differently, our results suggest that clinic
directors provide combinations of these five service-delivery models that
change in emphasis over time depending on community/patient needs.

The reasons for choosing delivery models included the recognition that
service models are constantly evolving in response to changing demands from
the community, funding sources, and national influence. Many respondents
cited patient need as a key driver in opting for expansion of services. These key
motivating factors did not vary significantly by clinic type. Table 6.2 provides
examples of how respondents discussed the evolution of their services, the
need-based approach to models, and the very real influences of grant requirements or fiscal constraints. Unlike their counterparts beyond the safety
net, respondents noted that changes in model type were frequently based on
adaptations to changing patient characteristics or funding opportunities rather

Table 6.1   **Percentage and Frequency of Predominant Health Care Service
Delivery Models Used by Safety-Net Organizations**

	FQHCs % (n)	Free clinics % (n)	Hybrids % (n)	Total % (n)
Model	N = 14	N = 11	N = 4	N = 29
Primary care	79% (11)	82% (9)	100% (4)	83% (24)
Medical home	71% (10)	45% (5)	50% (2)	59%(17)
Preventive	43% (6)	18% (2)	75% (3)	38% (11)
Urgent care	29% (4)	27% (3)	0% (0)	24% (7)
Referral	21% (3)	18% (2)	25% (1)	21% (6)

Source: Author interviews

than to market pressure or competition. Quotations used in table 6.2 are labeled by clinic type, although they are exemplary of respondents in many SNOs.

Federally Qualified Health Centers

Of the FQHCs sampled, 57 percent (8 of 14) stated that they used more than two models for service delivery to meet the community's needs and to meet federal grant requirements for funding and FQHC designation. The most commonly cited models were primary or preventive care and medical home. With primary care as the historical cornerstone of FQHCs, it is no surprise that many said they operate as medical homes. For example, one respondent noted that "medical home" is increasingly being recognized as the term for the model of service delivery for FQHCs, while another added that "we are a medical home just because there are multiple service providers working in close proximity and in collaboration."

Tellingly, several respondents indicated that using the term "medical home" was a semantic rather than a substantive device (that is, form over substance). "We don't have a sign that says [medical home] . . . but we provide the services that make us a medical home." One respondent added, "I hate to say

Table 6.2   Reasons Cited for Choosing Delivery Models

Rationale	Examples
Evolved	"The clinic started as family practice and evolved from there"—FQHC
	"We evolved into it. [Medical home model] became the thinking as they got more into managed care."—Hybrid
	"Initially [we were] just going to be a walk-in clinic for immediate needs. As patients with chronic diseases expanded, [we] became both a medical home and primary care provider."—Free Clinic
Need	"I think it comes back to Day 1—the need of the community, what they were needing at the time, which was primary care. It sort of evolved from there."—FQHC
	"[The clinic] was established to be a primary care clinic from the beginning. [I'd] expected it to be more of an urgent care model, but by accepting the patients they did with those criteria, you have patients with primary care needs."—Hybrid
Requirement/ resource constraint	"The charge to FQHCs is of primary and preventive medicine"—FQHC
	"[The model was selected based on] what we were able to supply. We knew we could supply referrals because we recruited specialists— they came out of the woodwork. We knew we had to provide the urgent care."—Free Clinic

Source: Author interviews

[we are a medical home] because FQHCs have always been medical homes [that] developed in the 1980s. When PCMH became trendy, we were urged from [the hospital] and others to jump on board. [The] idea of PCMH is a laundry list of what you could do that could be helpful." More cynically, one respondent noted that "[they] called themselves primary care until they said they were a medical home . . . they've been doing all that for years."

A consistent theme among FQHC respondents was that the model is constantly evolving. "We had people that didn't know what the hell they were doing. So when someone said no, you can't do that—we said why not? And we just did it. Pretty soon, you deal with domestic violence issues, ambulatory care that turns into primary care and that turns into patient-centered primary care, etc. There were people in this community, myself included, who didn't know better." Likewise, a respondent noted that medical-home adoption "happened early on. [It] wasn't deliberate–it's just how it was developed. It was a philosophy—a patient should have a person they can come and see."

In one community, respondents viewed urgent care as an add-on to primary care as the natural evolution of the centers: "[It's] evolved. [It] was always primary and preventive and has become urgent care walk-in seven days a week." Urgent care was not a core delivery model for most FQHCs, but for one, community need drove development of urgent care services because of a "younger population, with a little bit of industry, more kids."

Other commonly cited service-delivery models that support the functions and mission of FQHCs include referral, urgent care, and triage. Referral models, for example, used with other models—such as preventive and primary care—help meet the needs of the community as well as meeting the requirements of FQHC designation.

Free Clinics

Much like FQHCs, free clinics choose services and models for service delivery based on available resources and the changing needs of their community. Free clinics and FQHCs share resource constraints influencing the types of services they are able to provide. Free clinics differ from FQHCs in several important ways. First, they rely in greater part on donations rather than federal grant funding to augment the organization's mission and, for some, on religious values in providing services.

The second key distinction between FQHCs and free clinics is the volunteer rather than employee base for services. As a result, the expertise and specialization of their volunteers greatly influence options for the types and styles of services that they provide. Leadership in free clinics also plays a greater role than for FQHCs in determining the choices the organization makes. One respondent described the leadership as being able to maximize "altruistic opportunism" to take advantage of relationships, networks, and fundraising skills to support the altruistic goals and mission of the organization.

The top service-delivery models for free clinics are primary care and urgent care. In most cases, these models have evolved over time. For one free clinic that considers itself a PCMH, it does so by virtue of its ability and need to provide multiple services as a safety-net organization. Several clinics provide preventive or referral services as a supplement to either their primary care or urgent care services. In several cases, urgent care was the initial model that has expanded to include preventive or primary care, especially in communities already served by an FQHC. But according to one clinic representative, "As patients seen with chronic diseases expanded, [we] became both a medical home and primary care facility."

Two free clinics viewed urgent care as central to their mission. At one, an FQHC was already serving the community so that residents had access to primary care. To fill a gap in the community, the clinic focused on providing urgent care. In the other case, primary care was simply beyond the capacity of the clinic, noting that "[we] want to continue urgent care; this was our mission from the beginning." Other models cited by respondents include preventive (two clinics), referral (one clinic), family practice (one clinic), and HMO (one clinic).

Hybrid Clinics

Given the relatively small number of hybrid clinics interviewed, identifying patterns in service-delivery models proved challenging. Nevertheless, the hybrid clinics sampled also used multiple models to provide their services. As with free clinics and FQHCs, hybrids have evolved over time to meet the needs of the community. The three hybrid model clinics described themselves as medical homes because (1) a medical home fits the way services are provided (for one health department, physical proximity to additional services, such as substance abuse, facilitates this relationship); (2) their goal is to be a primary care medical home; and (3) they evolved into medical homes to balance cost and services. Limited resources constrain development into full-service medical homes. Preventive care is provided in conjunction with primary care, and one hybrid is able to use group, triage, and referral service models, although "referral is very limited."

Alternative Models

In the past three to five years, approximately 60 percent of the FQHCs (n = 8) and free clinics (n = 7) and 50 percent of hybrids (n = 2) had discussed alternatives to their existing service models (table 6.3). Across eight different FQHCs, we found three different approaches to weighing alternative service-delivery models: (1) alternative models were generally considered because the assessment of models is a part of regular operations and seen as integral to adapting to the changing needs of the community; (2) the FQHC wanted to provide new models/services (for example, integrated health care to include behavioral health, or group health); and (3) new models were considered in relation to clinical outcomes to improve efficiencies.

For free clinics, considerations were similar for FQHCs in determining how or whether to expand services. Alternatives were weighed in the context of expanding their capacity or improving existing services. In deciding not to change, factors such as the existence of other safety-net clinics or disruption of existing services played heavily: "One reason we haven't [applied for FQHC status] is that there are two FQHCs within five miles of the community. We've chosen not to go that route. With two other facilities that are so close by, would that make for a successful application for us? In addition to that, it comes back to whether a change like that would lead to us doing our true mission, i.e., serving the uninsured. If we're bringing in more with insurance, it decreases our capacity to treat those that don't have it." A further consideration for free clinics that is perhaps unique to this group is balancing benefits and challenges when operating with a volunteer staff in contrast to an employed staff.

Three respondents from two hybrid health centers discussed their potential alternatives, suggesting that the choice of models is dynamic rather than fixed. "We like to think our models will change as our community changes." Another said that although we like the medical-home model, "We just can't afford it." But the following quote suggests openness to flexibility and change: "[We are] trying to move to an FQHC, which would mean an expansion of services and providers."

Table 6.3   **Safety Net Organizations Considering Alternative Health Care Delivery Models**

	FQHCs % (n)	Free clinics % (n)	Hybrids % (n)
Model	N = 14	N = 11	N = 4
Yes	57% (8)	64% (7)	50% (2)
No	29% (4)	18% (2)	50% (2)
Don't know	14% (2)	18% (2)	0% (0)

Source: Author interviews

Discussion

No clear organizational model or best practice emerges as optimal, either in the literature or in our qualitative study. In most of our interviews the organizational model combined various services and evolved to meet changing community needs. For FQHCs, federal guidelines shape the services and delivery structure, free clinics are reliant on their leadership and volunteer base, and hybrids try to be everything to the communities they serve. The clinics in our sample are using multiple models and require flexibility to adapt to changing populations. All of our respondents indicated a desire to expand services without compromising existing services. In short, our results suggest that the care delivery model is a second-order consideration based on a pragmatic understanding of the needs in the communities they serve.

Medical Care Home

For SNOs in our sample, the PCMH is a novel way of describing the services they have been providing for years. Subsequent analysis and research may determine whether they are posturing, showing political savvy, or making a serious attempt to reshape how they provide primary care. While the goal may well be a medical home, the reality for most (though clearly not all of our sample clinics) may be something more akin to standard forms of primary care. Limitations on continuity of care and referrals are serious obstacles to compliance with medical-home criteria. Our sense from interviews is that the concept of a PCMH in SNOs remains aspirational and is tenuous in practice.

Does the Model Matter?

Our study was only able to obtain basic information about how sample clinics organize and why. Our results do not allow us to draw firm conclusions as to the desirability or efficacy of particular types of delivery models. It is nonetheless legitimate to ask whether it really matters how clinics, especially free clinics, are organized. On a practical level the answer is probably no, it does not matter. Free clinic directors (and perhaps FQHCs as well) are thankful they can just get through the day. Focusing on organizational models is a luxury they have little time to consider. To be sure, boards of directors would be the appropriate venue for considering the issue, but many boards of directors as currently constituted may lack the expertise to determine the most effective organizational strategy (Jacobson et al. 2005).

At least in theory, the type of model could make an enormous difference in efficiency, targeting the community's needs, operating to achieve maximum use of resources, connecting patients to the community's health services, and better quality of care. Trying to be all things to a particular population may not be an optimal strategy. Arguably the most important attribute predicting efficiency in service delivery is being part of a formal or informal system (at least for improved referral capacity) (Dalton et al. 2009). Therefore, further research and demonstration projects could address the extent to which the organizational model matters. For instance, a demonstration project could select a few discrete models based on consultation with clinic directors and other experts, develop metrics of expected performance, and assess the results. Doing so would require clinics to agree to implement a new care delivery model with minimal disruption of current services.

Strategies for Free Clinics after Insurance Reform

Assuming that efforts to repeal the ACA fail, Congress has placed a large bet on FQHCs to absorb the primary care needs of previously uninsured populations. In the process, free clinics have essentially been excluded from federal financial support. As an afterthought among policymakers, free clinics face even more daunting problems than they did before the ACA. Although the study was not designed to examine the post–health reform roles of FQHCs and free clinics, we can offer some general observations of what some of the options may be for free clinics that follow insurance reform's implementation in 2014.

To begin with, free clinics will remain an important part of the health care safety net. It is unrealistic to expect that FQHCs will have the capacity to serve all of the newly insured people, and some will no doubt prefer the continuity with the free clinic they already know. Nonetheless, the expansion of FQHCs likely means that free clinics will be increasingly squeezed for resources and their patients further marginalized.

To avoid becoming irrelevant, free clinics have several options. First, they can seek compacts with nearby FQHCs to form a system to provide primary care. This has the advantage of spreading the increased demand for primary care across provider types. It would also permit experimentation with different organizational structures within the system. Equally important, a regional compact could experiment with clinics' providing complementary services. Not all clinics need to provide the same array of services. For instance, one clinic might focus on chronic care while another would handle referrals. Specialization within a region could improve overall quality of care but would require careful evaluation. A potential barrier is that networking would require FQHCs to share some of their resources with free clinics.

Second, and discussed more generally in the following, free clinics can form their own regional networks to share resources, technology, best practices, and operating strategies. To do so, free clinics would need to overcome the fierce independence that they have demonstrated to date. This strategy may be particularly salient for clinics located in areas that lack FQHCs.

Third, free clinics must consider moving toward a hybrid clinic model where they would accept Medicaid and other forms of health insurance but would also serve all who lack insurance or resources to pay. This, too, would be a hard decision for free clinics to make. After all, what characterizes the concept of free clinics is that they are mission-driven entities serving poor communities. Taking reimbursement would severely compromise this vision. If the alternative, however, is becoming extinct, free clinics might be willing to consider evolving toward hybrids.

Policy Recommendations

Regardless of whether clinics adopt a particular model, public policy should support some specific strategies. First, public-health nursing should be expanded to help staff both FQHCs and free clinics. While the current nursing shortage certainly makes this difficult to achieve, states should take advantage of funding available through the ACA to develop public-health nursing programs. Graduates should be given broad scope of practice authority to work as primary care providers in clinics. States should be willing to provide financial incentives to nurses who are willing to work in clinics. Expanding nurse-based clinics would help alleviate the primary care shortage and limit the need for physician volunteers.

Second, clinics need to expand their telemedicine capabilities. This would require subsidies to establish electronic capacity not just for patient records but also for physician/nurse telemedical practice. Although it may be difficult to reach a certain percentage of the low-income population, over time an increasing percentage of the population will have access to the Internet and requisite technologies. For both efficiency and practical reasons, telemedicine should be an important strategy for clinics. It would help reduce no-shows. Persistent no-shows and people who have limited ability to travel to the clinic could instead be scheduled for a telemedicine appointment.

Third, policymakers need to encourage alternative delivery models and workforce requirements for the safety-net population, as they have with retail clinics. For example, Rosenthal and colleagues (2010) make a compelling case for an expanded primary care workforce of community health workers. As they note, doing so requires a set of minimum competencies as well as expected education and training levels and is certain to face political pushback from other health care professionals. Another analysis argues for the expansion of primary care medical residency training programs to be located in community health centers (Rieselbach, Crouse, and Frohna 2010). This is a good idea, but it is not sufficient. The program should include NPs and PAs (Jacobson, Parker, and Coulter 1998).

Finally, policymakers and clinic directors should explore regional strategies. Similar to the ideas set forth in Weinkle, Feinstein, and Kanel (2010), we suggest that the provision of care to low-income persons should be thought of as a social problem to be addressed regionally. Doing so could improve referral patterns, assign patients to the most appropriate clinic, and facilitate administration. One requirement for an effective and efficient regional strategy would be the development of a regional administrative support system to develop a common database, analyze data, develop and test best practices, develop and measure quality of care metrics, and provide general administrative support to clinics and their boards of directors.

A regional strategy makes sense conceptually but faces serious barriers. For one thing, free clinics are fiercely independent and have resisted collaborations, both with other free clinics and with FQHCs. Based on our recent interviews, we believe that directors of free clinics are likely to be much less resistant than in the past because they now recognize that survival and improved patient care depends on closer collaboration across organizations. For another, competition between FQHCs and free clinics, while rarely voiced publicly in our interviews, is an impediment to a regional strategy involving all types of SNOs. Differing attitudes toward providing care for uninsured populations might make it difficult, for instance, to execute contracts between free clinics and FQHCs as Weinkle, Feinstein, and Kanel envision (Chapin and Fetter 2002). Aside from the resources needed to implement and sustain an administrative support system, clinics would inevitably be concerned about ceding their autonomy to an entity that would be accountable to all the clinics in the network, but not to a clinic's board of directors or the community.

As part of its Safety Net Medical Home Initiative, the Commonwealth Fund is sponsoring regional coordinating centers (partnering with sixty-five SNOs) to test these ideas. An additional intervention would be to design a regional compact between FQHCs and free clinics to determine potential economies of scale and whether the compact would work in practice.

For SNOs, this is an exciting and challenging environment that offers opportunities for improving access to and quality of care for uninsured and underserved populations. In a fluid delivery and policy environment, SNOs will need to experiment with different organizational models to meet the primary care needs of their patient populations. Rigorous evaluation of the multiple models likely to emerge will help identify the most effective organizational strategies for SNOs to follow.

Acknowledgments

We appreciate the financial support we received from the University of Michigan's Center for Health Care Transformation and Research and the executive vice president for medical affairs. We also received excellent research support from Katherine Bradley, MHSA; Lauren Daaku, MPH 2012; Heather Kofke-Egger, MS-HSR; Natalia Maska, MHSA; Catherine Oakar, MPH; and Rushyal Shyamraj, MHSA.

Notes

1. We define the health care safety net as those organizations and programs in both the public and private sectors that have a legal obligation or a commitment to provide direct health care services to the uninsured, underinsured, and other underserved groups.
2. Rosenbaum, Shin, and Darnell (2004) examine FQHCs and conclude that "for every one insured, low-income patient that a health center is able to treat, there are an average of four additional low-income, uninsured persons." Felt-Lisk, McHugh, and Howell (2002, 282) add, "The free clinics offer an alternative for patients who are unsuccessful or simply not comfortable seeking care from other providers, including other safety-net providers."
3. While the list of services is suggestive, it is difficult to extrapolate to the preferred model because the data are presented as aggregate percentages that cannot be used to identify specific models (Darnell 2010, table 3, 949).
4. Urgent Care Association of America, "New to Urgent Care" http://www.ucaoa.org/resources_newtourgentcare.php.

References

Allison, M. A., L. A. Crane, B. L. Beaty, A. J. Davidson, P. Melinkovich, and A. Kempe. 2007. "School-Based Health Centers: Improving Access and Quality of Care for Low-Income Adolescents." *Pediatrics* 120, no. 4: e887–894.

Backer, L. A. 2007. "The Medical Home: An Idea Whose Time Has Come . . . Again." *Family Practice Management* 14, no. 8: 38–41.

Barr, M. 2006. "The Advanced Medical Home: A Patient Centered, Physician-Guided Model of Health Care." A Policy Monograph of the American College of Physicians. http://www.aanp.org/NR/rdonlyres/9D238E9C-DE64–4D30-BDA6-AA370370D2E4/0/MedicalHomedocument.pdf.

Blewett, L. A., J. Ziegenfuss, and M. E. Davern. 2008. "Local Access to Care Programs (LACPs): New Developments in the Access to Care for the Uninsured." *Milbank Quarterly* 86, no. 3: 459–479.

Bynum, A. B., C. A. Irwin, C. O. Cranford, and G. S. Denny. 2003. "The Impact of Telemedicine on Patients' Cost Savings: Some Preliminary Findings." *Telemedicine Journal & E-Health* 9, no. 4: 361–367.

Chapin, J., and B. Fetter. 2002. "Performance-based Contracting in Wisconsin Public Health: Transforming State-local Relations." *Milbank Quarterly* 80, no. 1: 97–124.

Clancy, D. E., S. B. Brown, K. M. Magruder, and P. Huang. 2003a."Group Visits in Medically and Economically Disadvantaged Patients with Type 2 Diabetes and Their Relationships to Clinical Outcomes." *Top Health Information Management* 24, no. 1: 8–14.

Clancy, D. E., D. W. Cope, K. M. Magruder, P. Huang, K. H. Salter, and A. W. Fields. 2003b. "Evaluating Group Visits in an Uninsured or Inadequately Insured Patient Population with Uncontrolled Type 2 Diabetes." *Diabetes Education* 29, no. 2: 292–302.

Clancy, D. E., C. E. Dismuke, K. M. Magruder, K. N. Simpson, and D. Bradford. 2008. "Do Diabetes Group Visits Lead to Lower Medical Care Charges?" *American Journal Managed Care* 14, no. 1: 39–44.

Cloeman, K., and K. Phillips. 2010. "Providing Underserved Patients with Medical Homes: Assessing the Readiness of Safety-Net Health Centers." *Commonwealth Fund* pub. 1395, vol. 85 (May). http://www.commonwealthfund.org/~/media/Files/Publications/Issue%20Brief/2010/May/1395_Coleman_providing_underserved_patients_med_homes_ib.pdf.

Dalton, V. K., P. D. Jacobson, M. A. Konig, and P. P. Holman. 2009. "Community Responses to Diabetes and Mental Care for the Uninsured Population in Michigan." *Journal of Health Care for the Poor and Underserved* 20:98–106.

Darnell, J. S. 2010. "Free Clinics in the United States: A Nationwide Survey." *Archives of Internal Medicine* 170:946–953.

Felt-Lisk, S., M. McHugh, and E. Howell. 2002. "Monitoring Local Safety Net Providers: Do They Have Adequate Capacity?" *Health Affairs* 21, no. 5: 277–283.

Friedberg, M. W., K. L. Coltin, D. G. Safran, M. Schneider, and E. C. Dresser. 2010. "Medical Home Capabilities of Primary Care Practices that Serve Sociodemographically Vulnerable Neighborhoods." *Archives of Internal Medicine* 170:938–944.

Guthmann, R. 2002. "My Visit to Urgent Care." *Journal American Board Family Practice* 15, no. 5: 423–425.

Hall, M. A. 2011. "Access to Care Provided by Better Safety Net Systems for the Uninsured: Measuring and Conceptualizing Adequacy." *Medical Care Research and Review* 68:441.

Hansen-Turton, T., S. Ryan, K. Miller, M. Counts, and D. B. Nash. 2007. "Convenient Care Clinics: The Future of Accessible Health Care." *Disease Management* 10, no. 2: 61–73.

Hjelm, N. M. 2005. "Benefits and Drawbacks of Telemedicine." *Journal of Telemedicine & Telecare* 11, no. 2: 60–70.

Institute of Medicine (IOM) Committee on the Changing Market, Managed Care, and the Future Viability of Safety Net Providers. Lewin, M. E., and S. Altman, eds. 2000. *America's Health Care Safety Net: Intact but Endangered.* Washington, DC: National Academies Press.

Jaber, R., A. Braksmajer, and J. Trilling. 2006."Group Visits for Chronic Illness Care: Models, Benefits and Challenges." *Family Practice Management* 13, no. 1: 37–40.

Jacobson, P. D., V. K. Dalton, J. B. Grand, and C. S. Weisman. 2005. "Survival Strategies for Michigan's Health Care Safety Net Providers." *Health Services Research* 40:923–940.

Jacobson, P. D., L. E. Parker, and I. D. Coulter. 1998. "Nurse Practitioners and Physician Assistants as Primary Care Providers in Institutional Settings." *Inquiry* 35:432–446.

Kalb, C. 2004. "Get Ready for E-medicine." *Newsweek* 144, no. 6: 53–54.

Kaplan, D. W., C. D. Brindis, S. L. Phibbs, P. Melinkovich, K. Naylor, and K. Ahlstrand. 1999. "A Comparison Study of an Elementary School-based Health Center: Effects on

Health Care Access and Use." *Archives of Pediatrics and Adolescent Medicine* 153, no. 3: 235–243.

Kramer, A. D, J. Mitchell, and K. Epplen. 2004. "Urgent Care Pharmacotherapy Clinic." *American Journal of Health-System Pharmacy* 61, no. 17: 1768.

Kruse, J. 2007. "Talking the Legislative Talk: The Patient-Centered Medical Home." *Annals of Family Medicine* 5, no. 6: 566–567.

Lin, D. Q. 2008."Convenient Care Clinics: Opposition, Opportunity, and the Path to Health System Integration." *Frontier of Health Services Management* 24, no. 3: 3–11.

Merritt, B., E. Naamon, and S. A. Morris. 2000. "The Influence of an Urgent Care Center on the Frequency of ED Visits in an Urban Hospital Setting." *American Journal of Emergency Medicine* 18, no. 2: 123–125.

Michigan Primary Care Association and Access to Health Care Coalition (MPCA and AHCC). 2004. "Michigan's Health Care Safety Net Providers: Current Capacity Assessment and Future Outlook." V. 4. Lansing, Michigan. http://www.mi.gov/documents/SAFETY_NET_White_Paper_149766_7.pdf.

Mundinger, M. O., R. L. Kane, E. R. Lenz et al. 2000. "Primary Care Outcomes in Patients Treated by Nurse Practitioners or Physicians: A Randomized Trial." *Journal of the American Medical Association* 283, no. 1: 59–68.

Pennachio, D. L. 2003. "Should You Offer Group Visit?" *Medical Economics* 80, no. 15: 70–72.

Pohl, J. M., V. H. Barkauskas, R. Benkert, L. Breer, and A. Bostrom. 2007. "Impact of Academic Nurse-Managed Centers on Communities Served." *Journal of the American Academy of Nurse Practitioners* 19:268–275.

Reschovsky, J. D., and A. S. O'Malley. 2008. "Do Primary Care Physicians Treating Minority Patients Report Problems Delivering High-Quality Care?" *Health Affairs* 27, no. 3: w222–231.

Rieselbach, R. E., B. J. Crouse, and J. G. Frohna. 2010. "Teaching Primary Care in Community Health Centers: Addressing the Workforce Crisis for the Underserved." *Annals of Internal Medicine* 152:118–122.

Robeznieks, A. 2007. "Of Primary Importance, Primary-Care Physicians Seek to Legitimize the 'Medical Home' Concept to Improve Quality, Costs—But Will Insurers Buy It?" *Modern Healthcare* 37, no. 45: 6–7.

Rosenbaum, S., P. Shin, and J. Darnell. 2004. "Economic Stress and the Safety Net: A Health Center Update, Washington." Washington, DC: Kaiser Commission on Medicaid and the Uninsured.

Rosenthal, T. C. 2008. "The Medical Home: Growing Evidence to Support a New Approach to Primary Care." *Journal of the American Board of Family Medicine* 21, no. 5: 427–440.

Rosenthal, E. L., J. N. Brownstein, C. H. Rush, et al. 2010. "Community Health Workers: Part of the Solution." *Health Affairs* 29, no. 7: 1338–1342.

Salinsky, S. 2004. "Necessary But Not Sufficient? Physician Volunteerism and the Health Care Safety Net." National Health Policy Forum Background Paper. Washington, DC.

Schmidt, R., R. Kolar, and C. Fairfield. 2007. "Convenient Medical Clinics Reshaping the Healthcare Landscape." *Healthcare Financial Management* 61, no. 6: 40–43.

Schoenbaum, S. C. 2007. "The Medical Home: A Practical Way to Improve Care and Cut Costs." *Medscape General Medicine* 9, no. 2: 28.

Silverman, R. D. 2003. "Current Legal and Ethical Concerns in Telemedicine and E-Medicine." *Journal of Telemedicine and Telecare* 9 (Suppl 1): S67–S69.

Starfield, B., and L. Shi. 2004. "The Medical Home, Access to Care, and Insurance: A Review of Evidence." *Pediatrics* 113(Suppl 5): 1493–1498.

Strange, K. C., P. A. Nutting, and W. L. Miller. 2010. "Defining and Measuring the Patient-Centered Medical Home." *Journal of General Internal Medicine* 25:601–612.

Stone, J. H. 2007. "Communication between Physicians and Patients in the Era of E-medicine." *New England Journal of Medicine* 356, no. 24: 2451–2454.

Thygeson, M., K. A. Van Vorst, M. V. Maciosek, and L. Solberg. 2008. "Use and Costs of Care in Retail Clinics Versus Traditional Care Sites." *Health Affairs* 27, no. 5: 1283–1292.

Weinick, R., and R. Betancourt. 2007. "No Appointment Needed: The Resurgence of Urgent Care Centers in the United States." *Journal of Urgent Care Medicine*, Nov., 35–38. http://jucm.com/2007-nov/update.shtml.

Weinkle, J., K. W. Feinstein, and K. Kanel. 2010. "Partnering Private Primary Care Practices with Federally Qualified Health Centers in the Care of Complex Patients." *Health Affairs* 29, no. 6: 1211–1213.

Wells, R., and B. Weiner. 2005. "Using the Balanced Scorecard to Characterize Benefits of Integration in the Safety Net." *Health Services Management Research* 18:109–123.

Wong, J. G. 1996. "Efficiency and Effectiveness in the Urgent Care Clinic." *Postgrad Medicine* 99, no. 4: 161–166.

Woodburn, J. D., K. L. Smith, and G. D. Nelson. 2007. "Quality of Care in the Retail Health Care Setting Using National Clinical Guidelines for Acute Pharyngitis." *American Journal of Medical Quality* 22, no. 6: 457–462.

Young, T. L., S. L. D'angelo, and J. Davis. 2001. "Impact of a School-Based Health Center on Emergency Department use by Elementary School Students." *Journal of School Health* 71, no. 5: 196–198.

Part II

Safety-Net Hospitals

Safety-Net Hospitals at the Crossroads

Whither Medicaid DSH?

A viable safety net depends heavily on hospitals. In addition to providing inpatient services, their emergency rooms deliver vast amounts of ambulatory care to low-income Americans. Not all hospitals are, of course, equal in this regard. Of the more than 5,700 hospitals in the United States, a much smaller number have been front and center in caring for the disadvantaged. These so-called safety-net hospitals face chronic fiscal stress brought on by serving large numbers of uninsured. Three decades ago, federal policymakers responded to this problem by taking steps to shore up funding for these institutions. Specifically, the Omnibus Budget Reconciliation Act of 1981 authorized state Medicaid programs to take into account the fiscal plight of hospitals that treat greater percentages of low-income individuals who are uninsured or enrolled in Medicaid. The legislation authorized states to provide disproportionate share hospital (DSH) payments to these institutions. Through different mechanisms, Congress also required Medicare to allocate DSH funds.

The landmark health care reform of March 2010 promises to reshape and curtail Medicaid DSH. In crafting the DSH portions of the Patient Protection and Affordable Care Act (ACA), two general perspectives animated federal policymakers. First, they fathomed that the states had historically used DSH as a platform for creative financing schemes to shift costs from themselves to the federal government. A highly technical intergovernmental politics of accounting had grown up around DSH, which left many federal officials with a jaundiced view of state behavior. Second, federal officials reasoned that the expansion of insurance coverage meant that safety-net hospitals would provide less charity care and that DSH would become less central to their fiscal solvency. Hence, the ACA calls for $18 billion in Medicaid DSH cuts through 2020.[1] It also pares Medicare DSH payments by $22 billion.

The ACA left many safety-net hospitals concerned about their future. During the health care debate in 2009, their advocates warned against the cuts in Medicaid DSH that the White House had negotiated with the American Hospital Association. While safety-net providers generally supported health care reform, they feared that reductions in DSH payments would erode their viability. The implications of the DSH modifications for the safety net will largely depend on the politics that unfolds over the next several years. The issue here involves the durability of the health reform legislation. Will the new law unleash positive feedback that entrenches it in the American health insurance regime? Or will subsequent elections and related political eddies create circumstances where federal policymakers repeal or otherwise vitiate it (Patashnik 2008)? If so, will the Medicaid provisions in general and its DSH components in particular survive? Beyond these large political questions, the unfolding story of DSH and the safety net will hinge substantially on the politics of the budgetary process and policy implementation. If safety-net hospitals face mounting fiscal woes, they may well strive to derail the DSH cuts envisioned in the new law. However, any such effort will unfold in a very difficult fiscal environment. With the federal deficit and debt exploding, the call for entitlement reform and further cuts may well gain steam. Beyond the budget process, discretion wielded during implementation by the federal and state governments will markedly shape which safety-net institutions get what, when, and how from DSH and Medicaid more generally. Executive branch politics will be pivotal.

We possess no crystal ball that enables us to predict DSH policy developments. But we can provide the provenance for insight by assessing the evolution of Medicaid DSH policy over nearly three decades as well as the challenges presented by health reform. This chapter opens with a review of DSH's transformation since its birth in 1981. The first decade of the initiative proved pivotal in forging a template for the program that became very difficult to revamp. DSH provides a particularly vivid example of what social scientists call path dependence. The chapter then turns to the issue of targeting—whether DSH monies flow to the most essential safety-net hospitals in greatest fiscal need. It opens by examining the variation in DSH spending among the states; it then considers targeting within their boundaries. We briefly compare the level of targeting achieved by Medicaid DSH to that fostered by Medicare. Having assessed the evolution of Medicaid DSH through the G. W. Bush administration, we turn to developments during the Obama years. Concerns about DSH voiced by key stakeholders in the processes leading to the passage of the ACA come under the microscope, as do pertinent provisions of the new law. We then assess four challenges that Medicaid DSH will pose for federal and state officials as implementation unfolds—challenges related to coverage, provider payment rates, targeting, and information. We conclude by suggesting means for casting additional light on Medicaid's contribution to the safety net.

The Evolution of Medicaid DSH

Medicaid DSH started slowly and after its first four years looked like a potential case of implementation failure. But with federal encouragement states woke up to its fiscal advantages. By the end of the initiative's first decade, many states had become aggressive fiscal entrepreneurs racing to obtain DSH dollars to fund hospitals, related institutions, and other needs. The take-off period also established DSH as a major vehicle for creative financing schemes by the states. Of even greater importance, the initial decade substantially froze in place the winners and losers in the competition for DSH dollars among the states. The program slouched into a pattern of de facto targeting among states that lacked a ready rationale in policy analysis. During the Clinton and G. W. Bush administrations, DSH politics featured a steady stream of intergovernmental sparring. Much of this revolved around federal efforts to clamp down on state efforts to use DSH to boost the federal share of Medicaid costs. But it also involved significant decisions concerning funding levels and related matters.

Take-off: From Indifference to Stampede to Template

Signed into law by President Ronald Reagan in 1981, Medicaid DSH did not immediately prompt aggressive action by the states to attract federal funds to bolster the safety net. It was not until 1985 when the federal bureaucracy promulgated a new rule governing contributions from providers that state interest in DSH intensified. The new rule allowed states to use targeted taxes or donations from providers to count toward their Medicaid match. Medicaid is an open-ended fiscal entitlement with states receiving a certain sum from the national government for every dollar they spend from their own coffers. The federal match depends substantially on a state's per capita income with the national government covering a minimum of 50 percent of a state's Medicaid costs in more affluent jurisdictions; the poorest states typically qualify for a federal match of 75 percent or more. The new administrative ruling provided states with a painless, illusory way to come up with their share of Medicaid funding. Action by West Virginia in 1986 set the pattern. Medicaid officials in that state struck a deal with hospitals to contribute some $22 million to the program. Given the state's low per capita income (and, hence, its higher federal match rate) this donation became officially tabulated as part of the state's expenditures on Medicaid and triggered more than $60 million in federal payments. State Medicaid officials then reimbursed the hospitals for their $22 million in donations. They used the remaining federal dollars, which they had essentially gotten for free, to pay for other Medicaid costs. Officials at the federal Health Care Financing Administration (HCFA) viewed the West Virginia approach as a fiscal gimmick that, left unchecked, would encourage states to skirt Medicaid law and artificially inflate the national government's share of program costs. But when HCFA moved to disallow the donation as an inappropriate interpretation of the 1985 rule, West Virginia officials appealed and prevailed in a federal district court (Thompson 1998, 38).

The West Virginia model rapidly spread to other states. By 1992 thirty-nine states had adopted programs using contributions by providers. Federal law officially specified that the national government would cover 57 percent of Medicaid costs overall, with states paying the rest. By the early 1990s some estimated that state manipulation of provider contributions had pushed the actual federal match rate well beyond 60 percent (Thompson 1998, 38).

The 1980s also witnessed another policy development that heightened state interest in DSH. The federal government had long capped the amount that state Medicaid programs could pay hospitals for certain services (the upper payment limit) at Medicare reimbursement rates.[2] In 1986 Congress approved a measure that appreciably increased what states could funnel to DSH hospitals. This development as well as state fiscal manipulation of provider contributions triggered an explosion in DSH spending. Between 1990 and 1992, federal and state outlays on DSH soared from $1.4 to $17.5 billion (Coughlin and Zuckerman 2003, 154; Frizzera 2009).

By the late 1980s the White House and HCFA committed themselves to staunching the flow of DSH dollars to the states. But slamming the door on creative financing and rapidly rising DSH costs proved far from simple politically. The National Governors Association (NGA), state Medicaid officials, and many safety-net providers stressed that efforts to curb DSH would hurt the poor. Their allies in Congress, which the Democrats controlled, resisted change. Tensions played out in a series of skirmishes between the G.H.W. Bush administration and Congress. HCFA attempted to issue administrative rules that would curtail state discretion to use provider contributions for the federal match. Congress responded by inserting provisions in the budget reconciliation acts of 1989 and then 1990 imposing a one-year moratorium on such rules.

Despite congressional opposition, HCFA issued a rule that broadly restricted state financial maneuvering in October 1991. Congressman Henry Waxman (D-CA) persuaded the House of Representatives to pass another moratorium on this rule through September 1992. By this point the Bush administration and the NGA had reached accord on legislation dealing with the subject. Their agreement broke the logjam, resulting in the passage of the Medicaid Voluntary and Provider-Specific Tax Amendments of 1991 (Thompson 1998, 38–39).

The new legislation contained three particularly important planks. First, with a few exceptions, it eliminated federal matching payments for provider donations. Second, it placed new restrictions on counting provider taxes as part of the state match. These taxes would count only if they were uniform across an entire class of providers (such as acute care hospitals) and did not involve back-door schemes to reimburse the institutions for the full cost of the tax they paid. Moreover, the provider taxes could not exceed 25 percent of a state's contribution to its share of Medicaid costs. Third, the new law signaled a sharp change in the way DSH would be considered within the overarching Medicaid entitlement. In essence, DSH would take on the accoutrements of a block grant. Rather than a function or service (such as outpatient care) with which states could determine how much they wished to spend and expect to receive a federal match, DSH would face a twofold cap. The 1991 law specified that national DSH spending should not exceed 12 percent of overall Medicaid outlays. Congress in this way sought to guard against the program increasingly becoming a vehicle for supporting institutions rather than for insuring low-income individuals. The new law also capped DSH spending by individual states using their federal allocations for fiscal 1992 as a base. This step did much to freeze in place the large variation in DSH spending among states up to that point. With funding no longer open-ended and a state-specific baseline established, low-DSH states that wanted to increase Medicaid funding for safety-net hospitals would face stiffer headwinds. The law galvanized a new process whereby the federal government would periodically publish a state-specific DSH allotment. Beyond that amount, the state would receive no federal match and would have to rely on its own resources to support safety-net hospitals.

DSH's initial decade proved enormously important for future policy developments. The case vividly testifies to the relevance of theories of path dependence and "institutional stickiness" (Pierson 2004). These perspectives emphasize that initial decisions shaping policy and program design often spawn networks and interests that benefit from them. The beneficiaries provide positive feedback and become defenders of the particular program configuration that has emerged. The original design tends to get locked in as the early winners fiercely resist modifications that would impose costs on them. Incremental changes tend to prevail unless highly unusual political circumstances combine to open a policy window for major transformation (Kingdon 1984).

The path DSH took in its first decade established an enduring template with several features. It clarified that DSH spending would not be an open-ended entitlement under Medicaid but would instead be subject to the play of the annual budget process. It made much more difficult any subsequent effort to target DSH funds to states that needed them the most for their safety nets. It also impeded states that had started slowly with respect to DSH from improving their plight. In Medicaid more generally, states with limited programs at one point have vast discretion to grow them over time. Some states have done so, rising from the back of the pack in Medicaid expenditures and enrollments to a position much closer to the front.[3] The 1991 legislation severely dampened prospects for this kind of fluidity in the case of DSH. Finally, the initial decade set the tone for a DSH politics rooted in state fiscal gamesmanship and federal mistrust. The legislative provisions of 1991 did not bring down the curtain on state financing schemes. Many states continued to see DSH as a vehicle through which they could do creative accounting to increase the federal share of Medicaid costs. For their part, federal officials believed that states could not be trusted to refrain from fiscal gimmickry or even to spend DSH funds on institutions that provided charity care. Representative Norman Lent (R-NY) did much to frame the flavor of enduring federal sentiments when in 1992 he likened states pursuing DSH to "embezzlers" illicitly draining the federal treasury (Thompson 1998, 39).

Intergovernmental Sparring Persists Under Clinton and G. W. Bush

The period from 1993 through 2008 witnessed continued intergovernmental jockeying for control over DSH. As Medicaid increasingly strained their budgets, state officials deployed new creative financing techniques to shift the program's costs to the national government. Federal regulators moved to thwart state gambits through new regulation, greater monitoring, and hard-nosed bargaining via the administrative process. In the meantime, a politics of the budgetary process played out that vacillated between cutting and restoring DSH.

Faced with the 1991 federal restrictions on provider donations and taxes, many states turned to another creative financing tool: intergovernmental transfers. The utility of this tool sprang from the fact that in many states public hospitals loomed large in serving Medicaid enrollees and the uninsured. A creative financing scheme typically entailed two steps. First, the state would use its discretion to reimburse public hospitals at the maximum Medicaid rate permitted under federal law (the upper payment limit). This would trigger the release of federal matching funds to the state. Second, the hospital would then retroactively accept reimbursement less than the upper payment limit and transfer funds back to the state. For example, the California Medicaid program paid supplementary amounts to certain county and University of California hospitals that operated emergency rooms and qualified for DSH. The federal government absorbed 50 percent of the cost of this payment. Subsequently, these institutions transferred some of the money back to the state treasury (Coughlin and Zuckerman 2003, 153, 167). By one estimate, by the early 2000s state legerdemain with intergovernmental transfers had raised the federal share of Medicaid costs three percentage points above what the law specified (Coughlin, Bruen, and King 2004).

Federal policymakers responded to state fiscal entrepreneurship in part through additional regulation. In 1993, for instance, Congress limited the amount of DSH funds that a particular hospital could receive to its annual uncompensated care costs for serving the uninsured and Medicaid enrollees. HCFA followed up in 1994 with a letter to state Medicaid directors that defined the method for calculating the hospital-specific DSH limit (Frizzera 2009).

While federal officials repeatedly dispatched missives to state Medicaid administrators on how to manage and account for DSH funds, they lacked the capacity to monitor compliance. In politics and administration, information is a major power resource; federal actors had very little of it in the case of state DSH practices. States had long faced a federal requirement to specify in their formal Medicaid plans the criteria used to designate DSH hospitals and their methods for paying them. But only in 1997 did Congress insist that states submit an annual report to the secretary of health and human services concerning DSH payments to each hospital. Still skeptical about the information many states submitted, Congress upped the ante in 2003, insisting that states submit independently certified audits of their DSH expenditures. The Bush administration formally promulgated additional reporting requirements just before it left office (US HHS 2008).

In addition to these activities, federal officials stepped up investigations of state fiscal practices involving DSH. From 1993 through 2008, the Government Accountability Office (GAO), an analytic arm of Congress, conducted at least fifteen studies of state DSH practices.[4] These studies frequently found states to be out of compliance with federal requirements. A GAO report issued in 2009, for instance, disclosed that 182 Texas hospitals had received more DSH funds than federal law allowed. This mirrored the finding of a federal inspector general in 2006 who had investigated ten states and found that nine of them had not complied with federal requirements concerning hospital-specific DSH limits (Frizzera 2009). Aside from particular findings on compliance, the numerous reports repeatedly decried the "illusory approaches" and "schemes" states employed. One study assessed state use of contingent-fee consultants to maximize federal Medicaid reimbursements (US GAO 2005). These investigations reflected and fueled the politics of intergovernmental mistrust around DSH and reinforced the framing of states as embezzlers.

In the 2000s the federal executive branch became more assertive in the sparring over DSH. The Centers for Medicare & Medicaid Services (CMS, formerly HCFA) opened up two new fronts in the struggle to fend off state fiscal maneuvers—one involving state plan amendments and the other, demonstration waivers. To participate in Medicaid, states must submit and obtain approval of a plan. Once in place, states frequently amend the document. In a given year, federal administrators typically receive hundreds of state amendments concerning such matters as Medicaid eligibility, payment practices, and service coverage. So long as the requested changes conform to Medicaid law, federal administrators routinely approve them. In 2003, however, the Bush administration decided to use this amendment process as a springboard for aggressive negotiations with the states over Medicaid financing. In August of that year, CMS told the states that any request to amend provider payment practices would trigger a more general analysis of their funding arrangements with respect to DSH and related matters. This posture sparked considerable intergovernmental bargaining. While the fiscal implications of CMS's assertive posture for DSH and Medicaid more generally remain unclear, twenty-nine states over a three-year period terminated financing practices that CMS deemed inappropriate (US GAO 2007, 5).

Negotiations of this kind also came to the fore with respect to state demonstration waivers authorized under Section 1115 of the Social Security Act. The 1990s had featured an unprecedented outpouring of these waivers as the Clinton administration embraced state requests to reinvent their Medicaid programs through managed care, coverage expansions, and other steps (Thompson and Burke 2007). Medicaid expenditures through waivers, rather than ordinary statutory channels, grew dramatically. As the demonstrations came up for renewal and as states proposed new waivers in the 2000s, the Bush administration often pushed them to trade Medicaid coverage expansions for a reduction in DSH. In 2005 Massachusetts became the poster child for this approach when it attempted to renew a comprehensive waiver launched during the Clinton years. CMS indicated it would not approve an extension unless the state ceased to use certain provider funding sources as part of its Medicaid match (Thompson and Burke 2007, 989). The resulting negotiation between federal and Massachusetts officials helped spur a comprehensive reform in the state that dramatically slimmed the ranks of the uninsured. To secure federal approval of the Medicaid waiver that undergirded the reform, Massachusetts virtually eliminated DSH payments to hospitals.

Trends in DSH Funding

While the federal government strove to curtail creative accounting by the states, the politics of the budgetary process yielded ebbs and flows for DSH. At times Congress wielded the budget knife. In 1997 it approved legislation that pared DSH allotments between 1998 and 2002. But resistance from the intergovernmental lobby and safety-net hospitals at times prompted Congress to reopen the federal purse. In 2000 new legislation postponed the DSH cuts slated for 2001 and 2002; in 2003 a Republican Congress approved a 16 percent increase in DSH funding and pledged to link future increases in DSH to the Consumer Price Index starting in 2010 (New Jersey Commission 2008, 111). The intergovernmental back-and-forth on DSH reflects an inherent political tension. On the one hand, federal policymakers want to close DSH loopholes and control funding in the interest of fiscal integrity and prudence. But mistrust of state financing schemes does not invariably trump the interest of congressional delegations in responding to requests from home-state governors and advocates for safety-net hospitals to support DSH.

However, any vacillation in the national government's orientation toward DSH should not obscure its diminishing role in Medicaid. Table 7.1 presents trends in DSH spending in constant dollars for the period from 1992 through

Table 7.1   **Trends in DSH Spending, 1992–2008 (2008 dollars)**

	DSH spending	DSH $ per poor person	DSH $ per uninsured person	DSH as a share of Medicaid expenditures (%)
1992	$27,093,253,862	$712.72	$701.15	11.4
2000	$19,544,687,035	$618.87	$505.25	7.9
2008	$17,738,530,492	$445.37	$382.79	5.2

Sources: Expenditure data are from Kaiser Commission on Medicaid and the Uninsured and Urban Institute Analysis of HCFA/CMS-64 data, 1992–2000; and from Kaiser State Health Facts, "Distribution of Medicaid Spending by Service, FY 2008," http://www.statehealthfacts.org/comparetable.jsp?typ=4&ind=178&cat=4&sub=47. Other data are based on the Bureau of Labor Statistics CPI calculator and the Current Population Survey.

2008 and as a share of overall Medicaid outlays.[5] The table also conveys trends in expenditures relative to those in poverty and the uninsured. Table 7.1 indicates that DSH spending from 1992 through 2008 declined by about 35 percent in constant dollars. As a share of all federal and state Medicaid expenditures, the drop was even more dramatic—from 11 percent in 1992 to 5 percent in 2008. DSH spending relative to the two measures of need—persons in poverty and uninsured—also fell. Expenditures per uninsured person evinced a particularly steep decline—nearly 50 percent. With slight variations, DSH funding to hospitals ebbed during both the Clinton and G. W. Bush administrations.

The Perils of Targeting

Data on aggregate expenditure trends with respect to DSH raise the issue of targeting. Do DSH monies overwhelmingly flow to states and institutions where in some sense they do the most good? Any attempt to answer this question quickly encounters a dense normative thicket. Informed observers can appropriately bring different values and preferences to the issue yielding diverse concepts of targeting. Indeed, there are several defensible versions of targeting in the context of American federalism (Stone 1988; Nathan 1993; Rich and White 1997). Need comprises one common criterion. This perspective holds that states with less wealth and greater proportions of poor residents should attract more federal funds per capita. Effort emerges as a second major criterion. According to this principle, states more willing to spend their own monies to bolster the safety net should attract more federal funds, adjusted for need (Gusmano and Schlesinger 2001, 49).

Along with establishing criteria for allocating DSH funds among states, targeting necessitates appropriate allocation of these monies within states. Need appears to be the most commonly accepted criterion for doing so. Defining and calibrating need within states presents many complexities.[6] For present purposes, however, we believe that targeting based on need is better achieved if states direct most of their DSH outlays to the most essential and fiscally dependent safety-net hospitals. By essential we mean those hospitals that play a major role in providing uncompensated care to the uninsured, Medicaid enrollees, and other disadvantaged people.[7] The concept implies that the elimination or major downsizing of an institution would in all likelihood severely threaten the access of the disadvantaged to quality care. By fiscally dependent, we mean those hospitals that achieve reasonable standards of efficiency and lack alternative sources of revenue to sustain their role in the safety net in the absence of Medicaid DSH. Given these criteria, the evidence suggests serious limitations to DSH targeting.

The Limits to Targeting among the States

As noted previously, the politics of the policy process had precipitated substantial disparities in DSH funding among the states by the time President Clinton took office. Table 7.2 fast-forwards to 2008 to capture important dimensions of this variation among states by placing them in quartiles based on DSH spending per poor person. The table also presents state-specific DSH expenditures per uninsured resident and the degree of change on each of the two metrics in constant dollars since 1992.

Two primary conclusions emerge from table 7.2. First, states vary greatly in their DSH expenditures. Six states spent well over $1,000 per poor person via DSH, with New Hampshire leading the way at $2,500. Five states surpassed $1,000 in outlays per uninsured person. In contrast, half the states (clustered in the moderately low–and low-DSH categories) spent less than $300 per poor person and per uninsured individual. DSH played a large role in a minority of states as a comparison of mean state effort for each quartile vividly illustrates. The mean of state DSH spending per poor person in the top group amounted to $1,140—more than three times the figure for the second quartile and well over ten times the amount for the bottom cohort. DSH outlays relative to the uninsured point to a similar pattern. In 2008 the top cluster of states averaged more than $1,000 in DSH spending per uninsured resident, well over three times the mean for states in the second quartile.

Second, state-specific data generally mirror the national trend toward a decline in DSH outlays and indicate that most of the early leaders sustained their relative advantage over other states. Thirty states moved downward on the poverty-related measure and thirty-two on the uninsured indicator from 1992 through 2008. States with increases tended to be in the third and fourth quartiles. Because these states started from such a minimal base in 1992, small increases in the two DSH expenditure measures show up as large percentage gains. These gains were not, however, sufficient to extricate themselves from their low rankings by 2008.

The trend data indicate that most states that had become DSH leaders in 1992 retained their positions. To be sure, all but four jurisdictions in the top quartile declined in DSH expenditures per poor person and all but three on the uninsured metric. Despite this erosion, they tended to preserve their high ranking. Seven of the twelve leaders in 2008 were also in the top quartile in 1992 (Connecticut, Louisiana, Missouri, New Hampshire, New Jersey, New York, and Rhode Island). In contrast five states fell from the top quartile between 1992 and 2008. Three (Maine, Michigan, and Pennsylvania) experienced relatively gradual declines to the second quartile while one (Kansas) dropped to

Table 7.2   Change in DSH Expenditures by State, 1992–2008

State	DSH expenditure per poor person 2008 ($)	% change 1992 to 2008 (based on 2008 $)	DSH expenditure per uninsured person 2008 ($)	% change 1992 to 2008 (based on 2008 $)
High DSH Effort				
Group Average	*1,139.62*		*1,058.17*	
New Hampshire	2,451.78	−60.3	1,677.53	−60.6
New Jersey	1,939.86	−6.9	1,271.17	−21.4
Rhode Island	1,727.76	65.4	1,854.18	35.7
Louisiana	1,224.94	−31.4	1,110.76	−43.4
New York	1,101.18	−34.9	1,106.85	−42.0
Connecticut	1,019.05	−45.9	819.99	−63.4
Missouri	858.69	−39.0	906.33	−41.1
District of Columbia	709.80	69.2	1,179.00	199.8
South Carolina	708.35	−26.6	625.19	−41.3
Vermont	657.90	13.6	634.81	−1.2
Indiana	641.55	31.0	748.75	42.9
Alabama	634.57	−27.6	763.52	−15.1
Moderately High DSH Effort				
Group Average	*372.58*		*335.20*	
Pennsylvania	597.58	−42.5	658.77	−53.6
Washington	479.88	−22.0	403.86	−39.1
Ohio	410.60	−17.0	488.39	−12.8
California	405.35	−37.2	317.53	−39.9
Michigan	381.92	−41.7	422.40	−52.6
Texas	380.49	−46.1	239.78	−57.1
Mississippi	371.76	6.3	376.06	−15.2
North Carolina	324.47	−31.1	293.42	−45.3
Maine	318.38	−75.0	367.18	−76.2
Colorado	306.28	−75.2	212.43	−79.8
Nevada	297.69	−47.4	169.93	−52.9
Wisconsin	285.85	1104.9	290.66	917.4
Alaska	283.29	0 in '92	117.15	0 in '92
Moderately Low DSH Effort				
Group Average	*218.72*		*207.85*	
West Virginia	279.47	−13.3	268.13	−42.5
Minnesota	275.29	140.3	313.73	70.9

(*Continued*)

Table 7.2   Change in DSH Expenditures by State, 1992–2008 (*Continued*)

State	DSH expenditure per poor person 2008 ($)	% change 1992 to 2008 (based on 2008 $)	DSH expenditure per uninsured person 2008 ($)	% change 1992 to 2008 (based on 2008 $)
Georgia	271.41	−30.5	235.39	−34.5
Kentucky	270.33	−51.1	286.98	−61.4
Hawaii	247.79	−46.6	316.06	−63.1
Kansas	233.47	−77.5	244.79	−76.8
Maryland	230.43	−22.3	165.68	−46.4
Virginia	216.64	−43.3	179.93	−27.4
Oregon	180.26	135.5	116.98	82.0
Tennessee	179.03	−76.7	177.69	−81.5
Iowa	176.88	718.5	178.13	638.8
Nebraska	142.55	406.6	127.01	303.3
Florida	139.86	2.2	91.59	−15.0
Low DSH Effort				
Group Average	*67.26*		*56.97*	
Illinois	124.20	−52.0	118.59	−61.2
Montana	123.77	7299.6	97.92	3918.5
Idaho	119.78	821.7	93.90	687.8
Arkansas	107.07	1084.7	91.38	1054.5
Oklahoma	104.47	85.5	101.54	114.2
Arizona	98.46	0 in '92	90.65	0 in '92
Utah	97.15	140.6	55.78	74.3
Delaware	68.64	0 in '92	59.87	0 in '92
North Dakota	16.61	7931.6	16.61	5435.3
South Dakota	13.23	1850.1	13.76	1966.3
Wyoming	2.39	−12.9	1.80	−25.3
Massachusetts	0.00	−100.0	0.00	−100.0
New Mexico	−1.38	−102.7	−1.13	−102.0
Total	445.37	−37.5	382.79	−45.4

Sources: Expenditure data are from Kaiser Commission on Medicaid and the Uninsured and Urban Institute Analysis of HCFA/CMS-64 data, 1992–2000; and from Kaiser State Health Facts, "Distribution of Medicaid Spending by Service, FY 2008," http://www.statehealthfacts.org/comparetable.jsp?typ=4&ind=178&cat=4&sub=47. Other data are based on the Bureau of Labor Statistics CPI calculator and the Current Population Survey.

Note: The percentage change controls for inflation. The 1992 and 2008 figures are in constant 2008 dollars.

the third cluster. Only Massachusetts plunged to the bottom quartile. As described earlier, Massachusetts officials agreed to give up all DSH monies in exchange for federal permission to use Medicaid funds to subsidize a major coverage expansion. Overall, a modest reduction in variation among the states occurred from 1992 through 2008. The coefficient of variation on DSH spending per poor person declined from 1.45 to 1.13; the comparable coefficient for the uninsured measure ebbed from 1.17 to 1.06. Still, the top quartile of jurisdictions in table 7.2 spent 48 percent of all DSH dollars in 2008, only slightly less than the 51 percent this quartile consumed in 1992.

To cast light on issues of targeting, table 7.3 compares the quartiles on certain indicators. To the degree that states in the higher quartiles of DSH effort are less affluent and have higher proportions of uninsured and poor people, the case for targeting based on need improves.[8] The data in table 7.3, however, do not reveal such a pattern. Modest differences exist among the different quartiles of states. In general, high-DSH states tend to have slightly lower proportions of poor and uninsured people within their boundaries. These states tend to be above average in per capita income and total taxable resources. In sum, one cannot explain the enormous variation in DSH effort among states by claiming that federal principles allocate monies to states in greatest need.

Targeting within States

While targeting among states appears limited, the question remains: once states receive a DSH allotment, do they direct these funds to the most essential,

Table 7.3   **Selected Characteristics of States by Quartile of DSH Spending per Person in Poverty, 2008**

	Q-1 High effort	Q-2 Moderately high effort	Q-3 Moderately low effort	Q-4 Low effort	National average
Mean state in poverty (%)	12.6	12.5	12.1	12.9	13.2
Mean state uninsured (%)	12.7	15.2	13.4	14.4	15.4
Mean state per capita income ($)	43,877	39,085	39,103	38,833	40,673
Mean state total taxable resources* ($)	58,948	52,190	51,771	55,949	54,757

Sources: Data are from the US Census Bureau, the Current Population Survey, the US Department of Commerce, Bureau of Economic Analysis, Regional Economic Accounts, the US Department of the Treasury, and the Bureau of Labor Statistics.

*2007 data in 2008 dollars

fiscally dependent safety-net institutions? Unfortunately, available data do not permit a definitive answer. Federal law, regulations, and other actions do not ensure that states will engage in finely honed targeting. Federal regulations generally require that hospitals with heavy volumes of Medicaid and charity patients are eligible for DSH. They also insist that, minimally, at least one percent of a DSH hospital's total inpatient days be attributable to Medicaid patients and that the institution have at least two obstetricians with staff privileges willing to serve Medicaid enrollees (New Jersey Commission 2008, 110). But these requirements leave state officials vast discretion to apportion DSH funds among hospitals. Targeting at times receives short shrift. State policymakers typically face substantial political pressures to spread DSH payments around to all hospitals even if some do not serve many uninsured individuals and Medicaid enrollees. Moreover, the creative financing schemes of some states mean that significant amounts of DSH monies failed to flow to safety-net hospitals. Instead, states used the federal funds they generated to subsidize other Medicaid services or simply to replenish the state treasury (Coughlin and Zuckerman 2003, 154, 158). As noted earlier, the federal government launched a belated effort to follow the DSH money trail in the 2000s through new reporting and auditing requirements. But a lack of transparency continues to shroud the DSH program and complicate efforts to gauge targeting.

States differ considerably in the ways they allocate DSH to particular hospitals. Consider, for instance, two states in the top quartile on DSH effort—Louisiana and New Jersey (see table 7.2). Both states experience substantial demand for charity care. Louisiana has one of the higher poverty rates in the country, at 22 percent; 18 percent of its populace lacks health insurance, above the national mean of 16 percent.[9] The core of Louisiana's safety net consists of ten public charity hospitals located across the state and operated by Louisiana State University. Discharge data from seven of these hospitals help illuminate their role. The proportion of patients without insurance who received treatment at each of these seven facilities ranged from 27 to 60 percent. The proportion discharged who were either uninsured or on Medicaid varied from 56 to 83 percent; this share amounted to more than 70 percent in six of the charity hospitals (Zaman, Cummings, and Spieler 2010, 24). To support these institutions, Louisiana has aggressively pursued DSH monies from the outset. Data on the fiscal solvency of these institutions are not readily available, but state officials believe that certain of these hospitals could not continue to operate in the absence of significant DSH payments (Robertson 2009).

In contrast to Louisiana, New Jersey primarily relies on private nonprofit hospitals to serve Medicaid enrollees and the uninsured. New Jersey is more affluent than Louisiana with a per capita income near the top of all states and a poverty rate of just over 10 percent. In terms of health insurance, the state does slightly better than the national mean, with those lacking coverage at 15 percent. Like Louisiana, New Jersey attracts considerable DSH dollars. New Jersey hospitals obtain DSH funding by submitting claims to the Medicaid fiscal agent in the state for the uninsured patients they treat. This agent "prices" charity care claims at Medicaid fee-for-service inpatient and outpatient rates. State officials then use this information in combination with a statutory formula to distribute DSH subsidies to hospitals. While the formula funnels appreciable monies to institutions that provide substantial charity care (DeLia 2007), it has drawn criticism for failing to do more to target safety-net hospitals. In this regard, a state commission chaired by health economist Uwe Reinhardt of Princeton University concluded that the formula had "interfered with a rational disbursement of funds" to "essential" hospitals that "serve a high fraction of individuals from vulnerable populations" (DeLia 2007, 36; New Jersey Commission 2008, 111–112). The commission noted that DSH subsidies often went to hospitals that did not need them to remain financially viable. Furthermore, the allocation methodology encouraged hospitals to devote more effort to documenting charity care rather than promoting public insurance enrollment through enhanced take-up efforts (New Jersey Commission 2008, 114).

The uncertainties about and limits to targeting discussed in this section should not obscure that great numbers of essential, fiscally stressed safety-net institutions receive substantial DSH funds and other Medicaid payments. Data collected by the National Association of Public Hospitals and Health Systems (NAPH) cast light on Medicaid's importance. NAPH members include some 115 public hospitals located in twenty-nine states and the District of Columbia. While not perfectly representative of safety-net hospitals, they encompass many large facilities in major urban areas serving ethnically diverse population, many of which are academic medical centers. A NAPH survey conducted in 2008 captured the extent to which their members disproportionately serve Medicaid enrollees and the uninsured. These two categories of patients accounted for more than half of all discharges in more than 60 percent of NAPH hospitals. Thirty-three percent of net revenues for these hospitals came from Medicaid, a figure that greatly exceeds that for hospitals in general. About one in five NAPH hospitals relies on Medicaid for more than 50 percent of net revenues, with the North Central Bronx Hospital in New York City leading the way at 80 percent. NAPH estimates that Medicaid DSH alone financed nearly 20 percent of the uncompensated care its members delivered (Zaman, Cummings, and Spieler 2010, xi, 24–25, 32–33). While data on the financial health of NAPH hospitals are not readily available, the association's president claims that without supplemental Medicaid and Medicare payments such as DSH, "most NAPH members would have been bankrupt years ago" (Zaman, Cummings, and Spieler 2010, ix).

Medicare DSH: Superior at Targeting?

While this chapter focuses on Medicaid, it deserves note that Medicare has also funneled substantial DSH funds to hospitals—a little over $10 billion in 2008 (US MedPAC 2010, 85). When policymakers created a new prospective payment system for Medicare in the 1980s, they worried that it would not adequately compensate hospitals that treated greater shares of low-income patients. In addition to having higher rates of uninsurance, this cohort might experience more acute, costly illnesses. The fact that Medicare also provides DSH payments to hospitals naturally raises the question of whether it has been more successful than Medicaid in targeting these monies to the most essential, fiscally dependent hospitals. If so, this would suggest that the dynamics of federalism make targeting particularly difficult in intergovernmental grant programs such as Medicaid. It would point to the possible superiority of a centrally administered federal program for funding the safety net.

Readily available data do not permit a precise comparison of targeting under Medicaid and Medicare DSH. But studies suggest that Medicare fares no better than Medicaid in this sphere. Medicare disburses DSH payments through a formula that alters the program's payment rates to reflect the degree to which the hospital serves low-income patients, adjusting for location and size. Officials calculate low-income patients by adding two ratios: (1) total Medicaid patient days as a percentage of all patient days, and (2) patient days for Medicare beneficiaries who receive Supplemental Security Income as a proportion of total Medicare patient days. Despite the use of this formula, many experts (such as Gusmano and Schlesinger 2001) believe that Medicare DSH fails to flow to hospitals in greatest need. In 2007 the US Medicare Payment Advisory Commission, an entity established by Congress to monitor and assess the program, found "little evidence of a relationship between the DSH payments hospitals receive and the amount of uncompensated care they provide" (50).

Like Medicaid DSH, Medicare allocations to the safety net have prompted skepticism among national policymakers. One study of Medicare's "collateral benefits" found that its failure to target funds effectively undermined its political support, especially among moderates and conservatives. As one observer put it, "The general perception on the Hill is that this has been a scam and a rip-off" (Gusmano and Schlesinger 2001, 54). Many saw the program as unjustified federal "pork" that flowed disproportionately to urban hospitals in districts represented by liberals (51–53). Given these sentiments, it is hardly surprising that the ACA not only cut Medicare DSH by 75 percent but also sought to promote better targeting of these funds.[10] It remains to be seen whether this will occur. At least for the present, Medicare's experience suggests that Medicaid's problems of targeting DSH funds do not simply flow from the dynamics of federalism. Instead, the DSH experience testifies to the general difficulty of achieving target efficiency within the American political system whether in programs administered by the national government or by the states.

DSH and Health Care Reform

The passage of the ACA modifies the playing field for Medicaid DSH. The debate leading to health reform's passage anticipated many of the challenges that DSH would face over the next decade.[11] The Obama administration and most members of Congress assumed that expanding insurance coverage to millions of Americans would reduce, if not eliminate, the need for Medicaid and Medicare DSH. In his radio address on June 13, 2009, President Obama asserted that health reform would yield a set of "common sense" changes, including reductions in DSH. As he explained, "If more Americans are insured, we can cut payments that help hospitals treat patients without health insurance" (Obama 2009). Similarly, during the Senate Finance Committee's markup of the health reform bill in September 2009, Senator Kent Conrad (D-ND) noted, "The reason we're able to make reductions in DSH payments is because there's going to be less uncompensated care. . . . When you cover 30 million more people with insurance there are then going to be much lower numbers for uncompensated care" (US Senate Finance Committee 2009a, 21).

This view did not go uncontested, however. Opponents of paring DSH raised four concerns. First, they pointed out that even with full implementation of the new law, groups such as the homeless and undocumented immigrants would continue to need free services from safety-net hospitals. Experts, such as John Sheils of the Lewin Group, testified that safety-net hospitals would face fiscal stress not only because these cohorts lacked insurance but also because many of them need special, costly care.[12] Sen. Jon Kyl (R-AZ) underscored that his state had a large immigrant populations and that DSH cuts would harm its safety net (US Senate Finance Committee 2009b, 386).

Second, opponents of cuts noted the role that Medicaid and Medicare DSH played in compensating hospitals for the higher costs associated with treating publicly insured patients and for inadequate Medicaid reimbursement rates. As Rep. Carolyn Maloney (D-NY) observed, "Historically, Medicaid hospital reimbursement rates, on average have been lower than the cost of providing care, and DSH payments were instituted to cover reimbursement shortfalls and uncompensated care costs. The need for DSH reimbursement will remain even after health care reform is passed since there will be millions of newly eligible individuals who will receive care through Medicaid" (US House of Representatives 2010, 567).

Third, several advocates and members of Congress expressed concern that retrenching DSH would harm rural hospitals. For instance, Charles N. Kahn III, the leader of the Federation of American Hospitals, claimed that "the statutory formula for determining DSH payments to hospitals provides lower payment to rural hospitals treating the same proportion of indigent patients than it does for larger urban hospitals." Rather than cutting DSH, Kahn favored payment equity for rural hospitals.[13] In a similar vein, Sen. Orrin Hatch (R-UT) observed that "caring for the uninsured creates a heavier burden on Utah hospitals because the state's DSH payment is so low. . . . Rural America is both poorer than urban America" and its residents "more likely due to employment conditions to lack health coverage. They are on the whole older. . . . Meanwhile, the rural hospitals that serve these communities are already struggling to survive" (US Senate Finance Committee 2009a, 376–378).

Finally, several advocates argued that the Massachusetts health reform provided a cautionary tale for those seeking to trim Medicaid DSH. Celia Wcislo of the Service Employees International Union testified: "In Massachusetts, the use of Medicaid Disproportionate Share funding to pay for coverage expansion has meant a dramatic cut" in payments to hospitals "that is devastating for the safety-net delivery system."[14] Patricia Gabow, the chief executive officer of the Denver Health and Hospital Authority and a leader in NAPH, voiced a similar claim. She argued that "the ongoing need for DSH support is well illustrated by Massachusetts' experience. Massachusetts paid for its coverage expansion with DSH dollars, assuming that hospitals would recover their costs with the new coverage options. Had payments for the newly-insured been adequate, this assumption may have proven true." But "safety-net hospitals in Massachusetts suddenly faced significant losses, and the state has been forced to use its economic stimulus dollars to make sure that [they] remain viable." Gabow argued for restructuring DSH payments "only after hospital losses on both the uninsured and Medicaid populations are substantially reduced."[15]

These and related concerns prompted NAPH, as a leading advocate for safety-net hospitals, to express strong reservations to Congress about the DSH provisions under consideration. NAPH leaders complained that they had been left out of negotiations between the American Hospital Association and the White House over the DSH cuts (Beaty 2009). While NAPH supported the ACA, it strongly preferred the House version rather than the Senate version of reform. The House bill called for a $10 billion cut in DSH over ten years, with most of the reductions occurring in 2019. In contrast, the Senate bill called for steeper declines that would begin sooner (Kaiser Family Foundation 2010, 26). Ultimately, NAPH persuaded 13 senators and 105 representatives to support the House version.

The final legislation reflected a compromise between the two houses of Congress. The total DSH reductions mirrored the Senate proposal but reflected House preferences for phasing them in at a slower pace. The ACA calls for saving $18 billion in Medicaid DSH through 2020, roughly a 20 percent cut.[16] Annual cuts will start with a modest half-billion-dollar reduction in 2014 and surge to $5.6 billion in 2019. The new law also signals that Medicaid DSH should undergo appreciable revision. It requires the secretary of health and human services to develop a methodology to allot DSH reductions among states.[17] It instructs the secretary to impose larger cuts on high-DSH states with lower percentages of uninsured people. The law also allows the secretary to impose greater reductions on states that have failed to target DSH payments to appropriate institutions (Kaiser Family Foundation 2010, 26). While providing some guidance, the ACA delegates vast authority to the federal executive branch and the states to determine who will get what DSH subsidies from Medicaid. In addition to retrenching Medicaid DSH, it pledges to pare spending on Medicare DSH by $22 billion, or about 75 percent, with the subsequent possibility of some restoration based on the numbers of uninsured and the amount of uncompensated care (US CBO 2010).

Key Challenges

The history of Medicaid DSH prior to the Obama administration and the concerns expressed during congressional deliberations leading to the ACA suggest that national and state stakeholders will face myriad challenges going forward. How they deal with them has significant implications for the safety net. Four challenges loom particularly large: (1) coverage—the proportion of uninsured who qualify for Medicaid and actually enroll; (2) payment—whether Medicaid reimbursement rates to hospitals decline, increase, or continue at current levels; (3) targeting—whether Medicaid manages to spend a higher proportion of DSH dollars on the most essential and fiscally dependent safety-net hospitals; and (4) information—whether the national government can monitor state DSH practices not only to curtail fiscal gimmicks but also to fathom better the specific providers that benefit.

The Coverage Challenge

In the debate leading to passage of the ACA, safety-net advocates warned that many people would remain uninsured. To the degree that the proportion of US residents who are here illegally grows, this problem will increase. Stress for safety-net hospitals will also tend to be more acute in states with larger percentages of undocumented residents. The ranks of the uninsured also seem sure to grow if the Republican majority elected to the House of Representatives in 2010 succeeds in delaying or vitiating the ACA.

Beyond these factors, take-up issues for those entitled to coverage under the ACA are very much in play. The law's requirement that individuals obtain insurance does not ensure compliance. To be sure, the Massachusetts experience suggests that the great majority of the uninsured will seek coverage. But state cultures and other characteristics vary widely. One cannot assume that Texas will mimic Massachusetts in response to the individual mandate. It deserves note that the large majority of those who could gain coverage from Medicaid will be exempt from penalties for failure to comply (Holahan and Headen 2010, 5). With respect to the state exchanges created by the new law, some individuals may calculate that their out-of-pocket costs for obtaining insurance are sufficiently high to justify remaining uncovered and paying a penalty. Probably more important, however, the fragmented enrollment structures of Medicaid interact with fluctuating enrollee incomes to create a take-up challenge. About half of the uninsured targeted for coverage under the ACA are adults with incomes up to 133 percent of poverty. As their incomes ebb and flow, people will be eligible for Medicaid at one point and the insurance exchanges (or other insurers) at another. States will need to display uncommon administrative acumen to avoid a churning of the rolls with individuals enduring spells of being uninsured as they transition from one source of coverage to the next. Many hospitals will have to endure the expense of having staff assigned to facilitate the enrollment of uninsured people when they show up on their doorsteps.

The Payment Challenge

The ACA does not explicitly deal with the Achilles' heel of Medicaid—the program's propensity in most states to reimburse providers at rates below Medicare and commercial insurers. To be sure, the new law requires states in 2013 and 2014 to establish payment rates for certain primary care doctors (those practicing family medicine, pediatrics, or general internal medicine) that achieve parity with Medicare rates. The federal government will absorb 100 percent of the added costs for these two years. This step may enhance the access of Medicaid enrollees to broader networks of primacy care providers over the short term and temporarily reduce their dependence on safety-net institutions.[18] But previous attempts to "mainstream" access to physicians for Medicaid enrollees suggest that safety-net institutions will continue to play a vital role (Grogan and Gusmano 2007). The ACA recognizes this likelihood by preserving the more generous Medicaid payment rates long mandated for federally qualified health centers. These centers have been pivotal in providing care to Medicaid enrollees and the uninsured. Still, the new law leaves open questions of Medicaid payments to hospitals and many other providers.

For two decades following its enactment in 1965, Medicaid reimbursed hospitals for their "reasonable costs" of serving enrollees—typically 95 percent of the Medicare rate. Increasingly, however, the devolution of authority over payment rates to the states and the rise of managed care altered this approach. The exact payment rates to hospitals have become more difficult to track as the great majority of nondisabled Medicaid enrollees under age sixty-five obtain coverage through managed care organizations. Some believe that these organizations have been aggressive and skillful in negotiating lower Medicaid payment to hospitals. But one cannot be sure because transparency concerning hospital reimbursement has declined since managed care plans often view the information as proprietary. Some evidence suggests, however, that Medicaid pays public safety-net hospitals less than 75 percent of what Medicare does (Zaman, Cummings, and Spieler 2010, 13–14). Some observers discount hospitals' claims about the inadequacy of Medicaid payments on grounds that these institutions are inefficient and could reduce expenses without compromising quality (Klein 2009). While this criticism contains a substantial germ of truth, it would be Panglossian to see efficiency gains as the antidote to low Medicaid payment rates. Hospital administrators cannot easily control many factors that boost costs, such as treatment norms that prevail among its affiliated physicians. Moreover, changes in medical technology and patient preferences along with the entrepreneurial quest by some physicians to maximize their incomes have often galvanized movement of more profitable procedures from hospitals to outside clinics and other ambulatory care centers (Berliner 2008; New Jersey Commission 2008). For example, between 2001 and 2003 the total number of cataract removals, colonoscopies, and arthroscopic knee surgeries performed in an outpatient setting in one large New York managed care plan increased by 15 percent while the number in hospitals declined by

24 percent (Berliner 2008). To the extent that hospitals lose more profitable procedures to ambulatory settings, their fiscal stress could well increase.

Hence, the politics of Medicaid payment in the states will shape whether DSH cuts threaten the hospital safety net. This politics will play out in annual struggles over state budgets. The extent to which safety-net institutions can forge potent coalitions to bolster Medicaid payment will be pivotal. Court action may also figure prominently in the struggle. Federal court decisions in the 2000s made it increasingly difficult for Medicaid providers and beneficiaries to sue successfully on grounds that the states had violated their rights under Medicaid law. But in 2008 and 2009 California providers persuaded the federal court of appeals in the Ninth Circuit to overturn that state's reductions in Medicaid reimbursement.[19] State officials reacted to this setback by mobilizing to protect their prerogatives to determine Medicaid payment rates and other program features. In 2010 the National Association of State Medicaid Directors sent a letter to federal Solicitor General Elena Kagan claiming that the California appellate court rulings would open the floodgates to other litigation. Twenty-two states filed a brief with the Supreme Court to hear California's appeal of the circuit court's decisions. Among other things, these officials sought to buttress the principle that state Medicaid programs cannot be sued in federal court over program cuts (Rosenbaum 2009; Baker 2010). The Supreme Court agreed to take the case and heard arguments in the fall 2011.

The Targeting Challenge

The ACA took modest steps to foster greater targeting of Medicaid DSH funds. The law primarily focused on the great imbalance among states. As noted earlier, DSH monies overwhelmingly flow to about ten high-DSH states. The ACA grants the secretary of health and human services considerable authority to apportion cuts among states but specifies that, all else equal, high-DSH jurisdictions should experience greater reductions. In considering this prospect, it deserves note that states with robust DSH programs have little to fear from the new health reform law over the short term. Major DSH cuts do not occur until late in the current decade. In theory, the federal executive branch could use its ample discretion under the ACA to unleash a bold offensive to reallocate and target DSH monies. But this would be difficult politically. The current cluster of high-DSH states includes highly populated ones from politically conservative and liberal areas of the country. With a considerable amount to lose, high-DSH states will tend to fight any executive initiative to cut their funds sharply. In turn, states that would benefit from redistribution may not gain enough new DSH funding to motivate them to wage a strong political battle on behalf of reallocation. The dwindling pool of DSH funds may well reinforce this proclivity.

The ACA recognizes that simply taking more money from high-DSH states will not facilitate greater targeting. It envisions lower cuts for states that continue to have higher proportions of uninsured people. It also affords the secretary of health and human services some discretion to pare DSH monies to states that do not "appropriately" target their allocations to the safety net. Taking into account the number of uninsured may well help states with high proportions of undocumented immigrants. Somewhat ironically, it also will reward poorly performing states—those with less will or capacity to achieve robust take-up rates for those who could qualify for Medicaid or other coverage. Efforts to boost the relative share of DSH going to states with more uninsured people may facilitate better targeting. But factors could intervene to thwart this outcome. If, for instance, states trim the ranks of the uninsured but also adopt penurious Medicaid payment rates, the fiscal stress of their safety-net hospitals may well increase. After all, uncompensated care derives substantially from both the number of uninsured patients and from Medicaid payments that fail to cover the cost of care. Also, reallocating DSH funds among states does not ensure that state Medicaid programs will channel the monies they receive to the most essential and fiscally dependent safety-net hospitals. The degree to which the national government will attempt to establish new criteria and regulations to shape within-state allocation decisions remains to be seen. Any such effort would probably spark resistance by the intergovernmental lobby, especially the National Governors Association.

The Information Challenge

Over DSH's three decades of existence, the federal government has slowly and incrementally moved to obtain more information about state DSH practices. It took seventeen years before Congress finally required states to submit annual reports that indicate which hospitals received DSH funds. By 2003 the level of mistrust in these reports reached a point that Congress required independently certified audits of state DSH expenditures. Investigations by GAO and other oversight agencies during the 2000s continued to raise questions about how states distribute DSH. The G. W. Bush administration was so skeptical about DSH that it worked through the waiver process to divert DSH dollars to coverage expansions.

Two concerns could animate federal efforts to reduce information asymmetry surrounding DSH. First, federal officials generally want to root out state fiscal gimmicks that increase the national government's share of program costs.

On balance, they have made some progress in this regard, though the ability of state administrators to exploit intergovernmental transfers to hike the federal match rate should not be ignored. Second, federal actors have sporadically evinced interest in whether DSH monies actually flow to institutions that provide the most uncompensated care. The ACA reinforces this thrust; it gives the executive branch more authority to take into account "inappropriate" targeting by a state in apportioning DSH reductions. The ability of the secretary of health and human services to implement this provision depends heavily on whether systems can be forged that substantially upgrade the information flowing to federal officials on the hospitals receiving DSH funds and their role in the safety net.

Of course, any quest by federal regulators to improve monitoring and oversight of state DSH practices poses complex questions. Issues of devolution and the appropriate balance of authority between the national government and the states lurk in the background. How far should the federal government go in imposing certain standards on the states? When do federal requirements become dysfunctional micromanagement? Will the value of more information exceed the cost of obtaining it? Stakeholders know that information does not come free and has power implications. It takes substantial commitment as well as money and other forms of capacity to develop a system that yields valid, timely, and comparable information about state targeting of DSH to the safety net. Even if federal policymakers increase their information, they may not be able to reach agreement on the normative criteria that should guide what the appropriate distribution of DSH funds means in precise, operational terms.

Conclusion

Among the many characteristics of Medicaid DSH in the decades prior to the ACA two stand out. First, the Clinton and G. W. Bush years witnessed steady erosion in DSH funding in constant dollars overall and relative to the numbers of poor and uninsured. The ACA reinforces but certainly did not originate this decline. While states and many hospitals greatly value DSH, it seems destined to play a diminished, if nonetheless significant, role in shoring up the safety net regardless of whether the ACA stays on track for implementation. Second, DSH matters greatly in a relatively small number of states. In this sense, DSH defies the common tendency in intergovernmental grant programs to spread money around to all states. In contrast, DSH benefits are highly concentrated in about ten jurisdictions. If this development represented the triumph of target efficiency, DSH might emerge as an all-too-rare achievement in American public policy. But, as this chapter has emphasized, the allocation of DSH funds among states hardly reflects highly calibrated targeting.

How the intergovernmental system responds to the four challenges facing DSH under the ACA and the ramifications for the safety net warrant continued scrutiny. Beyond efforts to understand the politics and evolution of DSH, we believe that certain overarching policy issues deserve additional analysis. One valuable research thrust would involve doing more to evaluate DSH as a kind of natural experiment where some states spend much more money than others. Controlling for key variables, do high- and low-DSH states differ in the access to quality health care services they provide to low-income people? Do high-DSH states have more vibrant safety nets? How do increases or declines in DSH monies in a state over time affect the safety net and alter access to health care for the poor? Variations in DSH and the safety nets among states provide a golden, if largely unexploited, opportunity to distill lessons from states as policy laboratories.

Efforts to respond to these and related questions intersect with issues of whether Medicaid DSH focuses excessively on hospitals relative to other elements of the safety net. In considering this matter, Medicaid's contribution to the financial viability of one major source of outpatient services for the disadvantaged—community health centers—should be underscored. About 75 percent of the patients seen at some 1,080 centers operating at more than 7,500 sites are uninsured or Medicaid enrollees. As of 2008, Medicaid accounted for 37 percent of the revenues the centers generated. The ACA provides an additional $11 billion to expand these centers and reaffirms the requirement that Medicaid reimburse them at more generous rates than it typically pays other providers. The number of patients served by centers is projected to catapult from nineteen million in 2009 to fifty million in 2019 (Rosenbaum et al. 2010, 2–3, 7). While Medicaid will continue to play a vital role in bolstering this element of the outpatient safety net, questions linger as to whether more DSH funds should target services outside hospitals. In some states, such as California, hospitals play a much less salient role in anchoring the safety net relative to office-based physicians and clinics. Does DSH adequately reward states like California? If not, should it be adapted to do so? These and countless other questions beg for attention.

Medicaid's substantial role under the ACA firmly roots health reform in class-based care. Virtually all national health insurance systems present issues as to whether low-income people have the same access to quality services as the more affluent, but these systems espouse the norm of equal treatment in principle. In contrast, the ACA explicitly counts on Medicaid to cover the bottom income tier. While Medicaid coverage conveys many benefits, it has not fulfilled its original promise to provide "mainstream" health care. Instead,

Medicaid enrollees have depended heavily (though not exclusively) on certain hospitals and other safety-net providers. This pattern seems destined to continue. Hence, those who shape Medicaid have a big stake in the safety net and in what the program can do to support it. In this regard, DSH certainly deserves ongoing consideration as one tool. But the time has come to think more broadly about Medicaid initiatives and options to shore up the safety net.

Acknowledgments

Frank Thompson gratefully acknowledges the Robert Wood Johnson Foundation Investigator Award Program for supporting his work on Medicaid in general and this chapter in particular. We extend special thanks to Jennifer Farnham of the Rutgers Center for State Health Policy and Meghan Cole, a graduate intern at the Hastings Center, for their assistance. Joel Cantor, Derek DeLia, David Mechanic, Claudine Swartz, and the other authors in this volume provided perceptive comments on an earlier draft. We alone remain responsible for any defects in the current version.

Notes

1. The Congressional Budget Office (US CBO 2010) officially scored the savings as just over $14 billion for ten years. But Congress authorized an additional $4 billion cut in 2020 as well (Kaiser Family Foundation 2010, 26).
2. Coughlin and Zuckerman (2003, 173) note that "the payment limit is not the price to be paid for each service provided, but rather a ceiling on total Medicaid expenses above which the federal government will not match" state expenditures. Upper payment limits apply to different classes of service such as nursing home care and inpatient hospital services.
3. Data from the Kaiser Commission on Medicaid and the Uninsured indicate that certain states, such as New Mexico and Arkansas, greatly increased their Medicaid effort in terms of enrollment and expenditures per poor person in the period from 1992 to 2008.
4. A list of these reports appears in US GAO 2009, 46–47.
5. These figures are adjusted for changes in the overall Consumer Price Index, not its medical care component. Had the latter been used, the decline would have been even greater.
6. Contrary to the position we take on DSH targeting, for example, one could make the case for formulaic systems that track and reward all hospitals for serving the uninsured and Medicaid enrollees. Done properly, this might give the disadvantaged more choice and spread the patient load. But the geographic concentration of the disadvantaged tends to place disproportionate burdens on some hospitals and make them more essential to the safety net.
7. For one effort to define and measure the concept of an "essential" hospital, see the New Jersey Commission 2008, 159.
8. Total taxable resources (TTR) is the US Treasury Department's estimate of state fiscal capacity. It is a more comprehensive measure of this capacity than either gross state product or state personal income. Instead it taps "the unduplicated sum

of the income flows produced within a state . . . and the income flows received by its residents . . . which a state can potentially tax. . . . In sum, TTR is a flow concept, a comprehensive measure of all the income flows a state can potentially tax" (Compson and Navratil 2006). These data on Louisiana and New Jersey are for 2010. See U.S. Census Bureau, *Current Population Survey. 2011. Annual Social and Economic Supplement.*

10. After the initial cut, subsequent Medicare DSH increases will take into account the level of uncompensated care provided and the proportion of the population without insurance. This provision goes into effect in fiscal 2014 (Kaiser Family Foundation 2010, 25).

11. Proposed changes to the Medicaid and Medicare DSH programs were discussed in committee hearings held by the House Energy and Commerce Subcommittee on Health; the House Health, Education, and Labor Committee; the House Ways and Means Committee; and the Senate Finance Committee. DSH also came up in the markup sessions on health reform of the Senate Finance Committee and several times in debate on the floors of the House and Senate.

12. Testimony before the House Energy and Commerce Committee, June 25, 2009. http://energycommerce.house.gov/Press_111/20090625/testimony_sheils.pdf.

13. Testimony before the US House Committee on Ways and Means, June 24, 2009: 4.

14. Testimony before the US House Committee on Education and Labor, June 23, 2009: 136.

15. Testimony before the US House Committee on Energy and Commerce, June 25, 2009.

16. This percentage is approximate and may exaggerate the reduction. It assumes that federal DSH expenditures in 2014 are the same as in 2010—about $11 billion; it further assumes that without the cuts these expenditures would amount to $77 billion from 2014 through 2020.

17. The ACA addressed specific state reductions through the following language (Subtitle G, Section 255, subsection (a)2(B), Pub. L. 111–148): "If the Secretary determines on the basis of the most recent American Community Survey of the Bureau of the Census, that the percentage of uncovered individuals residing in the State is less than that percentage of such individuals determined for the State for the preceding fiscal year—(I) if the State is a low-DSH State described in paragraph (5)(B), the applicable percentage is equal to the product of the percentage reduction in uncovered individuals for the fiscal year from the preceding fiscal year and 25 percent; and (II) if the State is any other State, the applicable percentage is equal to the product of the percentage reduction in uncovered individuals for the fiscal year from the preceding fiscal year and 50 percent."

18. However, the two-year nature of the increase may well cause some physicians to refrain from taking on Medicaid enrollees for fear they will be "stuck" with them if fees go back down.

19. For an overview, see Rosenbaum (2009). She underscores the importance of the Supreme Court's 2002 decision, *Gonzaga v. Doe*, in undermining provider and beneficiary claims that they had federally enforceable individual rights under Medicaid. The California providers based their claim on the Supremacy Clause of the US Constitution—the principle that federal law takes precedence over state law.

References

Baker, S. 2010. "States Seek Justice Dept. Help in Urging Supreme Court to Hear Medicaid Suit." *InsideHealthReform.com*, June 29.

Beaty, P. 2009. "Will Safety Net Hospitals Survive Health Reform?" *Health Care on MSNBC.* Sept. 8. Accessed Mar. 15, 2010. http://www.msnbc.msn.com/id/ 32672409?ns/health-health_care/.

Berliner, H. S. 2008. "The Movement of Services Out of the Hospital." *International Journal of Health Services* 38, no. 4: 625–639.

Compson, M., and J. Navratil. 2006. "An Improved Method for Estimating The Total Taxable Resources Of the States," Research Paper No. 9702. http://www.treasury.gov/ resource-center/economic-policy/Documents/wpnewm.pdf.

Coughlin, T., B. K. Bruen, and J. King. 2004. "States' Use of UPL and DSH Financial Mechanisms." *Health Affairs* 23, no. 2: 245–257.

Coughlin, T., and S. Zuckerman. 2003. "States' Strategies for Tapping Federal Revenues: Implications and Consequences of Medicaid Maximization." In *Federalism and Health Policy*, ed. J. Holahan, A. Weil, and J. M. Weiner, 145–178. Washington, DC: Urban Institute Press.

DeLia, D. 2007. "Evaluation of the Hospital Charity Care Program in New Jersey." New Brunswick, NJ: Rutgers Center for State Health Policy.

Frizzera, J. 2009. "History of the Medicaid Disproportionate Share Hospital (DSH) Program, 1981–2009." PowerPoint presentation at a conference of the National Health Policy Forum: Washington DC. June 15, 2009.

Grogan, C. M., and M. K. Gusmano. 2007. "Healthy Voices, Unhealthy Silence: Advocacy and Health Care Policy for the Poor." Washington, DC: Georgetown University Press.

Gusmano, M., and M. Schlesinger. 2001. "The Social Roles of Medicare: Assessing Medicare's Collateral Benefits." *Journal of Health Politics, Policy and Law* 24, no. 1: 37–80.

Holahan, J., and I. Headen. 2010. "Medicaid Coverage and Spending in Health Reform: National and State-by-State Results for Adults at or Below 133% FPL." Washington, DC: Kaiser Commission on Medicaid and the Uninsured.

Kaiser Family Foundation. 2010. "Focus on Health Reform: Side-By-Side Comparisons of Major Health Care Reform Proposals." Washington, DC. March 24.

Kingdon, J. 1984. *Agendas, Alternatives, and Public Policy.* Boston: Little, Brown.

Klein, E. 2009. "Does Medicare Pay Below 'Cost?' (Wonky!)." *Washington Post*, July 1.

Nathan, R. 1993. *Turning Promises into Performance: The Management Challenge of Implementing Workfare.* New York: Columbia University Press.

New Jersey Commission on Rationalizing Health Care Resources. 2008. "Final Report." Trenton, NJ: Department of Health and Senior Services.

Obama, B. 2009. "Health Care Reform, the Key to Our Fiscal Future." Weekly Radio Address, June 13. Washington, DC: The White House.

Patashnik, E. M. 2008. *Reforms at Risk.* Princeton, NJ: Princeton University Press.

Pierson, Paul E. 2004. *Politics in Time.* Princeton, NJ: Princeton University Press.

Rich, R. F., and W. D. White, eds. 1997. *Health Policy, Federalism, and the American States.* Washington, DC: Urban Institute Press.

Robertson, C. 2009. "Louisiana, with Its Special History, Has Big Stake in Health Care Debate." *New York Times*, Dec. 20.

Rosenbaum, S. 2009. "Medicaid Payment Rate Lawsuits: Evolving Court Views Mean Uncertain Future for Medi-Cal." Issue Brief. Oakland: California Health Care Foundation.

Rosenbaum, S., E. Jones, P. Shin, and J. Tolbert. 2010. "Community Health Centers: Opportunities and Challenges of Health Reform." Washington, DC: Kaiser Commission on Medicaid and the Uninsured.

Stone, D. 1988. *Policy Paradox and Political Reason.* New York: HarperCollins.

Thompson, F. J. 1998. "The Faces of Devolution." In *Medicaid and Devolution: A View from the States*, ed. F. J. Thompson and J. J. DiIulio Jr., 14–55. Washington, DC: Brookings Institution.

Thompson, F. J., and C. Burke. 2007. "Executive Federalism and Medicaid Demonstration Waivers: Implications for Policy and Democratic Process." *Journal of Health Politics, Policy, and Law* 32, no. 6: 971–1004.

US Congressional Budget Office (US CBO). 2010. Letter to the Honorable Nancy Pelosi, Speaker, US House of Representatives. March 20.

US Department of Health and Human Services (US HHS). 2008. "Medicaid Program; Disproportionate Share Hospital Payments; Final Rule." *Federal Register* Dec. 19. 73, no. 245: 77903–77951.

US Government Accountability Office (US GAO). 2005. "Medicaid Financing: States' Use of Contingency-Fee Consultants to Maximize Federal Reimbursements Highlights Need for Improved Federal Oversight." GAO-05–748. Washington, DC.

———. 2007. "Medicaid Financing: Federal Oversight Initiative Is Consistent with Medicaid Payment Principles but Needs Greater Transparency." GAO-07–214. Washington, DC.

———. 2009. "Medicaid: Ongoing Federal Oversight of Payments to Offset Uncompensated Hospital Care Costs Is Warranted." GAO-10–69. Washington, DC.

US House Committee on Education and Labor. 2009. "The Tri-Committee Draft Proposal for Health Care Reform," June 23. Washington, DC: Government Printing Office.

US House Committee on Energy and Commerce. 2009. "Reforming the Healthcare System: Written Statement by Patricia A. Gabow, M.D.," June 25. Accessed Nov. 15, 2011. http://republicans.energycommerce.house.gov/Media/file/Hearings/Health/062509_health_reform_discussion_draft_day3/Patricia%20Gabow%20Testimony%206.25.09.pdf.

US House Committee on Ways and Means. 2009. *Health Reform in the 21st Century: Proposals To Reform the Health System. (June 24)* Washington, DC: Government Printing Office.

US House of Representatives. 2010. "Remarks by Representative Carolyn Maloney (D-NY) on the Patient Protection and Affordable Care Act." *Congressional Record* Apr. 15; LexisNexis, 111th Congress, 2nd Session, 156 Cong Rec E 567.

US Medicare Payment Advisory Commission (MedPAC). 2007. *Report to the Congress*, March. Washington, DC: MedPAC. www.medpac.gov/documents/Mar07_EntireReport .pdf.

———. 2010. *A Data Book: Healthcare Spending and the Medicare Program*. Washington, DC: MedPAC. http://www.medpac.gov/documents/Jun10DataBookEntire Report.pdf.

US Senate Finance Committee. 2009a. "Continuation of the Open Executive Session to Consider an Original Bill Providing for Health Care Reform," Sept. 24. http://finance .senate.gov/hearings/hearing/?id=d8083e61-f98b-0204–3389–428e5a1a78e7.

———. 2009b. "Roundtable Discussion on Comprehensive Health Care Reform." Washington, DC: Government Printing Office.

Zaman, O. S., L. C. Cummings, and S. S. Spieler. 2010. "America's Public Hospitals and Health Systems, 2008." Washington, DC: National Association of Public Hospitals and Health Systems.

The Safety-Net Role of Public Hospitals and Academic Medical Centers

Past, Present, and Future

Public hospitals and academic medical centers (AMC) have long played an important role as safety-net providers in the United States. These institutions frequently offer outreach services to uninsured and Medicaid populations as well as an array of health and social services, either directly or through collaborative arrangements. Public hospitals and AMCs have faced many challenges over the years in maintaining their safety-net roles, especially given their need to balance these roles against others they have in the community, such as research, teaching, and patient care. However, many have demonstrated their resilience to these stresses.

This chapter examines the historical context that has led public hospitals and AMCs to serve as an important component of the health safety net and how their role in the safety net has been shaped by the challenges they have faced. Drawing on interviews we undertook with key stakeholders of safety-net institutions, the chapter also explores how the Patient Protection and Affordable Care Act (ACA) will affect these institutions and their ongoing roles in the community, including how these institutions will likely build on their existing efforts to address future challenges. The questions and uncertainties that exist for public hospitals and AMCs as health care reform is implemented is also explored.

Historical Context: Public Hospitals and AMCs as Safety-Net Institutions

Public hospitals in the United States have a long tradition of serving individuals who do not have the means to pay for their care. This role dates back to the

1700s when the first US public hospital opened to provide shelter and charitable health services for the poor (Lewin and Altman 2000). These facilities also were the training ground for physicians because they provided patients for physicians to hone their medical skills and understanding. As medicine became more advanced, public hospitals remained but, like private hospitals, became more focused on curative treatment rather than the warehousing of sick individuals. In addition, as medical education advanced and educational standards became more specific, large AMCs arose, some of which had their historical roots in the original public hospitals.

In 2008 the American Hospital Association (AHA) annual survey data indicated that there were 1,105 public hospitals nationwide and 305 hospitals listed as teaching hospitals affiliated with the Association of American Medical College's Council on Teaching Hospitals. Holahan and colleagues (2008) reported that hospitals provided $35 billion in uncompensated care in 2008, largely to poor and uninsured individuals. The National Association of Public Hospitals and Health Systems (NAPH), which represents those public and private hospitals that have large safety-net commitments, had approximately 140 hospital members in 2008. Data reported by NAPH (2010a) indicated that 16 percent of their members' costs of providing hospital care was uncompensated compared to 5.8 percent for all hospitals nationwide in 2008. NAPH members represented only 2 percent of the nation's acute care hospitals but delivered 19 percent of nationwide uncompensated care.

The continuing, and in fact growing, role of public hospitals and AMCs in the safety net is largely due to several unique characteristics of these institutions. The geographic location of urban public hospitals and AMCs makes them convenient sources of care for indigent populations. These institutions are frequently located in the central city, often near poor neighborhoods. In part, their location reflects historical decisions by local officials to place them in areas where services were limited, and also it may reflect the decisions of poor individuals to live near these facilities (Gaskin and Hadley 1999; Hadley and Cunningham 2004). Additionally, these institutions tend to offer a broad range of services given their teaching missions, including the public, social, and specialty services that are used by uninsured and Medicaid populations (Gaskin 1999; Zuckerman et al. 2001; Bazzoli et al. 2005; Horowitz 2005). Lewin and Altman (2000) noted that AMCs may be the only, or among the few, hospitals offering highly specialized services in a community that are used by both insured and uninsured (such as organ transplant, high-risk obstetrics care). Recognizing the special needs of the populations they served, public hospitals and AMCs developed outreach and culturally sensitive services over time for their uninsured populations, provided primary care services through their emergency departments or affiliated clinics, coordinated referral and specialty services, and collaborated with local agencies to address social and behavioral issues (Lewin and Altman 2000; Jones and Sajid 2010). In doing so, they have become places that low-income and uninsured individuals have grown to trust in addressing their needs and making them feel less marginalized.

Growing reliance of poor and vulnerable populations on public hospitals and AMCs has also occurred as private community hospitals reduced their safety-net involvement due to market pressures. Several studies have found that private community hospitals have dropped certain unprofitable services frequently used by the uninsured, such as psychiatric emergency services, high-risk pregnancy, and mental health and substance abuse (Zuckerman et al. 2001; Bazzoli et al. 2005; Horowitz 2005). Chen and colleagues (2009) found that short of dropping these services, private nonprofit hospitals reduced the volume of unprofitable services provided to uninsured patients during a period in which the number of uninsured grew. Bazzoli and colleagues (2006a) found that hospitals with lower commitments to providing indigent care reduced their uncompensated care over time when public and private reimbursement constraints were substantial. This necessarily implied a shifting of this care to public hospitals and AMCs as institutions of last resort for patients in need. Weissman and colleagues (2003) support this notion in that they found the market share of uninsured patients at teaching hospitals grew in the 1990s relative to other hospitals in their service areas and that these increases occurred primarily in urban areas with high levels of managed care penetration.

Growing Strains on the Hospital Safety Net

Public hospitals and AMCs have faced many stresses and challenges over time in their safety-net roles. In part, these pressures represent general market phenomena that affect all community hospitals. Total Medicare margins for hospitals have declined over time, from 5.2 percent in 2000 to -7.2 percent in 2008 (MedPAC 2010). As a result, there are fewer funds available to cross-subsidize Medicaid and uninsured losses. Certainly, private sector payment-to-cost ratios have been increasing, but it is impossible to shift the full burden of uninsured and public sector losses to one payer group (Dobson, DaVanzo, and Sen 2006). For safety-net providers, commercial payers represent a small share of their payer mix, only about 25 percent, as measured based on gross charges, among NAPH (2010a) survey respondents.

There also has been growing competition for highly profitable services over time due to the growth of niche providers (such as ambulatory surgery centers, diagnostic centers, cardiac and orthopedic specialty hospitals). Some of these profitable services were once the primary domain of public hospitals and AMCs (Cunningham, Bazzoli, and Katz 2008; Hall 2010). Coupled with this is the increasing growth of specialized facilities in areas outside of central cities, which reduces traditional travel of patients to high-tech, central-city facilities, especially among well-insured suburbanites (Bazzoli, Gerland, and May 2006b).

However, some pressures have been unique to the safety-net institutions. Between 1987 and 2008 the number of uninsured individuals grew from thirty-one to forty-six million (US Census Bureau 2009). In the current economic recession, Dorn and colleagues (2008) reported that for each 1 percent increase in the unemployment rate, the number of uninsured increased by 1.1 million. Since the start of the recession, NAPH (2010b) reported that its members have experienced a 23 percent increase in the number of uninsured patients treated and a 10 percent increase in uncompensated care to low-income populations. There has also been growing heterogeneity in the composition of the uninsured over time. The number of Hispanic uninsured has increased markedly by 143 percent between 1987 and 2008, whereas African American uninsured increased by 24 percent and white, non-Hispanic uninsured by 17 percent over this period (US Census Bureau 2009, 2010). Although they share the common trait of lacking insurance, the health and social needs of different uninsured groups are likely to vary, as are outreach approaches adapted to cultural differences.

In addition, sources of support upon which public hospitals and AMCs have grown to rely to cover a portion of uncompensated care costs have been quite volatile. One of these primary sources is Medicaid disproportionate share hospital (DSH) payments, which Hadley and colleagues (2008) suggest covered 30 percent of hospital uncompensated care costs in 2008. Federal policymakers often have targeted Medicaid DSH as a way to reduce federal deficits, especially given the perception that state governments have used various schemes to reduce state outlays and fund non-Medicaid projects under the guise of providing DSH support to hospitals (see Gusmano and Thompson, chapter 7, this volume). The 1997 Balanced Budget Act in particular included large cuts to this program on the order of $10.4 billion over the 1998–2002 period (CBO 1997). These DSH reductions represented the major sources of federal Medicaid savings, accounting for 61 percent of total Medicaid gross savings over five years. Although some of these original cuts were later delayed or rescinded, Medicaid DSH support has continued to decline over time.

Expansion of Medicaid managed care was also once viewed as a threat to safety-net provider survival (Norton and Lipson 1998; Lewin and Altman

2000). However, as events played out, public hospitals and AMCs in some states became vital players within Medicaid managed care plans (Lewin and Baxter 2007). In some cases, state governments implemented regulations that required health plans to include traditional safety-net organizations in their managed care networks so that these essential providers were not left out. In other cases, though, especially as commercial insurers dropped out of Medicaid managed care, public hospitals and AMCs stepped up to the plate, developing their own provider networks and the infrastructure to operate provider-sponsored plans (Holahan et al. 1998; Gray and Rowe 2000).

Public hospitals and AMCs are finding that they are increasingly involved with care that could have been avoided if other sources of social and health services were available for the indigent. There have been increased social admissions and services provided as other public and private sources of services decline. In particular, as options for psychiatric care diminish through the closure of state facilities, more individuals in need of these services have relied on public hospital and AMC emergency departments (Lewin and Baxter 2007; Cunningham, Bazzoli, and Katz 2008). In addition, evidence indicates that there has been increased incidence of preventable hospital admissions among the uninsured and Medicaid populations, and some have suggested that this is likely due to increasing difficulty in their ability to access primary care services in their communities (Gaskin and Hoffman 2000).

Hospital Safety-Net Response and Adaptation

Although public hospitals and AMCs have faced many stresses, many of them have shown great resiliency and creativity in responding to these pressures. Much of this action has been borne out of financial necessity. However, their responses and adaptations have in many ways led to beneficial improvements in patient care delivery. In addition, adaptation at public hospitals and AMCs has benefited from supportive local, state, and federal policies that have provided the funds or infrastructure to facilitate innovation.

A prime example of how public hospitals and AMCs have adapted is the development of their own Medicaid managed care plans. As noted earlier, some public hospitals and AMCs seized on opportunities as states shifted more of their Medicaid populations to managed care plans and as commercial health plans in some states dropped out of this market. As public hospitals and AMCs developed new plans, they recognized the need to create stronger relationships with other providers in the community, especially community health centers and private physicians so that sources of primary care could be included and integrated. The medical-home concept was an important foundation in several of these efforts as a means to link Medicaid patients with a personal primary care physician or health provider who provides continuing and coordinated care for these individuals. NAPH (2010c) identified forty-six medical-home programs at thirty-seven member hospitals in 2009. Public hospitals and AMCs also realized that linkages with private hospitals in some instances were important because these institutions were able to deliver certain care at lower cost.

Institutions such as Denver Health and Harborview Medical Center in Seattle, Washington, were early innovators in this regard. Denver Health established itself as an independent public authority that then went about aligning other hospitals, physicians, local health departments, and school-based clinics to become one of the largest Medicaid health maintenance organizations (HMO) in the nation (Gabow 1997). Harborview Medical Center developed relationships with the University of Washington Medical Center and created an HMO to serve the Aid to Families with Dependent Children population that included linkages with the university's physicians and primary care providers in an array of clinics (Norton and Lipson 1998). These programs served as models for other safety-net institutions; a 1998 NAPH survey reported that 67 percent of its members and 69 percent of surveyed teaching hospitals were developing similar strategies to partner with other health care organizations (Solloway and Darnell 1998).

Although the impetus for these actions may have been largely due to financial and market pressures, Medicaid patients benefited from the new models of care that were being developed. Public hospitals and AMCs were convenient, regular sources of care for these patients. Through the actions of these institutions, a broader array of physician and hospital services were made available to them. Risk-based contracting necessitated that safety-net providers think more carefully about how to manage chronic care rather than simply provide fragmented, episodic care. Access to community-based physicians also meant that patients could obtain more immediate medical services and not have to experience long wait times in the emergency department for routine care. Medicaid patients, especially in the early days of managed care in some states, were now financially attractive, and private and public health plans competed for their loyalty, which inevitably meant competition based on better customer service.

The provider collaboration and networks developed for Medicaid managed care also created a foundation for another wave of innovation, namely the development of managed care programs for uninsured patients of safety-net hospitals (NAPH 2005). This transition was in many ways a natural in that the infrastructure needed to operate a Medicaid managed care plan could be used to also support a similar program for uninsured populations. In addition, the health and social needs of the uninsured population shared similarities to those within the Medicaid population. Also, spurring these efforts on was the availability of federal grant money under the Healthy Community Access Program during the Clinton administration to develop local integrated and collaborative programs to serve the uninsured and underinsured populations. The W. K. Kellogg Foundation also sponsored a national demonstration program through the AHA's Health Research and Educational Trust to support the development of twenty-five collaborative community care networks largely focused on serving unmet needs of disadvantaged populations (Bogue and Hall 1997). In addition, Qualis Health, the Commonwealth Fund, and the MacColl Institute supported safety-net development of medical-home demonstration projects in 2009 (NAPH 2010b).

Public hospitals and AMCs involved in these initiatives recognized that these managed care models could mitigate losses they were experiencing from the uninsured receiving care in their emergency departments. Private physicians and community health centers could provide routine primary care more economically rather than having uninsured patients overcrowd and receive expensive emergency department care for basic health problems. Early provision of primary care also could reduce the need for subsequent emergency department visits and preventable hospitalizations, which also create unreimbursed expenses for public hospitals and AMCs.

Although some federal and foundation monies were available to develop programs for the uninsured, these sources of financial support are small in scale and highly variable. Public hospitals and AMCs, especially public sector AMCs, rely in part on state and local tax appropriations for financial support of their programs, but the extent of this support is highly dependent on the financial situation of state and local governments. Public hospitals and AMCs also use their own financial resources—namely their net patient revenues, financial reserves, non-operating income, and donations—to pay community-based physicians, other hospitals, and other providers. While at first blush this may seem illogical, it is important to recognize that this strategy may reduce the financial losses that public hospitals and AMCs experience. In other words, it may be more economical to "buy" services in the market for qualifying patients rather than to "make" similar patient care internally. Given this reliance on the bottom line, managed care programs for the uninsured are inevitably small in terms of the number of uninsured individuals served and are highly variable from year to year because funding depends on what resources involved institutions can muster (Andrulius and Gusmano 2000).

Despite small scale, public hospitals and AMCs that have well-structured programs typically report success. Hall (2010), in his study of Denver Health, noted that uninsured in the program in 2008 had similar numbers of physician, clinic, and emergency room visits as compared to national data from the National Ambulatory Care Survey. Gardner and Kahn (2006) reported that county programs for the uninsured in California, many of which involved safety-net hospitals, expanded access to care for the uninsured, especially for children. Reductions in the use of emergency department visits as well as increases in physician visits are frequently reported by public hospitals and AMCs with these uninsured programs (Gill et al. 2005; NAPH 2010c).

Health Care Reform and the Future of
Public Hospitals and AMC Program Efforts

The ACA presents an array of new challenges and opportunities for public hospitals and AMCs as they transform to meet the demands of a potentially new health care environment. We interviewed representatives from three public hospital and AMC health systems to gain their perspectives on how the ACA may affect their current programs, especially their Medicaid managed care plans and programs for the uninsured. We contacted representatives with Virginia Commonwealth University Health System, Denver Health, and Parkland Health and Hospital System in the fall of 2010, and the following four questions formed the basis for discussion:

1. Given your current programs for Medicaid managed care and for the uninsured, what challenges do you see resulting from the new health care reform law? What opportunities do you see?
2. Do you feel that your existing programs might be good platforms for developing accountable-care organizations (ACOs) as envisioned in the new reform law? Why or why not?
3. What concerns do you have about capacity (especially in terms of physician networks and/or hospital services) as more individuals become enrolled in Medicaid? What actions are you undertaking now to deal with future capacity issues?
4. What concerns do you have about financing care, especially for the residual uninsured, as the new health reform law is implemented?

Perhaps the biggest challenge apparent through these discussions was the current uncertainty about the future of the ACA given the political environment. Although the new law specifies an implementation timetable, the ACA continues to be debated and the possibility exists that key provisions of the law will be repealed or amended in ways that are unclear. Such changes might affect whether individuals will face an insurance mandate, how individuals will be able to obtain health insurance coverage, whether subsidies available for health insurance purchase will make coverage affordable, sources and amounts of financial support for various provisions of the act, and/or the timing of ACA implementation. Representatives of the three public hospital and AMC systems noted the challenge of trying to plan for the future given this uncertain environment. They also commented on the current struggle that exists to meet increasing indigent care needs in their communities at a time of strained state and local budgets and growing difficulty in maintaining balance in their patient care delivery, teaching, research, and community roles.

If the ACA is implemented as planned, the fifty-seven million individuals who would have been uninsured in 2019 without the health reform law are expected to divide into three groups, as illustrated in table 8.1, with eighteen million covered as a result of Medicaid expansions, sixteen million covered through the new health insurance exchanges, and twenty-three million remaining uninsured (US Office of the Actuary 2010). Most of these reductions in uninsured and increases in coverage would take place in 2014, the first year of the individual health insurance mandate. Our interviews identified that each of these transitions presents opportunities and challenges to public hospital and AMC health systems.

In relation to Medicaid expansions, interviewees agreed that this would be positive and would result in continued growth in their Medicaid managed care plan enrollment. Ultimately Medicaid expansions could lead to reductions in uncompensated care demands and simultaneous expansion in revenue inflows. Another positive aspect of Medicaid expansions is that many individuals who currently participate in existing public hospital and AMC managed care programs for the uninsured would be covered through Medicaid. These individuals already have some degree of integration within these systems of care that will serve as a starting point for further integration into a Medicaid managed care delivery model. However, several challenges were noted. First, the types of individuals in existing managed care programs for the uninsured differ from those currently enrolled in Medicaid managed care and thus have different health needs. In particular, new Medicaid managed care enrollees will more often be adults rather than children and will have more chronic care needs. Interviewees noted that they had efforts under way to identify distinct patient groups in their current uninsured programs who are likely to become eligible for Medicaid; they planned to develop tailored educational approaches to engage these individuals and better integrate them into their health system.

Another challenge being confronted is the need to retool the existing structure of public hospital and AMC health systems to meet growing patient need for services as they enroll in Medicaid. In particular, interviewees were beginning to identify more dispersed locations to deliver primary care in their communities and were evaluating the primary care capacity needed to support these locations. This was viewed as vital so that newly insured individuals do not continue to use emergency departments as a readily available place to obtain routine care.

Table 8.1   **Estimated Effects of Patient Protection and Affordable Care Act by 2019: Summary of Primary Opportunities and Challenges**

Baseline estimate* of uninsured (without ACA): 57 million	Insured through Medicaid expansions: 18 million	**Opportunities:** Reduce uncompensated care; increase revenues; increase enrollment in public hospital and AMC Medicaid managed care plans; maintain existing relationships with some uninsured who will become eligible
		Challenges: Expand availability of services; increase primary care capacity; address differences in service needs for current vs. newly enrolled; motivate patient behavior change
	Insured through employer or state health insurance exchanges: 16 million	**Opportunities:** Reduce uncompensated care; increase revenues; capture new enrollees through public hospital and AMC insurance product offered in health insurance exchange; maintain existing relationships with some uninsured who will become eligible
		Challenges: Expand availability of services; increase primary care capacity; address differences in service needs for current vs. newly enrolled; motivate patient behavior change; market insurance products to newly insured; improve customer service
	Residual uninsured: 23 million	**Opportunities:** None identified
		Challenges: Predict the number of uninsured who will rely on particular institutions; address problem of convincing public officials to financially support care provided to illegal immigrants; address uncertainty about internal financial resources; deal with growing burden of care if other hospitals limit safety-net involvement

*Estimate from US Office of the Actuary 2010

Interviewees noted the need to look beyond the traditional physician office and community health centers to alternative sites of care, such as miniclinics and urgent care centers, to improve access and reduce emergency room use. It was noted that relationships with these alternative sites not only can accommodate increased demand for health care services but also provide options for individuals who may not perceive the need to have a consistent medical home.

One of the biggest challenges noted by interviewees was aligning sufficient physician capacity to meet future health needs for an expanded Medicaid population, certainly in relation to primary care but also to specialty services. Interviewees noted the need to develop more extensive and diffuse physician partnerships. In particular, there is the need to increase the number of clinic locations within a health system's service area, increase hours of operation, expand physician capacity, and, in some cases, expand geographically beyond the existing service area. One factor that complicates these efforts is the historically low Medicaid payments to primary care physicians and specialists. For health systems that currently employ physicians, this was viewed as less of an issue than for health systems that wish to continue reliance on community-based physicians in private practice. Developing a relationship model that in some way acts as a middle ground between a staff model and private practice may be needed to gain the involvement of sufficient numbers of physicians to serve a larger Medicaid managed care population. Other strategies involve working with medical schools to increase medical school enrollment, encouraging students to pursue primary care, and developing and expanding opportunities to train resident physicians in the community.

Another concern noted was the importance of expanding capacity to manage chronic illness. Chronic illness management is vital so that Medicaid managed care programs are able to live within their financial budgets. Although public hospitals and AMCs have some experience in chronic care management through their Medicaid managed care plans and programs for the uninsured, these efforts will likely need to be ramped up or more diffusely spread over a wider network of providers. In addition, effective management strategies for a largely adult population may need to be added to the mix of strategies currently in use by their Medicaid managed care programs.

The estimated sixteen million otherwise-uninsured individuals who could gain access to coverage through health insurance exchanges create some opportunities and challenges similar to those of the Medicaid expansions. However, unique opportunities and challenges were also noted. The primary opportunity, as mentioned earlier, is the potential to reduce some uncompensated care burden and replace this with new sources of revenue. The mix of individuals

in the new privately insured, however, will likely have even greater heterogeneity than those who will become eligible for Medicaid. In particular, some
of the new private insureds may have participated in structured programs for
the uninsured, which typically have an income limit of 200 percent of the federal poverty level, but are ineligible for Medicaid expansions because the ACA
limit is 133 percent of the federal poverty level. Other new privately insured
individuals may have relied on public hospitals and AMCs for care but did not
develop relationships with these institutions because they used them for
episodic care. Trying to understand the distinct groups within this milieu is
complicated, as is thinking about how their health care decisions will be
affected by the ACA and newly gained coverage.

Another opportunity expressed by the public hospital and AMC interviewees related to the future health insurance exchanges. All saw potential for
their current Medicaid managed care plans to be transformed into products
that could be sold through the exchange and might represent low-cost options
for small businesses and lower income individuals. Although these plans
might have reputational issues if labeled as Medicaid plans, in some ways this
marketing bridge has already been crossed through approaches used to enroll
children in State Children's Health Insurance Plans, which also originally had
the connotation of "public" plans. Representatives from the three systems indicated that their organizations were seeking to learn more about the exchanges
and how they could be involved.

Other concerns expressed about the new privately insured paralleled
many of those identified for Medicaid expansions, namely the need to expand
coverage areas, sites of care, and primary care capacity. In addition, the importance of patient education and new management practices were brought up,
especially for individuals who enroll in managed care products of the public
hospitals and AMCs. In essence, the newly insured—whether they qualify
for Medicaid or are able to obtain coverage through the health insurance
exchanges—need to develop new ways to access the health system. The diversity in this population will require new management strategies both clinically
(given the array of illnesses they will present) and administratively (such as
enhanced procedures to ensure that copayments are collected at the point of
service in the emergency room and other departments). One concern raised
specific to the new privately insured was the need to improve customer
service, especially if an array of options is available to them through the
health insurance exchanges.

Another big challenge noted by the public hospital and AMC representatives related to the residual uninsured. As noted in table 8.1, despite national

reform, a projected twenty-three million will remain without coverage. Although the organizations studied have developed managed care plans for these populations, the future of these programs is uncertain. They are largely funded through state and local tax revenues and the financial bottom line of public hospitals and AMCs. The ultimate effect of the ACA on the financial resources of public hospitals and AMCs is unclear. Certainly there may be reductions in uncompensated care as more individuals gain coverage and enroll in Medicaid. These newly insured will also bring new sources of revenues to public hospitals and AMCs. However, interviewees recognized that they will likely experience sharp reductions in Medicaid and Medicare DSH funds. Also, there is recognition that some newly insured individuals might only be able to afford high-deductible health plans, which may leave them exposed to high health bills that they cannot afford. These individuals might disproportionately seek care at public hospitals and AMCs if other health providers are reluctant to treat them given the type of coverage they have. In addition, changes in state and local financial support for the uninsured are also unclear. It may be difficult to convince state and local officials to continue to financially support uncompensated care and programs for the uninsured if the bulk of the residual uninsured are illegal immigrants.

There is also substantial uncertainty about exactly how many uninsured individuals will rely on individual public hospitals and AMCs when the ACA is fully implemented. Although some estimates of the illegal immigrant population are possible based on existing hospital information, it is unclear how US citizens and legal residents will respond when insurance mandates are in force. How many will opt not to obtain coverage and thereby face penalties despite the mandate? Interviewees indicated that they lack a methodology to predict these numbers. It is hard to discern how much uncompensated care burden will remain for public hospitals and AMCs and whether the enhanced revenue flows from ACA will offset these residual burdens.

Another area of discussion with public hospital and AMC representatives was the development of ACOs as envisioned under the ACA. The exact form and requirements of these organizations are unclear at this stage and subject to a series of demonstration projects under way by the Centers for Medicare and Medicaid Services through its Center for Medicare and Medicaid Innovation. It is envisioned, though, that these organizations will provide a broad range of preventive, primary, acute, chronic, and long-term care. They also will be accountable to their communities for assessing health needs and reporting provider performance, and fiscally accountable in terms of operating with risk-sharing or capitation (Shortell and Casalino 2010). When asked if their current Medicaid managed care and programs for the uninsured represented good platforms on which to develop future ACOs, all interviewees indicated that this was the case but with important caveats. One concern is aligning sufficient primary care capacity, which reflects issues discussed earlier. Interviewees also raised concerns about infrastructure investments, especially expanding health information technology. Although interviewees noted that their institutions had made great strides in implementing and using advanced health information technology within the walls of their organizations, they realized that they would need to link to a broader network of health providers in the community.

Although interviewees recognized some of the steps needed to transform to the ACOs of the future, garnering the financial resources to support this transition was a major issue. Interviewees indicated interest in pursuing funding through existing federal and foundation demonstration programs. Potential avenues to develop necessary capacity and test the effectiveness of their programs include the Center for Medicare and Medicaid Innovation programs noted here and participation in the Health Innovation Zones concept developed by the Association of American Medical Colleges. Pediatric safety-net demonstration programs were also identified as opportunities for financial support to expand and test existing programs as public hospitals and AMCs transition to ACOs.

It is clear that public hospitals and AMCs will confront a number of opportunities and challenges as the ACA unfolds over the next few years. There is recognition that, although there is much promise as many uninsured individuals become covered, there are potential new stresses that may result. The experience in Massachusetts, which implemented similar reforms, makes clear that stresses on safety-net institutions do not necessarily lessen even as more individuals become covered. Despite the increase in the number of insured, safety-net hospitals in Massachusetts have had to balance the loss of traditional safety-net hospital support (primarily the loss of Medicaid DSH), the concentration of low-income individuals in their institutions as other hospitals cut back safety-net involvement, and sharp reductions in Medicaid payments that were implemented to offset state costs for expanded Medicaid eligibility (NAPH 2009). These kinds of countervailing forces will be important as public hospitals and AMCs nationwide navigate the new health care environment that materializes.

Acknowledgments

Research support for the development of this chapter was provided by NIH Grant R01 HL082707: Safety Net Hospitals and Minority Access to Care, awarded by the National Heart, Lung and Blood Institute of the National Institutes of Health. We also thank Betsy Carrier from the National Association of Public Hospitals and Health Systems, LeAnn Donovan of Denver Health, and Sharron Phillips from Parkland Hospital and Health System for their helpful input on the issues that will confront public hospitals and academic health centers as health care reform is implemented.

References

Andrulius, D., and M. Gusmano. 2000. "Community Initiatives for the Uninsured: How Far Can Innovative Partnerships Take Us?" New York: New York Academy of Medicine.

Bazzoli, G. J., A. Gerland, and J. May. 2006b. "Construction Activity in US Hospitals." *Health Affairs* 25, no. 3: 783–791.

Bazzoli, G. J., R. Kang, R. Hasnain-Wynia, and R. C. Lindrooth. 2005. "An Update on the Safety-Net Hospitals: Coping with the Late 1990s and Early 2000s." *Health Affairs* 24, no. 4: 1047–1056.

Bazzoli, G. J., R. C. Lindrooth, R. Kang, and R. Hasnain-Wynia. 2006a. "The Influence of Health Policy and Market Factors on the Hospital Safety Net?" *Health Services Research.* 41, no. 4, Pt 1: 1159–1180.

Bogue, R. J., and C. H. Hall. 1997. *Health Network Innovations.* Chicago: American Hospital Publishing.

Chen, H. F., G. J. Bazzoli, and H. M. Hsieh. 2009. "Hospital Financial Condition and the Provision of Unprofitable Services." *Atlantic Economic Journal* 37, no. 3: 259–277.

Congressional Budget Office (CBO). 1997. "Budgetary Implications of the Balanced Budget Act of 1997." Washington, DC. December. http://www.cbo.gov/ftpdocs/3xx/doc302/bba-97.pdf.

Cunningham, P. J., G. J. Bazzoli, and A. Katz. 2008. "Caught in The Competitive Crossfire: Safety-Net Providers Balance Margin and Mission in a Profit-Driven Health Care Market." *Health Affairs* 27, no. 5: w372–w382.

Dobson, A., J. DaVanzo, and N. Sen. 2006. "The Cost-Shift Payment 'Hydraulic': Foundation, History, and Implications." *Health Affairs* 25, no. 1: 22–33.

Dorn, S., B. Garrett, J. Holahan, and A. Williams. 2008. "Medicaid, SCHIP and Economic Downturn: Policy Challenges and Policy Responses." Kaiser Commission on Medicaid and the Uninsured. April. Available at http://slides.kff.org/chart.aspx?ch=360.

Gabow, P. A. 1997. "Denver Health: Initiatives for Survival." *Health Affairs* 16, no. 4: 24–26.

Gardner, A., and J. G. Kahn. 2006. "Increasing Access to Care for the Uninsured: Considering the Options in California Counties." *Journal of Health Care for the Poor and Underserved* 17 (Nov.): 830–50.

Gaskin, D. J. 1999. "Safety Net Hospitals: Essential Providers of Public Health and Specialty Services." New York: Commonwealth Fund, Feb.

Gaskin, D. J., and J. Hadley. 1999. "Population Characteristics of Markets of Safety-Net and Non-Safety-Net Hospitals." *Journal of Urban Health* 76, no. 3: 351–370.

Gaskin, D. J., and C. Hoffman. 2000. "Racial and Ethnic Differences in Preventable Hospitalizations across 10 States." *Medical Care Research and Review* 57 (Supplement 1): 85–107.

Gill, J. M., H. B. Fagan, B. Townsend, and A. G. Mainous. 2005. "The Impact of Providing a Medical Home to the Uninsured: Evaluation of a Statewide Program." *Journal of Health Care for the Poor and Uninsured* 16, no. 3: 505–535.

Gray, B., and C. Rowe. 2000. "Safety Net Health Plans: A Status Report," *Health Affairs* 19, no. 1: 185–193.

Hadley, J., and P. Cunningham. 2004. "Availability of Safety Net Providers and Access to Care of Uninsured Persons." *Health Services Research* 39, no. 5: 1527–1546.

Hadley, J., J. Holahan, T. Coughlin, and D. Miller. 2008. "Covering the Uninsured in 2008: Current Costs, Sources of Payment, and Incremental Costs." *Health Affairs* 27, no. 5: w399–w415.

Hall, M. A. 2010. "The Costs and Adequacy of Safety Net Access for the Uninsured: Denver, Colorado." Robert Wood Johnson Foundation. http://www.rwjf.org/files/research/safetynetdenver201006.pdf.

Holahan, J., S. Zuckerman, A. Evans, and S. Rangarajan. 1998. "Medicaid Managed Care in Thirteen States." *Health Affairs* 17, no. 3: 43–63.

Horwitz, J. R. 2005. "Making Profits and Providing Care: Comparing Nonprofit, For-Profit, and Government Hospitals." *Health Affairs* 24, no. 3: 790–796.

Jones, A. S., and P. S. Sajid. 2010. "A Primer on Health Care Safety Nets." Robert Wood Johnson Foundation. http://www.rwjf.org/files/research/49869.pdf.

Lewin, M. E., and S. Altman. 2000. *America's Health Care Safety Net: Intact but Endangered.* Washington, DC: Institute of Medicine, National Academies Press.

Lewin, M. E., and R. J. Baxter. 2007. "America's Health Care Safety Net: Revisiting the 2000 IOM Report." *Health Affairs* 26, no. 5: 1490–1494.

Medicare Payment Advisory Commission (MedPAC). 2010. *A Data Book: Healthcare Spending and the Medicare Program.* MedPAC: Washington, DC. June. http://www.medpac.gov/documents/Jun10DataBookEntireReport.pdf.

National Association of Public Hospitals and Health Systems (NAPH). 2005. "Managing Care for Uninsured Patients: Five Success Stories from America's Public Hospitals and Health Systems." Washington, DC: NAPH. July. http://www.naph.org/Publications/managingcareforuninsuredpatients.aspx?FT=.pdf.

———. 2009. "Massachusetts Health Reform: Lessons Learned about the Critical Role of Safety Net Health Systems." Washington, DC: NAPH. Apr. http://www.naph.org/Publications/MA-Health-Reform-Issue-Brief.aspx?FT=.pdf.

———. 2010a. "America's Public Hospitals and Health System, 2008: Results of the Annual NAPH Hospital Characteristics Survey." Washington, DC: NAPH. Feb. http://www.naph.org/Main-Menu-Category/Publications/Safety-Net-Financing/Characteristics-2008.aspx?FT=.pdf.

———. 2010b. "Safety Net Health Systems: An Essential Resource during the Economic Recession." Washington, DC: NAPH. Feb. http://www.naph.org/Publications/Recession-Brief-Feb-2010.aspx?FT=.pdf.

———. 2010c. "Safety Net Hospitals Establish 'Medical Homes.'" Washington, DC: NAPH. Feb. http://www.naph.org/Publications/Medical-Homes-Brief.aspx?FT=.pdf.

Norton, S., and D. Lipson. 1998. "Public Policy, Market Forces, and the Viability of Safety Net Providers." Occasional Paper No. 13. Washington, DC: Urban Institute.

Shortell, S. M., and L. P. Casalino. 2010. "How the Center for Medicare and Medicaid Innovation Should Test Accountable Care Organizations." *Health Affairs* 29, no. 7: 1299–1304.

Solloway, M., and J. Darnell. 1998. "The Impact of Medicaid Managed Care on Essential Community Providers." Portland, ME: National Academy for State Health Policy.

US Census Bureau. 2009. "Income, Poverty and Health Insurance Coverage in the US: 2008." Report P60–236(RV). Washington, DC: US Census Bureau. Sept. http://www.census.gov/prod/2009pubs/p60–236.pdf.

———. 2010. "Health Insurance Historical Tables-Original Series, Table HI-1, 2010." http://www.census.gov/hhes/www/hlthins/data/historical/original.html.

US Office of the Actuary, Centers for Medicare and Medicaid Services. 2010. "Estimated Financial Effects of the Patient Protection and Affordable Care Act as Amended." https://www.cms.gov/ActuarialStudies/Downloads/PPACA_2010–04–22.pdf.

Weissman, J. S., D. J. Gaskin, and J. Reuter. 2003. "Hospitals' Care of Uninsured Patients during the 1990s: The Relation of Teaching Status and Managed Care to Changes in Market Share and Market Concentration." *Inquiry* 40, no. 1: 84–93.

Zuckerman, S., G. J. Bazzoli, A. Davidoff, and A. T. LoSasso. 2001. "How Have Safety Net Hospitals Coped during the 1990s?" *Health Affairs* 20, no. 4: 159–168.

The Declining Public Hospital Sector

Public hospitals have long served as the backbone of the health care safety net, caring for the poor, uninsured, and racial and ethnic minorities, as well as providing critical regional services. In major metropolitan areas, public hospitals provide more than 20 percent of emergency and 33 percent of outpatient visits, as well as 60 percent of burn and 36 percent of trauma care. Medicaid and uninsured patients account for more than 50 percent of all public hospital visits (NAPH 2009). In rural areas, they are major components of local health systems, representing nearly 40 percent of hospitals. Public hospitals have also traditionally provided extensive outpatient services, community public health programs, and culturally and linguistically appropriate care.

Under health reform, there will continue to be a need for safety-net hospital services. It has been estimated that, following the implementation of health reform, 23 million Americans will still be uninsured and 16 million will be covered by Medicaid or the State Children's Health Insurance Program, populations historically reliant on public hospitals (CBO 2010).

In the wake of the 2008 recession, state and local governments have been under financial pressure, which has in turn threatened the financial stability of public hospitals. State and local budget crises have prompted large cutbacks in funding for many institutions while the number of uninsured and those covered by Medicaid have grown at record rates (Hartocollis 2010; KFF 2010; Skipp 2010; Sun and Mummolo 2010).

Prior to the economic downturn, public hospitals were already battling financial and political pressures to survive in an increasingly cost-driven health care market, and many were closed or converted to private ownership

(Lewin and Altman 2000). When considering future changes in health care and implications for access to care, particularly for the most vulnerable Americans, it is important to understand the trends in the decline of the public hospitals that are major providers of safety-net care. In this chapter, we examine the shifts in US public hospital supply from 1983 to 2003. We focus on hospital closures and conversions to private ownership, and regional and rural-versus-urban differences. We also examine the countertrend of development of new public hospitals. We describe the role of these institutions in their respective communities and augment the analysis of the trends with the discussion of individual cases.

The Characteristics of Public Hospitals at the Beginning of the Period of Decline

There were 5,894 community hospitals in the United States in 1980; 1,801 (31 percent) were public, 3,337 (56 percent) were nonprofit, and 756 (13 percent) were for-profit. By 2009 the number of community hospitals had declined by 15 percent to 5,008, largely the result of mergers and closures, with some offsetting development of new hospitals. The number of public hospitals, however, had declined by 39 percent to 1,092, in sharp contrast to the 13 percent decline in nonprofit hospitals and 32 percent increase in for-profits (based on author calculations from American Hospital Association Annual Survey of Hospitals, 1980 and 2009).

For a detailed analysis of the decline in hospitals, we focus on the twenty-year period of 1983–2003, for which we have confirmed changes in ownership in the American Hospital Association (AHA) annual survey data. For these years, we have reviewed change of ownership data that would signal a hospital conversion from public to nonprofit or for-profit. Where the data reported to the AHA were anomalous (such as one year in a new ownership status, or ping-ponging back and forth for several years) we confirmed conversions using ownership data from the Medicare cost report, directly contacting the hospital, contacting state licensure officials, or reviewing web-based resources when a hospital had closed or could not confirm the date of ownership changes. We also focus on general medical and surgical hospitals. We have augmented the AHA annual survey data with county level data from the 1980, 1990, and 2000 censuses.

In 1983 there were 5,671 general nonfederal hospitals, of which 1,691 were public, 3,224 nonprofit, and 756 for-profit (table 9.1). There were strong regional differences in numbers and the mix of ownership types, with the Northeast (New England and the Middle Atlantic) hospitals being overwhelming nonprofit (88 percent), with only 7.5 percent public and 4.5 percent for-profit. The South had the largest proportion of both public and for-profit hospitals (38 percent and 23 percent, respectively) and smallest proportion of nonprofit hospitals (39 percent). In the Midwest and West, public hospitals constituted 30 percent of hospitals, with nonprofits dominating, but a larger share of the Western hospitals were for-profit than in the Midwest (18 percent compared to 3 percent).

The distribution of ownership is consistent with the patterns described by Rosemary Stevens (1989) in *In Sickness and in Wealth: American Hospitals in the Twentieth Century*. In her review of the development of hospitals in America, she notes that the first hospitals established in the United States were nonprofits, and rivalry among ethnic immigrant groups and exclusion of physicians from newly arrived immigrant communities from medical staffs at more established hospitals encouraged the establishment of voluntary hospitals in the Northeast and Midwest. Public hospitals, often established with exclusive missions of care for the poor, also developed during that early period.

The second half of the nineteenth century saw the development of anesthesia, aseptic surgery, X-rays, and effective drug and antibiotic therapies. Hospitals, now much safer and offering unique services, became places where the well-to-do, not just the poor, were treated, and the industry began to grow rapidly. For-profits thrived in this environment and were more than half of all hospitals in 1910. For-profits and public hospitals were more likely to be created in rural areas such as the South and in the West, where voluntary hospitals did not exist, and where sparse or new populations meant that the voluntary community organizations that might sponsor hospitals were not well established.

Table 9.1   **General Hospital Ownership, by Region, 1983**

	Ownership			
Region	Public, *n* (%)	Nonprofit, *n* (%)	For-profit, *n* (%)	Total, *n* (%)
Northeast	61 (7.5)	718 (88.2)	35 (4.3)	814 (100)
Midwest	500 (29.9)	1,132 (67.7)	43 (2.6)	1,675 (100)
South	812 (38.2)	827 (38.9)	488 (22.9)	2,127 (100)
West	318 (30.1)	547 (51.9)	190 (18.0)	1,055 (100)
Total	1,691 (29.8)	3,224 (56.9)	756 (13.3)	5,671 (100)

Source: Author calculations from American Hospital Association Annual Survey, 1983.

The Depression led to a major collapse in the for-profit hospital sector, which did not have access to community capital or philanthropy, but for-profit numbers remained relatively higher in the South and West. The creation of the federal Hill–Burton program to fund hospital construction following World War II provided grants for nonprofit and public hospitals, further reducing the role of for-profits. The regional distribution of investment in public versus nonprofit hospitals through Hill–Burton was very different, however, with the well-established nonprofit sector dominating hospital investment in the Northeast while investment in public hospitals was more likely in areas with weaker philanthropic traditions or rapid population growth.

Public hospitals in 1983 were distinctive in other ways beyond their distribution across states (table 9.2). They were much more likely to be nonurban (72 percent compared to 49 percent for all hospitals). They were relatively small, 123 beds on average compared to an average of 218 beds for nonprofit hospitals (but a similar 125 for for-profits). The smaller size was a function of their large concentration in nonurban areas, as the average size of public hospitals in urban areas was 256 compared to 295 for nonprofit hospitals and 147 for for-profits. Hospitals in 1983 were more focused on inpatient services than contemporary hospitals are, deriving only 16 percent of their gross revenues

Table 9.2   **Characteristics of General Hospitals, by Ownership, 1983**

Characteristic	Public	Nonprofit	For-profit	Total
Nonurban (%)	72	40	33	49
Sole hospital in county (%)	47	20	13	27
Average inpatient beds (n)	123	218	125	177
Average inpatient beds (urban counties) (n)	256	295	147	262
Revenues from outpatient (%)	17	17	12	16
Medicare days (%)	45	46	47	46
Medicaid days (%)	14	11	7	11
County Medicaid market share (%)	67	39	25	45
Ratio of Medicaid market share to overall market share (%)	112	98	98	102
County Medicaid market share (urban counties where the public hospital is not the sole hospital) (%)	28	17	7	17
Ratio of Medicaid market share to overall market share (urban counties where the public hospital is not the sole hospital) (%)	143	97	95	103

Source: Author calculations from American Hospital Association Annual Survey, 1983.

from outpatient services, and public and nonprofit hospitals had comparable levels of outpatient services.

The safety-net status of public hospitals is apparent in several key measures from the AHA survey. Forty-seven percent were the sole hospital in their community, compared to 20 percent of nonprofits and 13 percent of for-profits. While the percentage of their inpatient days attributable to Medicare patients was comparable to that in nonprofits and for-profits, 14 percent of their days were attributable to Medicaid patients, compared to 11 percent in nonprofits and 7 percent in for-profits. Their Medicaid market share was 67 percent for all the counties in which they were located, compared to 39 percent for nonprofits and 25 percent for for-profits. They disproportionately served Medicaid patients, with their Medicaid market share 12 percent higher than their overall market share. This disproportionate service to Medicaid patients is not an artifact of their rural location or sole county-hospital status. When this analysis is limited to urban counties in which publics are not the sole hospital, their percentage of Medicaid market share averaged 28 percent compared to 17 percent for nonprofits and 7 percent for for-profits. Their Medicaid market share was 43 percent higher than their overall market share for these counties. The 1983 public hospitals disproportionately served the Medicaid population.

The Decline in Public Hospitals 1983–2003

Of the 1,691 hospitals that were public and open in 1983, fewer than 60 percent remained by 2003 (figure 9.1). Nineteen percent (318) had closed and 23 percent (390) converted (figure 9.2). Conversions outpaced closures between 1983 and 1986 and again from 1992 to 2001, with closures exceeding conversions in the late 1980s and early 1990s.

Rates of closure and conversion differed across regions (figure 9.3). The West and Midwest were more likely to maintain public hospital services. In the Northeast, more than 35 percent of the facilities were closed outright, and fewer than half of the original institutions remained in 2003. There were far fewer public hospitals in the Northeast overall (28, compared to 496 in the South). In the South, public hospitals were more likely to undergo privatization rather than closure, particularly for-profit conversion (7 percent versus 2.8 percent for all other regions).

Rates of closure and conversion also differed between urban and nonurban areas. In urban areas, 25 percent of public hospitals closed. Of the hospitals that closed, 67 percent were the sole public hospital in the county, which underscores the fact that these closures reflected decisions by the public

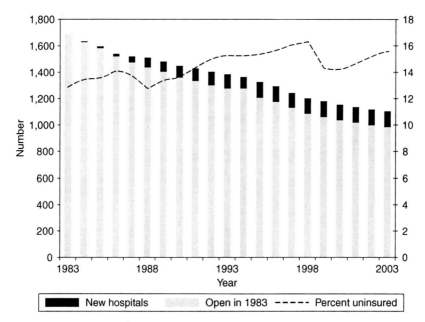

Figure 9.1 Decline of Public Hospitals and Openings of New Public Hospitals, 1983–2003

Source: Author calculations from American Hospital Association Annual Survey with author corrections of ownership data

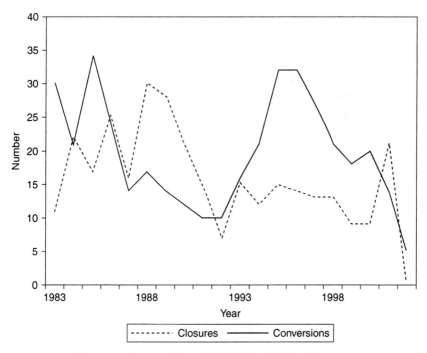

Figure 9.2 Closings and Conversions of Public Hospitals, by Year, 1983–2003

Source: Author calculations from American Hospital Association Annual Survey with author corrections of ownership data

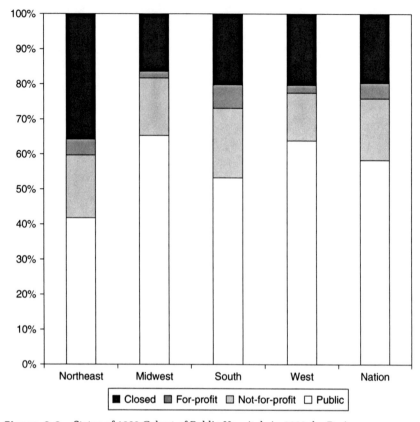

Figure 9.3   Status of 1983 Cohort of Public Hospitals in 2003, by Region

Source: Author calculations from American Hospital Association Annual Survey with author corrections of ownership data

hospital owners to abandon these services rather than trim or reconfigure a public system. These hospitals provided an average of 23 percent of the Medicaid inpatient care for the county prior to closure. They also provided disproportionately more Medicaid care in their respective areas, with their market share of Medicaid inpatient days 62 percent higher, on average, than their share of total inpatient care for the county.

Most of the urban hospitals that closed were relatively small, but there are some notable exceptions. St. Louis City Hospital, a 485-bed facility, closed in 1984. John L. Doyne Hospital, formerly the Milwaukee General Hospital, a 445-bed facility, closed in 1995. Financial losses at the hospitals that the local governments were no longer willing to underwrite and significant future required capital investments were key precipitating factors in decisions to close both hospitals. Provision was made in both closings to shift some of the local health funding from inpatient care to outpatient care through networks of private clinics. In the St. Louis case, this transition was at the center of the decision to close the hospital.

In the Milwaukee case, the transition to funding outpatient care was less direct. Initially, the assets of Doyne Hospital were transferred to a nonprofit hospital constructed on the same campus and with which the county had contracted for some specialty services. The county entered a two-year "preferred provider" contract with the nonprofit hospital using funds from a state General Assistance Medicaid Program (GAMP) block grant to pay for the contract. After two years, the contract was ended and the GAMP program was restructured to focus on primary care in clinics and private physicians' practices. Hospital provision of uncompensated and charity care, half of which was provided by Doyne prior to its closing, became dispersed among Milwaukee's hospitals, with many of these nonprofits seeing substantial increases in the demand for charity care.

The experience of these hospitals—closures encouraged because of financial difficulties or bankruptcy and large levels of future capital spending, limited provision for alternatives for inpatient care, shifts in public funds to outpatient care—are also seen in many of the other urban public hospital closings. There have been no assessments to date of the impact of these closings on health care use or health outcomes of the former patients of closed hospitals.

In urban areas, there also was a substantial number of public hospital conversions to nonprofit, or less commonly, for-profit status. Twenty-eight percent of urban public hospitals converted, and when this percentage is added to that of hospitals that closed, more than half of urban public hospitals closed or converted between 1983 and 2003. As was the case with the hospitals that closed, the overwhelming majority of converting hospitals (79 percent) were the sole public provider in the county prior to conversion. These hospitals accounted for 28 percent of their county's Medicaid inpatient care on average, and their share of Medicaid inpatient days was 29 percent higher, on average, than their share of total inpatient care for the county.

Nonprofit conversions or mergers are among the most prominent and visible changes in the public hospital landscape. Among the most notable have been the conversions of Tampa General Hospital, University of Tennessee Medical Center, Grady Memorial Hospital in Atlanta, and the North Broward Hospital System in Florida, as well as the merger of Boston City Hospital and Boston University Medical Center into Boston Medical Center, and the merger and conversion of Cambridge Hospital and Somerville Hospital into the Cambridge Health Alliance.

Many of the same issues arose in these conversions that were present in urban closures. While not all were present in each conversion, common issues were imminent large repairs or capital costs, or ongoing operating losses, sometimes with local desire to shift financing from hospitals to outpatient services or from direct institutional support to support for individuals and families. Also motivating these conversions was the belief that the governance structure and inflexibilities associated with public purchasing and other management functions increased costs, made creating efficiencies difficult, and slowed response to changing market conditions, including contracting with managed care. There was a perception in some cases that being labeled a government hospital reduced the willingness of insured patients to seek care at the facility.

Also common among the conversions were the issues that had to be resolved in moving the conversion forward. Key among these were governance structure and any continuing role for government in hospital governance, openness and transparency in operations, the nature and extent of ongoing public funding for indigent care and other public services, leasing versus transfer of the building and other physical assets (which affects funding for capital improvements), and transitioning of public employees. Part of the calculation about the wisdom of conversion was the implication of ownership changes for Medicaid reimbursement because some states restrict disproportionate share hospital (DSH) payments to public hospitals. The most successful hospital conversions have found ways to stop losses, stabilize funding, constrain costs, and position the converted hospital better in the market for privately insured patients. In the cases of many less-celebrated conversions, financial challenges have continued postconversion. It should also be noted that several prominent public systems, such as Denver Health, have succeeded in these areas without conversion.

There are no clear distinctions between urban communities that closed or converted a public hospital and communities that maintained public ownership. Those communities with closures and conversions were more likely to have lower poverty rates in 2000 than those in which the hospital remained open and public (closed: 12.6 percent; privatized: 11.6 percent; public: 13.1 percent). While these differences are statistically significant, they are modest, and there is little evidence that a community's poverty influenced the decision to close or convert a public hospital. Rather, the differences in choices made across urban communities about closing, converting, or maintaining public ownership of hospitals appear to be influenced by local political culture, the general public support for the public mission, beliefs of policymakers regarding how inflexible public management was, and how much management improvement could be realized under alternative governance, financial resources at the local level, and state programs to support hospitals with high volumes of Medicaid and indigent patients.

We have conducted regression-based analyses to identify factors that might explain whether a public hospital was likely to close or convert. We found that disproportionate Medicaid share among urban hospitals increased the risk of closure while offering more specialty services (perhaps reflecting a larger role in the health care of privately insured patients) reduced the risk of closure. A higher proportion of revenues from Medicaid increased the likelihood of conversion in urban areas.

In nonurban areas, more than one-third of public hospitals closed or converted, with 17 percent closing and 20 percent converting. Of the hospitals that closed, 39 percent were the sole hospital in the county and an additional 37 percent were the sole public hospital. In counties with multiple hospitals available, these hospitals provided an average of 34 percent of the area's Medicaid inpatient care prior to closure, although their Medicaid share was not substantially higher than their overall market share. Of the hospitals that converted, 64 percent were the sole hospital in the county. The remaining 36 percent provided an average of 47 percent of the county's Medicaid inpatient care prior to privatization, although their Medicaid share was only 6 percent greater than their overall market share.

In our multivariate analysis, we found that higher market competition, lower share of revenues from Medicare, smaller size, and lower occupancy rates among rural hospitals were all associated with closure. Each of these is likely to reduce the operating margin of the hospital, reducing its attractiveness as an acquisition or financial viability as a converted hospital. No specific variables were associated with conversion, which suggests that the decision to convert a local public hospital in a rural area or to maintain it as a public facility was heavily influenced by local circumstances and policy preferences.

The 2000 poverty rate was higher in areas that lost a public hospital, compared to those that retained a public hospital. The poverty rate in counties that closed a public hospital was 17 percent, versus 15 percent in areas in which the public hospital remained open. While the difference was statistically significant, it is relatively small. Poverty rates were also higher (16 percent) in areas in which the public hospital was converted to a private facility.

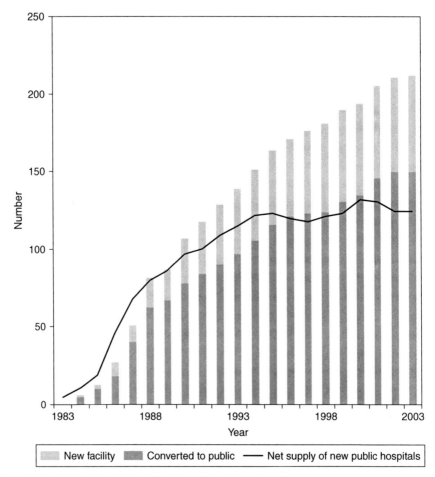

Figure 9.4   Development of New Public Hospitals, 1983

Source: Author calculations from American Hospital Association Annual Survey with author correction of ownership data

The Modest Countertrend in the Establishment of New Public Hospitals

During 1983–2003, 212 new public hospitals emerged (see figure 9.1). More than 70 percent (150) of these consisted of conversions from existing privately owned hospitals; the remaining hospitals were new facilities (figure 9.4). Of the conversions, approximately three-quarter were of nonprofit hospitals, one-quarter for-profit. In many of these cases, the private hospital was in financial difficulty and was considering closing. Existing public systems often acquired the hospital rather than the hospital being acquired as a freestanding facility. The intent of the systems appears to be to maintain services in the community or expand their local reach. However, many of these hospitals subsequently closed or converted back to private ownership; only 125 were still public and open in 2003. The same forces acting on the public hospitals in 1983 operated on those built or converted to public hospitals after that year. And the financial and operational challenges that led nonprofit and for-profit owners to divest the hospital were not always correctable by the new public owners.

Implications for a Future with Health Reform

The number of US public hospitals dropped substantially throughout the 1980s and 1990s, and this contraction in supply far exceeded the rate of decline seen in the overall US hospital industry. However, these trends were not uniform across the United States. Many public hospitals in the Northeast closed, which suggests that the private sector has borne a relatively larger burden of safety-net care in this region. In the South, the tendency toward for-profit conversion raises concerns about access to care for vulnerable groups, given research showing that former public hospitals provide less uncompensated care following conversion to for-profit ownership (Needleman 1999).

For rural areas, public hospital closure may threaten services for an entire community because many of these hospitals were the sole providers in their respective counties. Even in areas in which the public hospital was not the sole county hospital, public hospitals cared for a large percentage of the Medicaid population prior to closure. We did not find that these hospitals provided a disproportionately higher share of Medicaid care, but in the absence of data on uncompensated care, we note that these hospitals may still have performed a critical safety-net function for the uninsured in the region. Communities most likely to have lost a public hospital also had higher poverty rates in 2000. Our findings suggest that rural areas with a relatively greater need for indigent care lost hospital services over this time period.

In urban areas, public hospitals that closed appeared to serve as safety-net providers. Many were the sole public provider in their respective areas and provided disproportionately more Medicaid care. At the same time, the urban areas that lost a public hospital had slightly lower poverty rates. Because these hospitals were relatively more "safety net"–like in character, this finding suggests that the hospitals were not closed in response to declining demand but other factors such as operating losses, high future capital needs, local frustration with the inflexibility of public personnel, procurement and management systems, and the ability of government to efficiently manage the hospitals.

Thinking about how these trends may interact with the implementation of health reform, new coverage expansions in rural areas may enable public hospitals to recoup costs for previously uncompensated care, potentially slowing the rate of closure or enabling those that privatize to maintain needed regional services. It is unclear to what degree the new legislation will benefit public hospitals in urban areas, which primarily serve disadvantaged groups. Prior expansions of public coverage programs led to private sector "cherry-picking" of healthy public patients, leaving public institutions to care for the sicker, more costly populations (Gaskin, Hadley, and Freeman 2001). New coverage expansions rely upon expanding Medicaid eligibility, but hospitals with a relatively greater Medicaid burden were more likely to close. Public hospital systems with extensive outpatient services may be better positioned to access global capitated payments under Medicaid, but large systems with the potential to create integrated inpatient and outpatient networks exist only in a handful of cities (CBO 2010). The stability of public hospitals in urban areas will likely hinge upon revisions in formulas for DSH funding.

Conversions have been the response to concerns about effective management while recognizing the need for the services public hospitals provide. Individual successes in high visibility conversions, such as that of Tampa General, have been reported, but there has not been a systematic study of how successful these conversions have been and which models of governance and financing support the continued safety-net mission of the converted hospitals.

Closure has been a move away from the commitment to provide the services or a judgment that the community cannot afford to bear the cost. Local commitment to public provision of hospital care and to the belief that government can manage such facilities effectively and efficiently has declined over the past several decades. If the general public perceives that greater coverage has been achieved as a result of health care reform, regardless of the remaining uninsured or the unwillingness of many private providers to accept Medicaid, local communities may no longer support using tax dollars to underwrite public hospitals. Public hospitals may face the expectation to become increasingly competitive and self-sufficient, even though their unique services will remain critical components of the health care system.

Acknowledgments

This study was supported by the Robert Wood Johnson Foundation Investigator Awards in Health Policy Research program and the Agency for Healthcare Research and Quality Predoctoral Training Awards.

References

Congressional Budget Office (CBO). 2010. "H.R. 4872, Reconciliation Act of 2010 (Final Health Care Legislation)." Washington, DC.

Gaskin, D. J., J. Hadley, and V. G. Freeman. 2001. "Are Urban Safety-Net Hospitals Losing Low-Risk Medicaid Maternity Patients?" *Health Services Research* 36:25–51.

Hartocollis, A. 2010. "City's Public Hospitals Fear Huge Loss in Subsidies." *New York Times*, Feb. 21.

Kaiser Family Foundation (KFF). 2010. "Medicaid Enrollment: June 2009 Data Snapshot." Menlo Park: Kaiser Commission on Medicaid Facts.

Lewin, M. E., and S. Altman. 2000. *America's Safety Net: Intact but Endangered.* Washington, DC: Institute of Medicine, National Academies Press.

National Association of Public Hospitals and Health Systems (NAPH). 2009. "Safety Net Health Systems: An Essential Resource During the Economic Recession." Washington, DC.

Needleman, J. 1999. "Uncompensated Care and Hospital Conversions in Florida." *Health Affairs* 18, no. 4: 125–133.

Skipp, C. 2010. "Miami Board Looks to Close Two Hospitals." *New York Times*, Mar. 5.

Stevens, R. 1989. *In Sickness and in Wealth: American Hospitals in the Twentieth Century.* New York: Basic Books.

Sun, L., and J. Mummolo. 2010. "Prince George's, Md., Health-Care System Remains Unsold." *Washington Post*, May 19.

Part III

Safety-Net Systems

Achieving Universal Access through Safety-Net Coverage

The United States has long been derided as the world's only industrialized country that falls well short of universal health care coverage. The 2010 Patient Protection and Affordable Care Act (ACA, or Affordable Care Act) will close approximately half the existing coverage gap but will leave more than twenty million people still uninsured. Can anything be done for the remaining uninsured that will bring us, finally, to some acceptable form of universal coverage? In particular, can safety-net programs be structured in a way that provides access to care sufficiently to approximate the goals of universal coverage?

To better understand this social policy landscape, this chapter undertakes a conceptual analysis of what exactly we mean by "universal," "coverage," and "access." Understanding the policy significance of these terms over a range of meanings might help crystallize social debate and reveal the most achievable path forward. Necessarily, this inquiry is heavily normative, or value laden, but it avoids being excessively philosophical or opinionated by rooting normative analysis in real-world systems that express and operationalize actual social values. Specifically, I gauge the adequacy of coverage or access according to existing insurance systems that are widely considered to be at least minimally acceptable.

My normative task is to identify the low-water markings of adequacy, rather than aim for pure equality. Idealistic aims can be useful to motivate improvements, but rarely are they fully achievable. My aim is more modest: to identify the nearest finish line of what might constitute some acceptable form of universal access. If we as a society are about to run out of gas in the drive for a fair and just health care system, knowing the shortest distance to this goal might help us finally push past rather than stall short of the line.

To identify norms for universality, we begin by looking abroad. Then returning to domestic soil, we explore whether acceptable coverage necessarily requires insurance, or instead whether coverage can be accomplished through direct-access safety-net systems. The chapter concludes with analysis of data measuring access to care in model safety-net programs.

Universality

Universality can be thought of as a percentage, consisting of a numerator and a denominator. The numerator is the easy part. We hope it can be as close as possible to 100 percent. European countries report covering from 98 to 100 percent of their population—which is similar to the 99 percent of people in this country aged sixty-five or older who are insured, thanks to Medicare. Thus, it appears we can agree on the numerator—that about 98–99 percent is close enough to count as "universal," or at least nearly so.

Population Denominator

More troubling is the population denominator. This immediately raises the socially divisive issue of immigration. European countries cover legal permanent residents on essentially the same terms as full citizens (Huber et al. 2008). Likewise, the ACA provides subsidies to resident immigrants on the same terms as citizens and requires them, like citizens, to purchase insurance if it is affordable. Legal immigrants are fully eligible and responsible because the basis of social solidarity is not citizenship, per se; instead, it is living in the same community under the same laws and contributing to the same tax base. Inclusion of legal immigrants is especially appropriate in a country such as ours whose population derives so substantially from its history of massive immigration.

Noticeably and notoriously excluded from US health reform, however, are undocumented (or "illegal") immigrants. From a demography point of view, they are part of the US population, but health reform provides them no subsidies and does not require them to purchase coverage. Accordingly, undocumented immigrants are expected to account for roughly a third of people in the United States who will remain uninsured following full implementation of national health insurance reforms. Should this sizeable portion of the community be included in the population denominator used to gauge universality?

Views are deeply divided on this difficult question of social justice. According to some philosophers and theologians, social justice should be judged by how we treat the most underprivileged people. Undocumented immigrants are underprivileged by income and by exclusion from the protections inherent in citizenship. However, there are passionate objections to extending full social benefits. Reasons include their basic lack of deservedness, xenophobia, fear of economic competition, and a desire to deter more illegal border-crossing.

Some social policy arguments on the other side of the debate are not wholly convincing. For instance, the call to protect ourselves from infectious disease is a reason that covers only a small portion of health care services. Similarly, maintaining health so immigrants will be more productive workers only extends to those who are in the workforce, and seems to call for contributions as much or more by employers as by society at large. Advocates also argue that unnecessary costs can be reduced through primary care services that prevent avoidable emergencies, noting that emergency services are available regardless of insurance. But this also justifies only a limited range of services, and the actual extent of cost avoidance is largely unproven (DeLia and Cantor 2009).

The limited force of these moral and public health arguments leaves supporters with two broad-based arguments for inclusion—one based on idealism and one on pragmatism. The idealistic position is that access to health care is a basic human right, one that is not contingent on the social circumstances of citizenship, residency, income, or legal status. Deservedness arises simply from the fundamental human condition, according to a basic moral compulsion (as expressed in, for instance, the Bible) to help anyone who is suffering or in need. Even prisoners, after all, have a constitutional right to a decent level of medical care. Although their claim to access is based on different considerations that arise from being in involuntary custody, the prisoner example demonstrates that compromised civic status does not necessarily negate basic human rights.

The pragmatic position is quite different. It admits that nonresidents may be less entitled to support, but it notes that excluding them imposes a burden on the rest of society. To exclude undocumented immigrants, they must be identified as such, which entails requiring legitimate citizens also to identify and validate themselves. Documenting citizenship is not a simple matter and so is not feasibly done in some circumstances, such as urgent care. Moreover, many citizens consider mandatory documentation to be offensive or intrusive, especially when it is required to access basic social institutions such as courts or elementary schools. This avoidance of documentation is one basis on which community health centers and other safety-net institutions often accept undocumented immigrants. Their policy is not necessarily one of purposeful inclusion so much as it is a policy against burdensome documentation for any patient. (Some safety-net programs require documentation of local residency, which is easily confirmed using a utility bill, as opposed to documenting citizenship status, which requires birth records.) For subsidized insurance, an interesting question to consider is whether a majority of citizens are sufficiently opposed to documenting their own legitimacy that they would want to dispense with the need for documentation altogether. If so, this pragmatic consideration might make moot the question of whether undocumented people deserve coverage.

Elsewhere in the world, though, this debate has been settled mostly against full inclusion. Because many countries register citizens automatically, it is easier to exclude those who lack documentation. Thus, few European countries provide full coverage to illegal immigrants (France, Portugal, and Spain are exceptions). Most provide them only urgent care, except for asylum seekers who are applying to convert to legal status. (For them, some European countries provide full coverage and some do not.) Following this international ethic of social justice, an acceptable level of universality would be achieved by covering all legal residents. For those who hold the view that illegal immigrants merit some but not full access, such as for urgent, contagious, and perhaps acute conditions, these immigrants would not count in either the denominator or numerator in measuring our progress toward universal coverage.

Coverage Numerator

Returning to the universality numerator, precisely what does coverage mean? Usually, it denotes enrollment in public or private insurance. However, actual enrollment may not be essential to be included in the numerator for two reasons. First, eligibility for insurance might suffice even without enrollment. Second, structured programs other than insurance might provide access that is roughly equivalent to insurance.

The first of these two points is fairly straightforward. Take, for instance, those who are eligible for Medicaid but have not enrolled, or those whose enrollment has lapsed. They are counted as uninsured yet they are covered in the sense that they might seek care at any point and could be enrolled automatically or retroactively. Thus, actual coverage is available at the point of service. Gaps in official enrollment certainly are not ideal since they indicate likely failure to receive optimal primary or preventive care, but it is difficult to maintain that eligible people who are not enrolled lack access to affordable care simply for lack of enrollment. If technical enrollment is not essential for meaningful coverage, then a substantial portion of uninsured people do in fact have a form of coverage and so should be counted in the numerator.

Beyond this somewhat technical qualification is a more fundamental point that gets to why insurance coverage matters to begin with. Being insured per se is not the ultimate social objective. Instead, insurance is a means to achieve the goal of affordable access to care. Properly understood, then, access does not always coincide with insurance. Bill Gates would have decent access even if he were uninsured, whereas Joe the Plumber might have impaired access even with insurance. Several factors can compromise access for insured people, such has high deductibles or copayments relative to income or assets, or a shortage of available providers—either in general or those who are willing to accept patients with a particular kind of insurance.

Rather than use insurance as a proxy for access, it is quite possible to measure access directly, regardless of whether people are technically insured or uninsured. The following section explores how this comparison might be done, but for now the key point is this: systems of direct access might in theory exist that provide a form of coverage that is roughly equivalent to, but is not the same as, insurance. Indeed, this is precisely the case in many European health care systems that include a substantial direct-service element for hospital and specialist care. Rather than use a social insurance system to reimburse private providers, these nationalized delivery systems provide care directly through government-owned facilities and employed physicians without a third-party insurance intermediary.

Direct-access systems also exist in the United States in several guises, including the Indian Health Service (IHS) and student health facilities on university campuses. The largest example of a direct-access system is the Veterans Health Administration (VHA). At its core, the VHA covers health problems related to military service, but the VHA has expanded to cover most or all medical problems for some categories of veterans, such as those near poverty, and it provides service throughout the country. It is widely accepted that VHA enrollment constitutes acceptable coverage despite the absence of an official insurance aspect (Congressional Budget Office 2007; Sales 2008; Longman 2010). VHA enrollment meets the individual mandate requirement in both Massachusetts and under the new federal law. Adequacy is acknowledged despite the fact that many veterans have little choice among providers and must travel long distances to receive care from the VHA's broadly dispersed network of facilities (Mooney et al. 2000; LaVela et al. 2004; Shen et al. 2008).

An equally strong case can be made that enrolling with well-structured safety-net access programs in local communities confers a form of coverage equivalent to insurance. Viewing delivery system structure as the essential feature of coverage, rather than the legal form of insurance, is consistent with the current push to create accountable care organizations and other better-coordinated delivery systems. These innovations shift the focus from the particular form of background insurance or financing to the actual structure of provider networks that deliver care. In fact, some safety-net access programs for the uninsured already have the very features that the ACA seeks to promote under Medicare and private insurance. A series of case studies I have done (Hall 2010c) documents that these model safety-net programs have the following essential elements of coverage for the uninsured: they screen patients for eligibility and provide a membership identification card; they assign patients to a primary care medical home; and they arrange for prescription drugs and referrals to specialists, hospitals, and diagnostic testing as needed.

When members of these model safety-net programs are surveyed about health insurance, they often do not realize that they are technically uninsured. Despite limited or no choice of providers, these programs' structure and content feel very much like insurance to their members. This perceived equivalence has been noted in several different studies around the country (Andrulis and Gusmano 2000; Silow-Carroll et al. 2001; Cook and Ormond 2007; Long et al. 2008; Hall 2011).

Purists might object that safety-net access programs do not provide the type of legal entitlement needed for true coverage. Insurance entails a legally enforceable promise of coverage for a defined standard of care, usually pegged to prevailing professional standards for what is medically appropriate. The legal framing of safety-net access programs is quite different. This, after all, is what distinguishes them from the managed care Medicaid programs that often are run side by side, using the same management structure and provider networks. Safety-net programs for the uninsured specifically disavow any insurance-like undertaking. Some warn that their services are limited by available funding. And some free clinics and volunteer physicians cannot even be sued for malpractice. Aside from emergencies (which are governed by the Emergency Medical Treatment and Active Labor Act), uninsured safety-net patients have few or no enforceable legal rights to receive the medical care they are provided.

But, again, much the same is also true in European health systems. Some are forced by budget constraints to explicitly ration treatment in various ways that limit the capacity to provide care at the optimal level for all conditions. Broadly stated legal rights to health care are operationalized in many European countries only through the political process and not through the legal system, which is why scholars characterize these rights as social rather than individual rights (Bell 1998; Jost 2007). In theory, this means that a particular patient's claim to a specific service depends on how the patient's need is weighed against the expected needs of all other patients over the course of the same funding cycle. In practice, this means that, in some countries (such as England), courts rarely or never intervene in administrative or medical decisions about how best to allocate limited resources. Nevertheless, the form of coverage provided by these direct-access, noninsurance systems is considered to be socially just under broad international norms.

The other lesson learned from international norms, and reinforced by scholarly analysis, is that two-tiered coverage systems can achieve acceptable social justice (Krohmal and Emanuel 2007; Beauchamp and Childress 2008). Other than Canada (which enforces a pure single-tier insurance system by prohibiting private insurance that duplicates public coverage), most countries with social insurance allow people to opt out of the baseline public program by purchasing their own private coverage. People who can afford to do so are motivated by the fact the private coverage is distinctly superior; it minimizes any rationing and circumvents queues for service. Similar to private education, this inequity does not undermine social justice as long as the baseline system is minimally decent.

In the view of leading philosophers and social theorists, the same logic should apply in the United States (Krohmal and Emanuel 2007; Beauchamp and Childress 2008). The major difference here from Europe is that our higher tier is not one that people opt into. Instead, as embodied in Medicaid and employer-based insurance, the higher tier exists as a matter of right and social obligation. The two-tier structure, then, would arise not by allowing some people to purchase more but by purposefully providing less to some people than others. However, this does not negate the possibility that a lower-tier safety net could provide minimally acceptable access that is sufficient to count in our universality numerator. Whether a particular program in fact does so turns on how access is measured, and how "minimally acceptable" is operationalized, which we next address.

Access Metrics

Benchmarks

Volumes could be written on defining and measuring decent access, but to cut to the chase: my approach gauges adequacy using access metrics from equivalent insured populations that, by broad consensus, have minimally decent coverage. This is how Medicaid, for instance, determines whether its payment rates are adequate—by comparing access measures for Medicaid with those for privately insured patients (MedPAC 2010). Any other approach to defining adequacy embroils us in endless debates over what access levels are in theory acceptable or ideally achievable. Obviously, not all insurance coverage is the same, and economists battle over what levels and types of coverage are best (e.g., Gruber and Levy 2009). But we are not aiming for "best possible," only for a passing grade. By broad consensus, existing types of insurance generally provide minimally acceptable levels of access. Therefore, if a safety-net program for the uninsured shows risk-adjusted access levels that are within the actual range for comparable US populations with public or private insurance, the program's coverage should be regarded as at least minimally adequate.

In essence, we reverse the proposed direction of analysis. Instead of using access measures to determine insurance adequacy, insurance coverage that is thought to be adequate can be used to gauge acceptable access. Starting with insurance that is generally regarded as acceptable, we look to the levels of access reported by covered populations who are similar in risk profiles in order to generate metrics for evaluating access levels under noninsurance programs. But what measures of access should we consult? There are many to choose from (Eden 1998; Hoffman and Paradise 2008).

Access theorists distinguish among potential access, perceived access, and realized access (Bashshur, Smith, and Stiles 1993; Gold 1998; Kasper 1998). Potential access constitutes having a place to go when people are sick. Perceived access is measured by questions such as whether people have experienced problems obtaining needed care. Realized access, in contrast, is measured through actual patterns of service utilization, such as number and frequency of medical visits.

Few of these measures have an accepted gold standard (Davidson et al. 2004; Ricketts and Goldsmith 2005; Blewett, Ward, and Beebe 2006). We might even disagree, for instance, over whether everyone should have at least one doctor's visit per year, but even if that standard were accepted, it hardly resolves the total number of visits a population should have, since that depends, of course, on how population needs are assessed. Similarly, we might hope that no one ever encounters difficulty receiving care that they deem necessary or desirable, but that idealism is probably not achievable; even if it were, the goal tells us nothing about what shortfall from perfection constitutes acceptable access. Even having a usual source of care requires further interpretation of what "usual" means and agreement on whether the criterion is satisfied for someone who sees many different doctors.

Moreover, when access deficiencies are detected, they cannot necessarily be blamed on lack of insurance. Instead, there might be systemic shortages of available providers in a geographic area or language, transportation, or other barriers that obstruct access regardless of insurance status. The best solution to these confounding issues and inevitable imperfections is to benchmark access measures based on the range of responses from people similarly situated who are covered by insurance that is generally regarded as adequate.

In comparing access for uninsured populations with access for insured populations, it may not be necessary or even desirable to match the insurance population metrics. Some insurance may be too comprehensive, producing excess utilization because of "moral hazard." And insurance may distort the distribution of services—for instance, away from primary and preventive care and toward high-tech interventions. Despite the imperfections, however, insurance-based access standards should be regarded as at least adequate (or sufficient, even if not necessary). Therefore, if a noninsurance direct-access system comes close to the range of access metrics for an insured population, the safety-net direct-access system should be judged as at least minimally acceptable.

To correctly compare insured and uninsured populations, it is essential to minimize differences in population and geographic characteristics that might drive responses to these measures. Otherwise, the comparison group might falsely look the same only because it is healthier or less demanding or because it faces fewer noninsurance barriers than the benchmarking group, or vice versa.

Another difficulty is that minor variations in survey wording and methodology can substantially affect responses. Therefore, it is important, when possible, for comparison data to come from the same source and to cover similar time periods and geographic regions. Whitmore (1997), for instance, shows that responses varied from 6 to 45 percent among five different surveys that asked similar questions about problems getting needed care. Cunningham and Whitmore (1998) report a variation in having no usual source of care from 23 to 43 percent of people in twelve different communities who responded to the same question from a single survey. McCarthy and colleagues (2009) and the State Health Access Data Assistance Center (2006) report similar variations even at the level of statewide averages for insured and uninsured.

Despite these imperfections, there is a broad range of benchmarks from insured populations to which one might look in gauging key access measures for the uninsured. Table 10.1 shows responses to standard access questions from a variety of national surveys or state-level surveys. Across a range of surveys, insured people who report no usual source of care tend to range from 10 to 20 percent nationally. Across states the range is wider, from 5 to 27 percent depending on the particular survey, year, and type of insurance. Similar variations are seen for insured people who had difficulty receiving needed care and who did not have a doctor's visit in the past year (or two). These surveys suggest that direct-access safety-net programs might satisfy minimal adequacy and thus count toward universal coverage under a fairly wide range of access metrics that fall well short of optimal or ideal access.

Findings

The $64,000 question, then, is whether in fact any safety-net programs actually do provide access at levels within these general ranges. On average, safety-net systems for the uninsured are clearly inferior, as well documented in several large, national studies (Hadley and Cunningham 2004; Ross, Bradley, and Busch 2006; Gresenz, Rogowski, and Escarce 2007). But that is not our inquiry here. Because the strength of safety nets varies widely from one location to another, we look to see whether there are particular locations where access measures for low-income uninsured compare favorably to national norms for insured populations.

Looking first at the most sophisticated studies, which control for relevant differences in comparison populations, encouraging indicators emerge from some studies. A study of Denver's safety-net delivery system that adjusted for health risk and demographics found few disparities in the quality and quantity of selected areas of care (cancer screenings and management of various chronic diseases) provided to insured versus uninsured patients during 1999–2001 (Eisert, Mehler, and Gabow 2008). A second Denver study compared service frequencies during 2001–2005 between patients who remained uninsured and those who became insured (Eisert et al. 2009). After adjusting for relevant risk factors, the two groups had no significant difference in the frequency of primary care visits and only small differences in urgent care and specialty visits. In a national study, Zuckerman and colleagues (2004) found that Native Americans served by the IHS fared as well as people with insurance for standard access measures, such as having a usual source of care and having had a medical or dental visit in the past year, controlling for differences in age, gender, education, poverty level, health status, and community size. And a comparison of foreign-born residents in the United States versus Canada found few differences in access to primary and preventive care, despite the universality of social insurance in Canada (Lebrun and Dubay 2010).

Elsewhere, local comparisons usually show that uninsured people do worse than insured populations living in the same area, even in areas with better safety-net systems (Stanley, Cantor, and Guarnaccia 2008). This does not resolve, however, whether the uninsured in some locations do as well as the insured in *other* locations, or nationally. Recalling that our guide is minimal adequacy and not perfect equity, a local comparison might hold a safety-net system to a standard that is too demanding if the insured population locally happens to enjoy especially good access. In fact, this raised bar is more likely in the very same communities that have the best safety nets. This is because safety nets have been shown to have spillover effects on the entire community, since they draw from a common pool of local providers and medical resources and therefore support or deplete resources that serve both insured and uninsured populations (Institute of Medicine 2003; Pauly and Pagan 2007). Because purely local comparisons may fail to detect superior safety net performance, it is also relevant to compare local measures with national standards, or with levels in other locations.

Unfortunately, little sound data exists for either local or national comparisons. One important challenge is to determine how accurately standard surveys identify the relevant safety-net population. Direct-access safety-net programs target uninsured people with low incomes—typically less than 200 percent of poverty. But the sample sizes in national or state population surveys often limit their ability to report reliable results stratified at this level of specificity for both income and insurance status. For these reasons, surveys typically provide tabulations for all low-income people, including those who are on Medicaid, or for all uninsured, including the roughly half who are not eligible for safety-net programs due to having higher incomes. Also, the capacity of safety-net programs is often constrained such that they can enroll only a portion of people in the area who are potentially eligible, so even targeted population surveys would be too broad to measure performance of particular programs. Finally, in areas that have better safety-net programs, these surveys probably misclassify some uninsured people as being insured, for reasons explained above. Therefore, they may be least accurate in the very locations that have the best programs.

With these caveats in mind, there are scattered indications that some safety-net systems provide access that is at least minimally acceptable, judged by comparison to the insurance norms shown in table 10.1. (All surveys discussed here refer to nonelderly adults.) In Denver 26 percent of uninsured respondents reported not seeking medical care in 2007–2008 due to costs, and 18 percent of low-income people (below 250 percent of poverty) reporting having no usual source of care (Hall 2010b). In the Boston metropolitan area 35 percent of the uninsured in 2002 had no doctor's visit (Kennedy 2003), and in Massachusetts statewide 23 percent of the uninsured failed to receive needed care due to costs in 2006 (Hall 2010a). For low-income Massachusetts residents (below 300 percent poverty), 21 percent had no usual source of care in 2006, and 25 percent had no doctor's visit that year (Long and Phadera 2009).

In San Antonio 30 percent of members enrolled with the county's safety-net program for the uninsured had no primary care visit in 2007 (Hernandez et al. 2009). In Asheville, North Carolina, 20 percent of uninsured people had no usual source of care, and 30 percent failed to get needed care in 2000: the statistics were better for people below 200 percent of poverty (7 percent lacked a usual source of care, and 19 percent failed to get needed care) (Professional Research Consultants 2000). In San Francisco 78 percent of uninsured enrollees in the safety-net program had a primary care visit in the fiscal year 2008–2009, and 86 percent had a usual source of care (Chazin et al. 2010). In post-Katrina New Orleans, low-income adult patients of community health centers, 72 percent of whom were uninsured, reported better or much better

Table 10.1   **Access Problems for Nonelderly Insured Adults Reported in Various National Surveys**

		General Question (%)		
Survey	Population	No usual source of care	Difficulty getting needed care last year	No medical visits in past year (or two)
CTS (2003, 1997)	Private insurance	11	8	19
	Medicaid	13	13	15
	Insured, range across 12 cities		12–18	
MEPS (2004, 2007)	Private insurance	16	4	29
	Medicaid	15–20	6	26–35
	Private insurance, low-income	22	5	37
BRFSS (2007)	Insured, median state	12	8	13 (2 yrs)
	Insured, bottom 5 states	22	11	18 (2 yrs)
	Insured, top 5 states	8	5	7 (2 yrs)
NHIS (1993, 1996, 2008)	Private insurance	12	14	15
	Medicaid	13	32	14
	Private insurance, low income	15		
	Low income insured, range across 29 communities	5–27	4–17	8–33
PRC (2008)	Insured	20		36

Sources: For additional detail, see National Center for Health Statistics 1997; Brown 2000; State Health Access Data Assistance Center 2006; Kaiser 2009; McCarthy et al. 2009; Professional Research Consultants 2009.

access measures in 2009 than did the population generally, both in New Orleans or nationally (Doty et al. 2010). Better access measures included the ability to get needed care, to afford care, and to schedule appointments. In San Mateo County, California, adults enrolled in the county's direct-access program in 2009 reported access similar to norms for insured populations for measures such as usual source of care, ability to get needed care, and doctor's visit in the past year (Howell et al. 2010), and in Williamsburg, Virginia, uninsured adults reported access to primary and urgent care in 2007 similar to that for adults covered by Medicaid (Rossiter, Jensen, and Blanco 2007).

In surveys of about thirty metropolitan areas nationally, one-fifth of the cities reported that fewer than 19 percent of low-income uninsured had problems getting needed care in 1995–1996 (Brown, Wyn, and Teleki 2000), or that fewer than 15 percent of low-income people had no usual source of care in 1999–2000 (Billings and Weinick 2003). In statewide surveys in 2006–2007, low-income people (<200 percent poverty) in the best-performing five states averaged 17 percent without a usual source of care, 16 percent who were unable to see a doctor due to costs, and 7 percent with no routine check-up in two years (McCarthy et al. 2009).

Again, these indications are hardly conclusive. They come from surveys whose wordings and methods differ, and they do not accurately target the most relevant population (low-income uninsured covered by safety-net access programs). Moreover, this has been a selective reporting of only the most favorable indicators. In most of these same locations, there are other access measures that fall outside the ranges shown in table 10.1 (Hall 2010c; Hall 2011). Therefore, absent more precise measures, it remains largely undetermined whether well-structured safety-net access programs can consistently provide access that counts as minimally decent coverage, as indicated by these population survey measures. Still, at least some programs are able to meet or approach benchmarks for insured populations, and we have a better appreciation for how to gauge improvements or deficits on all such programs.

Conclusion

The ACA will still leave more than twenty million people without health insurance, well short of true universal access. But if open-access providers can also be supported in serving a safety-net function for the remaining uninsured, perhaps a workable compromise could be devised that would bring us to a minimally acceptable form of coverage that combines insurance with well-structured direct-access programs. Of the 7 percent of the US population estimated to remain without insurance, roughly a third will be eligible for

Medicaid and another quarter will be undocumented immigrants (Congressional Budget Office 2010; CMS Office of the Actuary 2010; Buettgens and Hall 2011). If adequate safety-net access were provided to even half of the remaining uninsured, we could be within sight of minimally acceptable coverage for at least 98 percent of legal residents—which is the international benchmark.

This goal is achievable but requires first that we understand how much safety-net capacity is required and how it should be distributed across rural and urban areas. Providers need active encouragement and financial support to take on these enhanced safety-net roles, and they must adopt well-defined policies about which patients they accept on a subsidized basis, and under what terms. These are tall orders to fill, so they should be placed with a clear and attainable goal in mind. This chapter's main objective is to help specify that goal. Understanding more concretely what constitutes universal coverage and acceptable access may help to motivate and guide efforts to patch the remaining holes left by the Affordable Care Act.

References

Andrulis, D., and M. Gusmano. 2000. "Community Initiatives for the Uninsured: How Far Can Innovative Partnerships Take Us?" *Grey Literature Report*. New York: New York Academy of Medicine.

Bashshur, R., D. G. Smith, and R. A. Stiles. 1993. "Defining Underinsurance: A Conceptual Framework for Policy and Empirical Analysis." *Medical Care Review* 50, no. 2: 199–218.

Beauchamp, T. L., and J. F. Childress. 2008. *Principles of Biomedical Ethics*. New York: Oxford University Press.

Bell, S. 1998. "Rationing the Right to Health." *Journal of Law and Medicine* 6:83–92.

Billings, J., and R. M. Weinick. 2003. "Tools for Monitoring the Health Care Safety Net." Agency for Healthcare Research and Quality. Rockville, MD: US Department of Health and Human Services.

Blewett, L. A., A. Ward, and T. J. Beebe. 2006. "How Much Health Insurance Is Enough? Revisiting the Concept of Underinsurance." *Medical Care Research and Review* 63, no. 6: 663–700.

Brown, E. R., R. Wyn, and S. Teleki. 2000. "Disparities in Health Insurance and Access to Care for Residents Across US Cities." Los Angeles: UCLA Center for Health Policy Research and New York: The Commonwealth Fund. http://www.healthpolicy.ucla.edu/Pubs/Publication.aspx?pubID=30.

Buettgens, M., and M. A. Hall. 2011. "Who Will Be Uninsured After Health Insurance Reform?" Princeton, NJ: Robert Wood Johnson Foundation. http://www.rwjf.org/coverage/product.jsp?id=49869.

Chazin, S., I. Friedenzohn, E. Martinez-Vidal, and S. A. Somers. 2010. "The Future of US Charity Care Programs: Implications of Health Reform." Hamilton, NJ: Center for Health Care Strategies, Inc.

Centers for Medicare and Medicaid Services (CMS) Office of the Actuary. 2010. "Estimated Financial Effects of the 'Patient Protection and Affordable Care Act,' as Amended." Baltimore: Department of Health and Human Services.

Congressional Budget Office. 2007." The Health Care System for Veterans: An Interim Report." Washington DC: United States Congress.

———. 2010. Letter to Honorable Harry Reid, Dec. 19, 2010. Washington, DC: United States Congress.

Cook, A., and B. A. Ormond. 2007. "Who Has Insurance and Who Does Not in the District of Columbia?" *Health Policy Brief No. 3.* Washington, DC: Urban Institute.

Cunningham, P. J., and H. H. Whitmore. 1998. "How Well Do Communities Perform on Access to Care for the Uninsured." Research Report No. 01. Washington, DC: Center for Studying Heath System Change. http://www.hschange.com/CONTENT/109/.

Davidson, P. L., R. M. Andersen, R. Wyn, and E. R. Brown. 2004. "A Framework for Evaluating Safety-Net and Other Community-Level Factors on Access for Low-Income Populations." *Inquiry* 41, no. 1: 21–38.

DeLia, D., and J. Cantor. 2009. "Emergency Department Utilization and Capacity." Princeton, NJ: Robert Wood Johnson Foundation.

Doty, M. M., M. K. Abrams, S. Mika, S. Rustgi, and G. Lawlor. 2010. "Coming Out of Crisis: Patient Experiences in Primary Care in New Orleans, Four Years Post-Katrina." New York: The Commonwealth Fund.

Eden, J. 1998. "Measuring Access to Care Through Population-Based Surveys: Where Are We Now?" *Health Services Research* 33, no. 3: 685–707.

Eisert, S. L., M. J. Durfee, A. Welsh, S. L. Moore, P. S. Mehler, and P. A. Gabow. 2009. "Changes in Insurance Status and Access to Care in an Integrated Safety Net Healthcare System." *Journal Community Health* 34, no. 2: 122–128.

Eisert, S. L., P. S. Mehler, and P. A. Gabow. 2008. "Can America's Urban Safety Net Systems Be a Solution to Unequal Treatment?" *Journal of Urban Health* 85, no. 5: 766–778.

Gold, M. R. 1998. "Beyond Coverage and Supply: Measuring Access to Healthcare in Today's Market." *Health Services Research* 33, no. 3: 625–652.

Gresenz, C. R., J. Rogowski, and J. J. Escarce. 2007. "Health Care Markets, the Safety Net, and Utilization of Care among the Uninsured." *Health Services Research* 42, no. 1 (Pt 1): 239–264.

Gruber, J., and H. Levy. 2009. "The Evolution of Medical Spending Risk." *Journal of Economic Perspectives* 23, no. 4: 25–48.

Hadley, J., and P. Cunningham. 2004. "Availability of Safety Net Providers and Access to Care of Uninsured Persons." *Health Services Research* 39, no. 5: 1527–1546.

Hall, M. A. 2010a. "The Costs and Adequacy of Safety Net Access for the Uninsured: Boston, Massachusetts." Princeton, NJ: Robert Wood Johnson Foundation.

———. 2010b. "The Costs and Adequacy of Safety Net Access for the Uninsured: Denver, CO." Princeton, NJ: Robert Wood Johnson Foundation. http://www.rwjf.org/files/research/safetynetdenver201006.pdf.

———. 2010c. "The Costs and Adequacy of Safety Net Access for the Uninsured." Princeton, NJ: Robert Wood Johnson Foundation. http://www.rwjf.org/coverage/product.jsp?id=49869.

———. 2011. "Access to Care Provided by Better Safety Net Systems for the Uninsured: Measuring and Conceptualizing Adequacy." *Medical Care Research and Review* 68:441.

Hernandez, G. B., L. B. Fornos, V. S. Mika, K. Urbansky, and R. Villarreal. 2009. "One Regional Health System's Innovative Steps to Deal with the Uninsured." *Journal of Health Care Finance* 36, no. 1: 70–84.

Hoffman, C., and J. Paradise. 2008. "Health Insurance and Access to Health Care in the United States." *Annals of the New York Academy of Sciences* 1136:149–160.

Howell, E. M., D. Hughes, S. Benatar, A. Klein, A. Palmer, and G. Kenney. 2010. "A Report on the Second Year of the San Mateo County Adult Coverage Initiative." San Mateo County Health System. Washington, DC: Urban Institute.

Huber, M., A. Stanciole, K. Wahlbeck, N. Tamsma, F. Torres, E. Jelfs, and J. Bremner. 2008. "Quality in and Equality of Access to Health Care Services." Brussels: European Commission." http://www.ehma.org/files/HealthQuest_en.pdf.

Institute of Medicine. 2003. *A Shared Destiny: Community Effects of Uninsurance*. Washington, DC: National Academies Press.

Jost, T. S. 2007. *Readings in Comparative Health Law and Bioethics*. Durham, NC: Carolina Academic Press.

Kaiser Commission on Medicaid and the Uninsured. 2009. "Low-Income Adults under Age 65: Many Are Poor, Sick, and Uninsured." Washington, DC: Kaiser Family Foundation. http://www.kff.org/healthreform/upload/7914.pdf.

Kasper, J. D. 1998. "Asking About Access: Challenges for Surveys in a Changing Health-care Environment." *Health Services Research* 33, no. 3: 715–739.

Kennedy, S. 2003. "Health Insurance Status of Massachusetts Urban Area Residents." Massachusetts Division of Health Care Finance and Policy. Boston: Commonwealth of Massachusetts.

Krohmal, B. J., and E. J. Emanuel. 2007. "Access and Ability to Pay: The Ethics of a Tiered Health Care System." *Archives of Internal Medicine* 167, no. 5: 433–437.

LaVela, S. L., B. Smith, F. M. Weaver, and S. A. Miskevics. 2004. "Geographical Proximity and Health Care Utilization in Veterans with SCI&D in the USA." *Social Science and Medicine* 59, no. 11: 2387–2399.

Lebrun, L. A., and L. C. Dubay. 2010. "Access to Primary and Preventive Care among Foreign-Born Adults in Canada and the United States." *Health Services Research* 45, no. 6 (Pt. 1): 1693–1719.

Long, S. K., and L. Phadera. 2009. "Health Insurance Coverage and Access to Care in Massachusetts: Detailed Tabulations Based on the 2009 Massachusetts Health Insurance Survey. Massachusetts Division of Health Care Finance and Policy." Boston: Commonwealth of Massachusetts. http://www.rwjf.org/coverage/product.jsp?id=49869.

Long, S. K., S. Zuckerman, T. Triplett, A. Cook, K. Nordahl, T. Siegrist, and C. Wacks. 2008. "Estimates of the Uninsurance Rate in Massachusetts from Survey Data: Why Are They So Different?" Massachusetts Division of Health Care Finance and Policy. Boston: Commonwealth of Massachusetts.

Longman, P. 2010. *Best Care Anywhere: Why VA Health Care Is Better Than Yours*. Sausalito, CA: PoliPointPress.

McCarthy, D., S. H. How, C. Schoen, J. C. Cantor, and D. Belloff. 2009. "Aiming Higher: Results from a State Scorecard on Health System Performance." New York: Commonwealth Fund Commission on High Performance Health Systems. http://www.commonwealthfund.org/~/media/Files/Publications/Fund%20Report/2009/Oct/1326_McCarthy_aiming_higher_state_scorecard_2009_full_report_FINAL_v2.pdf.

Medicare Payment Advisory Commission (MedPAC). 2010. "Report to the Congress: Medicare Payment Policy (March 2010)." http://www.medpac.gov/documents/Mar10_EntireReport.pdf.

Mooney, C., J. Zwanziger, C. S. Phibbs, and S. Schmitt. 2000. "Is Travel Distance a Barrier to Veterans' Use of VA Hospitals for Medical Surgical Care?" *Social Science and Medicine* 50, no. 12: 1743–1755.

National Center for Health Statistics. 1997. "Access to Health Care Part 2: Working-Age Adults." Washington, DC: Centers for Disease Control and Prevention. http://www.cdc.gov/nchs/data/series/sr_10/sr10_197.pdf.

Pauly, M. V., and J. A. Pagan. 2007. "Spillovers and Vulnerability: The Case of Community Uninsurance." *Health Affairs* 26, no. 5: 1304–1314.

Professional Research Consultants. 2000. "The Health of Buncombe County." Omaha, NE: Professional Research Consultants, Inc. http://www.buncombecounty.org/common/health/HealthOfBuncombeCounty2000.pdf.

———. 2009. "PRC National Health Report." Omaha, NE: Professional Research Consultants, Inc.

Ricketts, T. C., and L. J. Goldsmith. 2005. "Access in Health Services Research: The Battle of the Frameworks." *Nursing Outlook* 53, no. 6: 274–280.

Ross, J. S., E. H. Bradley, and S. H. Busch. 2006. "Use of Health Care Services by Lower-Income and Higher-Income Uninsured Adults." *Journal of the American Medical Association* 295, no. 17: 2027–2036.

Rossiter, L., C. Jensen, and M. Blanco. 2007. "Targeted Survey on Access to Physician Care in Medically Underserved Areas in the Foundation's Geographic Area." Williamsburg, VA: Schroeder Center for Healthcare Policy.

Sales, A. E. 2008. "The Veterans Health Administration in the Context of Health Insurance Reform." *Medical Care* 46, no. 10: 1020–1022.

Shen, Y., A. Hendricks, F. Wang, J. Gardner, and L. E. Kazis. 2008. "The Impact of Private Insurance Coverage on Veterans' Use of VA Care: Insurance and Selection Effects." *Health Services Research* 43, no. 1 (Pt 1): 267–286.

Silow-Carroll, S., S. E. Anthony, P. A. Seltman, and J. A. Meyer. 2001. "Community-Based Health Plans for the Uninsured: Expanding Access, Enhancing Dignity." *Community Voices*. Battle Creek, MI: W. K. Kellogg Foundation. http://www.community voices.org/Uploads/nu2eq555sghyrq45gcxhn0ew_20020828081946.pdf.

Stanley, A., J. C. Cantor, and P. Guarnaccia. 2008. "Holes in the Safety Net: A Case Study of Access to Prescription Drugs and Specialty Care." *Journal of Urban Health* 85, no. 4: 555–571.

State Health Access Data Assistance Center. 2006. "The Coverage Gap: A State-by-State Report on Access to Care." Princeton, NJ: Robert Wood Johnson Foundation. http://www.rwjf.org/files/newsroom/CoverageGap0406.pdf.

Whitmore, Heidi H. 1997. "Access to Health Care: Bridging the Gap between Policy and Research." Issue Brief No. 08. Washington, DC: Center for Studying Health System Change. http://hschange.org/CONTENT/73/.

Zuckerman, S., J. Haley, Y. Roubideaux, and M. Lillie-Blanton. 2004. "Health Service Access, Use, and Insurance Coverage Among American Indians/Alaska Natives and Whites: What Role Does the Indian Health Service Play?" *American Journal of Public Health* 94, no. 1: 53–59.

Public Coverage Expansions and Private Health Insurance Crowd-Out

Implications for Safety Nets

What Is Crowd-Out?

Historically, high numbers of individuals without health insurance have meant that the United States must deliver care to roughly 15 percent of the population through a fragmented health care safety net that includes Medicaid, federally qualified health centers, and a variety of sources of free care, such as free clinics (Department of Health and Human Services 2005). The severe economic downturn that began in 2007 and resulted in record high unemployment, combined with a private health insurance sector that is dominated by employer-supplied insurance, has resulted in an additional 5.6 million Americans without health insurance as of 2010 (Holahan 2010). High unemployment, and therefore high rates of uninsurance, is projected to persist if not increase through 2011. Unemployment is expected to remain high for several more years (Federal Reserve 2010).

For these reasons, enactment of the Patient Protection and Affordable Care Act (or Accountable Care Act, ACA) in 2010 seemed a potentially well-timed expansion of access to both private and public health insurance. However, as this chapter is being written in late 2010, there is credible political discussion of repealing all or parts of the act. If ACA opponents are successful, the need for adequate and comprehensive safety-net care is likely to be higher than at any time since enactment of Medicare and Medicaid in 1965. This may be further exacerbated by reductions in federal aid to states and shrinking state revenues resulting from political efforts to reduce deficit spending in response to recent US fiscal and economic problems.

Unfortunately, expansions in the safety net or publicly financed care are not without controversy. Underlying discussions about repeal of ACA and previous attempts to expand publicly provided care is an idea that lies at the heart of American economic thought: that the private sector is more efficient at producing and providing goods and services than the public sector. "Efficient" means the private sector produces more at lower cost and in the right mix and amounts—where "right" is determined by consumer preferences as revealed in their market purchases, constrained only by their budgets and prevailing prices. For this reason, the public sector and publicly provided health care, such as that supplied by safety-net providers or financed by the Medicaid program, are viewed by some with skepticism at best and with near hostility in the extreme. The idea of private sector efficiency or superiority drives much of the dialogue about both. It also gives rise to lawmaker and private interest group concerns that any expansions of the public sector will crowd out or displace the private sector. It is therefore no surprise that a considerable literature has arisen devoted to assessing the extent to which federal Medicaid and State Children's Health Insurance Program (SCHIP) eligibility expansions "crowd out" private provision and private financing of health care.

"Crowding-out" is a term that originated in macroeconomics where it is used to describe the effect of federal budget deficits on private investment spending (Krugman and Wells 2006). All else held constant, government borrowing to finance deficits tends to increase interest rates, thus raising the price of private borrowing and reducing private investment. Another form of macroeconomic crowd-out arises when government demand for goods and services bids up wage rates among firms and industries that provide the goods and services. This will tend to affect other private firms that draw from the same labor markets, causing them to face more sharply rising production costs. Over time, if an economy is at full employment, both forms of crowd-out will tend to shrink private sector output and raise private sector prices, reducing consumer welfare.

To the extent that the private sector has all the good (that is, efficient) qualities of competitive markets populated with fully informed rational consumers, then crowd-out will be harmful to individuals and to the public interest. It interferes with the efficient allocation of private capital and resources to sectors of the economy where demand and productivity are highest, thereby slowing economic growth. The important thing to note in this macroeconomic conceptualization of crowding-out is that the harm inflicted depends critically on at least three assumptions: the economy's being at full employment; the private sector's being competitive and, therefore, efficient (that is, no externalities, information asymmetries, or agency problems, and price is a reliable signal of marginal social cost); and consumers being rational and fully informed in some meaningful sense that permits them to accurately evaluate quality and prices of goods and services they purchase and to accurately assess future risks and returns to investment of present dollars and time. When these criteria are met, crowd-out results in welfare losses, costs that are borne by society and the individuals within it. When the criteria are not met, it is difficult to know whether expansion of the public sector will result in a welfare loss (Lipsey and Lancaster 1956).

Crowding-out appears to have taken on a slightly different meaning when it was first used by Cutler and Gruber (1996) to describe consumer substitution of public for private insurance as Medicaid eligibility expanded during the late 1980s. In this context, it is conceptualized as a reduction in public policy "bang" for each public "buck" expended on expanding public program eligibility to reduce the number of uninsured. For the most part, this meaning preserves the underlying conceptualization of crowd-out as something that negatively impacts social welfare. Cutler and Gruber measure crowd-out in health insurance markets as the reduction in probability of private insurance coverage, expressed as a share of total Medicaid uptake, as Medicaid eligibility is expanded.

Thus, public provision or subsidy of health insurance or medical care that results in increased access for previously uninsured individuals or families is viewed as a gain. However, if the gain is partially offset by a decrease in privately insured individuals, who are assumed to be substituting public programs or public insurance for private insurance, this is viewed as a loss. Under the substitution assumption, the loss is (1) to taxpayers who must now pay for previously privately insured services; (2) to policymakers who were trying to close the uninsured gap with dollar-for-dollar reductions in uninsurance rates; and (3) to private health insurers who lose revenues from individuals and families who substitute away from private insurance. Because the first and the last of these three are transfers from one entity to another, they do not necessarily reflect output-reducing economic "losses" in the commonly used sense of the term. Assessing welfare losses becomes difficult because individuals and families who substitute public for private insurance presumably also gain something.

Other researchers have used the term crowd-out to describe the phenomenon of different rates of public and private take-up when Medicaid is expanded. Some appear to have implicitly associated efficiency losses with the term. Rask and Rask (2000), in a study that examines the impact of public hospitals on private insurance coverage, state that there are costs associated with what is in effect a transfer from the private to the public sector, but they do not specifically identify the costs. Typical efficiency losses due to substitution away from the private sector might include increased transaction costs, higher prices, and lower quality. However, these are not discussed. This may be because in a "second-best" market such as health care (which economists consider to be less than socially optimal), there is no guarantee that a move from private insurance to public insurance represents such losses—that is to say, that there is a welfare loss in the Paretian sense (Lipsey and Lancaster 1956; Frick and Chernew 2009). Moreover, there is some evidence that Medicaid expansion may produce efficiency gains in terms of reductions in primary-care-preventable hospital admissions (Dafny and Gruber 2000; Aizer 2007). The value of such gains, to the individuals who experience them and to taxpayers and insurance beneficiaries who otherwise underwrite some or all of the costs of more expensive hospital care, should at least in part offset some of the losses associated with program expansion and crowd-out.

As can be seen, "crowding-out" is a term that implies a societal loss: in the macroeconomy due to loss of efficiency; in health care due to erosion of a policy goal of reducing the number of uninsured or increasing the number with access to health care per public dollar expended. In this chapter, I examine the literature on crowding-out in health insurance markets as erosion of a policy goal of an expanded health safety net that is ultimately aimed at improving social welfare. I provide a review of studies that have examined the issue and discuss their findings, starting first with Medicaid crowd-out of private insurance, and then considering crowd-out by safety-net programs for the uninsured. I conclude by discussing ways in which the concept of crowding-out in the context of health and social safety nets could be refined to ensure that the policy goal of improving social welfare is accurately conceptualized and comprehensively assessed.

How Medicaid Expansions Could Crowd Out Private Insurance

Employer Effects

One way that expansions in Medicaid eligibility might cause individuals or families to substitute away from private insurance is if employers cut benefits or increase employee contributions as public insurance becomes more generous. To date there has been little evidence of the former. Cutler and Gruber (1996) found some evidence consistent with this in a sophisticated econometric analysis of Medicaid crowd-out using the 1987–1992 Current Population Survey (CPS). Shore-Sheppard, Buchmueller, and Jensen (2000) and Buchmueller, Cooper, and Vistnes (2005) also find supporting evidence, as does Marquis (2005), who looked at safety-net effects on employer health benefit decisions using data from a large survey of employers. However, in all cases, the effects are quite small, which suggests that any crowd-out originates among families, not among employers. A more recent study from Massachusetts, the nation's only laboratory for universal health insurance, provides strong evidence that, at least as part of comprehensive health reform, employers not only continue to support health reform but more firms offer coverage (Long and Stockley 2009). Of course, there is no way of knowing at present whether the Massachusetts experience would generalize to other US states or the nation as a whole.

Consumer Effects

The other way in which public health insurance expansion might lead to private health insurance crowd-out is that individuals or families drop or fail to take up private insurance even in the absence of private insurance price rises or benefits cuts as public insurance eligibility expands to include them. However, eligible families can simply fail to enroll in Medicaid despite expansion in program eligibility. Card and Shore-Sheppard (2004) provide evidence that low take-up of Medicaid, rather than crowd-out of private insurance, is the causal mechanism for low expansion effects.

Unfortunately, it is methodologically challenging to distinguish between a voluntary shift from private to public insurance (crowding-out) and an involuntary shift due to loss of employment. Table 11.1 presents a simplified depiction

Table 11.1   **Counterfactual and Observed Insurance Status Changes with and without Public Program Expansions**

Person	Private insurance status in the absence of program expansions		Private insurance status after program expansions	
	Year 1	Year 2	Year 1	Year 2
1	Yes	No	Yes	No
2	Yes	No	Yes	No
3	No	No	No	No
4	No	Yes	No	Yes
5	Yes	Yes	Yes	*No*
6	Yes	Yes	Yes	Yes
Average	66%	50%	66%	33%

of the difference in these two processes. In this six-person example, we imagine the world as it would be without a public program expansion. This is the "counterfactual" that we do not observe experimentally when public programs are expanded. In table 11.1 we see that if we could have observed the world as it would have been without the public expansion, between years 1 and 2, persons 1 and 2 would have lost health insurance, possibly due to business-cycle effects or for personal reasons. Person 3 would have remained uninsured, person 4 would have obtained private insurance, and persons 5 and 6 would have retained their private insurance in year 2. The rightmost two columns of table 11.1 depict what is actually observed after a public program expansion in year 2. As you can see, most of our six individuals have the exact same insurance status in year 2 in this scenario as they did without the Medicaid expansion. However, person 5 in year 2 opts out of private insurance, presumably because of the expansion in eligibility. Person 5 is an example of crowd-out, and it is person 5 who must be identified and distinguished from persons 1 and 2 who would have lost or opted out of private insurance even in the absence of the expansion. The literature that I review has recognized this difficulty and has employed credible techniques, notably instrumental variables (IV) regression as well as other statistical approaches, in an effort to discriminate between the two causal mechanisms. For reasons discussed in the following, I am not confident that use of IV methods has successfully isolated the self-chosen (sometimes called endogenous) effects from the background macroeconomic business-cycle effects.

Business-Cycle Effects

More recent work by Reschovsky, Strunk, and Ginsburg (2006) using the Community Tracking Study Household Survey indicates that business-cycle effects on private employers are important. They find that changes in job quality that fluctuate with the business cycle, not Medicaid and SCHIP expansions, have large impacts on both employer offers and employee take-up of private health insurance. In fact, the authors liken publicly sponsored health insurance programs to a form of automatic stabilizer that plays a countercyclical role in dampening downturns in productivity and aggregate demand. Shore-Sheppard (2008) also provides compelling evidence that declines in private insurance coverage are due to these macroeconomic trends.

Establishing Causality between Medicaid Expansion and Private Insurance Crowd-Out

Establishing a causal link between Medicaid expansion and individual or family decisions to terminate private insurance because they now qualify for a public program such as Medicaid is difficult (Swartz 1996). Because Medicaid is a state-federal program, state expansions of eligibility criteria beyond federally mandated minima are likely to be endogenous. This means that they are likely to be chosen or designed by state lawmakers and, therefore, highly correlated with unobserved state macroeconomic and state-resident characteristics that may vary over time and that may also influence state-level trends in insurance coverage and individual decisions about purchase of private insurance. Thus, there is no guarantee that a federally mandated expansion will result in changes that are uncorrelated with state program characteristics, mainly because the federal mandate will tend to expand services more in states with more restrictive policies. For this reason, the magnitude and effects of an expansion that originates at the federal level may still capture endogenous state-level traits that will tend to bias estimates of private sector crowd-out, particularly if job quality and employment in those same states are more sensitive to business-cycle fluctuations. Estimates of Medicaid eligibility effects are then more likely to be biased by unobserved (and therefore uncontrolled) variables correlated with both Medicaid benefit expansions and state or individual characteristics that determine Medicaid use.

Despite these caveats, federal expansion of Medicaid eligibility during the late 1980s appeared to offer the possibility of a natural experiment that would allow researchers to investigate the extent to which the mix of public and private insurance coverage changed in response to a presumably exogenous policy change (Currie and Gruber 1996a). Unfortunately, there is evidence that, due to a concurrent business-cycle downturn, the policy change was preceded by dramatic nationwide declines in private health insurance coverage as unemployment increased (figure 11.1) (Shore-Sheppard 2008). Consequently, individuals who left private coverage and ended up covered by Medicaid must be viewed against a backdrop in which this was already occurring at an increasing rate even as Medicaid coverage was being expanded.

The seminal study of Medicaid crowd-out is that of Cutler and Gruber (1996), which estimated statistically significant and practically important crowd-out on the order of 50 percent (as a share of Medicaid uptake). To reduce bias from endogenous individual and family choice data, they used individual and family data from the 1987–1992 CPS and employed instrumental variables (IV) regression using an instrument developed in previous work by Currie and Gruber (1996a, 1996b). For the IV method to yield unbiased and precise coefficient estimates, it requires an "instrument" regressor that is highly correlated with the variable of interest (in this case, individual or family Medicaid or SCHIP eligibility) but uncorrelated with unobserved state,

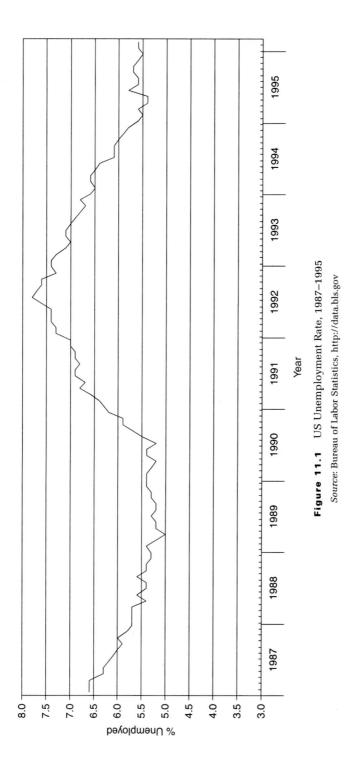

Figure 11.1 US Unemployment Rate, 1987–1995

Source: Bureau of Labor Statistics, http://data.bls.gov

business cycle, and individual-level determinants of federal-state expansions and individual insurance purchase decisions (Bound, Jaeger, and Baker 1995). The instrument then should identify the families or individuals who drop private insurance in response to the public expansion (for example, person 5 in table 11.1). This requires that the instrument be correlated with voluntary movement from private to public insurance and uncorrelated with involuntary movement from private to public insurance. In the case of nonlinear regression, restrictions on functional form through use of interaction terms may also provide identification (or at least capture unobserved time-varying state-level determinants of public program uptake that, if uncontrolled, may produce spurious estimates of crowd-out) (Shore-Sheppard 2008).

The instrument used by Gruber and Cutler was constructed to correlate with individual or family Medicaid eligibility but to be uncorrelated with other individual or family traits associated with insurance choice. It measured average state-year Medicaid eligibility applied to a national population standardized for race and age. This should also have the effect of purging the eligibility measure of correlation with state-specific population characteristics that might correlate with a state's political climate. There are potential problems with the instrument, however. One is that the year-state-age specific instrument could still be correlated with macroeconomic business-cycle trends. During the 1987–1992 period, a recession began in July 1990, with unemployment continuing to climb well past Election Day in November 1991 (see figure 11.1). Since private health insurance coverage is largely determined by employment and income in the United States, it is highly likely that much of the loss in private health insurance during this period was involuntary (for example, persons 1 and 2 in table 11.1) rather than a strategic attempt to substitute public for private insurance. The methods and language employed by Cutler and Gruber appear to assume that all changes from private to public coverage were voluntarily chosen. Yet a reasonable counterfactual would be that some people involuntarily dropped private insurance when they lost their jobs. It is not clear that the instrument used would identify only those who opted out of private insurance or into public insurance voluntarily.

Another potential problem with Cutler and Gruber's 1996 analysis, and with IV methods generally, is that, like all instruments, the variable used assumes that all families or individuals regardless of age, time period, and contemporaneous observed insurance status respond to the eligibility expansions in the same average way (Heckman 1997). However, there likely would be some variation in average response both over time and across age and insurance groups because of time-varying national economic trends and because of variations in age-coverage of federal mandates and state-specific expansions (see also Yazici and Kaestner 2000 for further discussion).

Shore-Sheppard (2008), using a slightly longer time period (1988–1996) and the same CPS March supplement data as Cutler and Gruber, provides evidence of differing responses to Medicaid expansions among children by age and time. Age-specific and state-specific differences in eligibility and coverage are apparent in raw data (see, for example, figures 2–5 in Shore-Sheppard 2008). When Shore-Sheppard estimated models that control for age-specific time trends, take-up and crowd-out estimates were substantially reduced. Shore-Sheppard also found evidence that later program expansions generated lower rates of public program take-up and private insurance crowd-out, which is consistent with the upturn in the business cycle during the later time period. As can be seen in figure 11.1, unemployment was falling from 1992 to 1995, which would be expected to result in higher uptake of private insurance and lower rates of uptake of Medicaid. (See also Ham, Li, and Shore-Sheppard 2009, figure 1, for evidence of business-cycle variation in children's health insurance coverage.)

I speculate that, in addition to providing identification, inclusion of age-specific time trends may also allow for better control of business cycle fluctuations that influence health insurance choice. The Shore-Sheppard (2008) results suggest that the instrument used by Gruber and Cutler is not uncorrelated with state macroeconomic trends and therefore may not yield unbiased estimates of consumer responses to Medicaid expansions. This is partly because it does not take into account age-specific time trends but also because it may be correlated with business cycle influences on insurance decisions by both families and employers.

Crowd-Out Estimates

The extensive literature that has built on Cutler and Gruber's seminal work has produced many often conflicting estimates of crowd-out by Medicaid/SCHIP. Table 11.2 duplicates and updates a table from Gruber and Simon's (2008) reexamination of crowd-out ten years after the original work by Cutler and Gruber. In what follows, I discuss selected articles and summarize the results from all studies included in table 11.2.

As noted, Cutler and Gruber (1996)—using 1987–1992 CPS data and a methodologically sound IV approach—established the initial crowd-out benchmark, that expansion of Medicaid coverage was offset by a roughly 50 percent decline in private insurance coverage. Dubay and Kenney (1997), also using CPS data from 1988 to 1992, found no evidence of crowd-out among

Table 11.2 Literature on Medicaid Crowd-Out

Article	Data Source	Methodology	Crowd-out Definition	Results
Cutler and Gruber (1996)	1987–1992 CPS	Instrument eligibility with simulated eligibility based on entire nation; control for state, year, age; consider family-level spillovers	(Reduction private insurance/growth public insurance) or (1 − [Change in uninsured/growth public insurance])	Children: 31–40% Family level: 50%
Dubay and Kenney (1996)	1988 & 1993 CPS	Change in insurance coverage of children relative to change for adult men	(Reduction private insurance/growth public insurance)	Below poverty: 15% 100–133%: 22%
Dubay and Kenney (1997)	1988 & 1992 CPS	Change in insurance coverage of pregnant women relative to change for men	(Reduction private insurance/growth public insurance)	Below poverty: 0% 100–133%: 27% 133–185%: 59%
Thorpe and Florence (1998)	1989–1994 NLSY	Measure movement from private insurance onto Medicaid among children with privately insured parents	% of those entering Medicaid with privately insured parents	16%
Blumberg, Dubay and Norton (2000)	1990 SIPP Panel	Compare change in insurance coverage of children made eligible by expansions to those not made eligible	% of children made eligible losing private relative to gaining public	4%
Yazici and Kaestner (2000)	1988 & 1992 NLSY	Compare change in insurance coverage of children becoming eligible to those not becoming eligible	(1 − [Change in uninsured/growth public insurance]) or (Reduction private insurance/growth public insurance)	55–59% or 5–24%
Aizer and Grogger (2003)	1995–2002 CPS	Compare change in insurance for those above AFDC eligibility vs. below, in states with adult expansion, before vs. after expansion	Coefficient on private coverage equation (no crowd-out calculations)	Statistically insignificant effect on private coverage for mothers and for children

Study	Data	Method	Measure	Estimate
Card and Shore-Sheppard (2004)	1990–1993 SIPP Panels	Compare changes in insurance coverage of children around income and age limits for eligibility	(Reduction private insurance/growth public insurance)	Below poverty: 0 100–133: 50%
LoSasso and Buchmueller (2004)	1996–2000 CPS	Instrument eligibility with simulated eligibility based on entire nation; control for state, year, age, state-year; interact with state waiting periods	(Reduction private insurance/growth public insurance)	Average: 50% Varies with state waiting periods
Ham and Shore-Sheppard (2005)	1985–1995 SIPP	Instrument eligibility with simulated eligibility based on all other states; control for state, year, age	(Reduction private insurance/growth public insurance)	No crowd-out
Hudson, Selden and Banthin (2005)	1996–2002 MEPS	Compare changes in children made eligible and remaining ineligible; instrument with simulated eligibility	(Reduction private insurance/growth public insurance)	Comparison: 25–55% IV: 39–70%, imprecise and unstable
Gruber and Simon (2008)	1996–2002 SIPP	Same as Cutler-Gruber in assigning simulated eligibility. Also use cross tabulation method like Card and Shore-Sheppard; however, income held fixed and considered endogenous to expansion	(1 – [Change uninsured/growth public insurance]) or (Reduction private insurance/growth public insurance)	47–92%
Shore-Sheppard (2008)	1987–1995 CPS	Same as Cutler-Gruber, but add additional controls—children only	(1 – [Change uninsured/growth public insurance]) or (Reduction private insurance/growth public insurance)	No crowd-out
Dave, et al. (2008)	1985–1991 NHDS	Same as Cutler-Gruber, but normed to state-specific sample	(Reduction private insurance/growth public insurance)	50%

poor pregnant women (incomes <100 percent of the federal poverty level [FPL]). However, they did find evidence to suggest that pregnant women with incomes between 100 and 185 percent of FPL substitute away from private health insurance to Medicaid. Using a slightly different measure of crowd-out, they attributed 27–59 percent of the expansion in Medicaid coverage among this group to women who had previously been covered by employer-sponsored private plans. They arrived at this estimate by comparing rates of leaving private insurance among near-poor pregnant women and near-poor men. A decline in employer-sponsored health insurance among near-poor men, who would not be covered by Medicaid expansions, was taken as evidence that not all loss of private coverage among near-poor pregnant women was a strategic response to Medicaid expansions. The difference in crowd-out by income group is consistent with Cutler and Gruber (1996), who also found evidence of smaller crowd-out for women and families below poverty but moderate crowd-out for pregnant women between 133 and 185 percent of poverty.

Thorpe and Florence (1998) examined the proportion of children with privately insured parents who switched to Medicaid as it was expanded. Their results indicate that only about 16 percent of children switched. This is in line with results obtained by Yazici and Kaestner (2000) using data from the 1988–1992 National Longitudinal Survey of Youth (NLSY) and a difference-in-difference analysis to compare insurance status between children who became eligible during that period and children who did not. They estimate that roughly 14 percent (5 to 24 percent, depending on how the comparison group of noneligibles is specified) of expanded Medicaid coverage among children is due to substitution away from private to public health insurance.

The strength of the Yazici and Kaestner study is the use of a rich longitudinal data set that allows them to identify more accurately children whose families became newly eligible, and to compare them with several control groups, including children whose families were not eligible. Use of longitudinal data provides some confidence about establishing causal links since actual changes over time within the same family can be observed more accurately. The study also provides some insight into possible problems with other studies. Specifically, when they attempted to use similar approaches to those of Cutler and Gruber (1996) and Shore-Sheppard (2008), they estimated extremely high and implausible crowd-out effects from the NLSY data. They concluded that the instruments used in IV regression methods employed by previous researchers are flawed.

Because of the obvious advantages of longitudinal data in observational studies, several subsequent studies have used the Survey of Income and Program

Participation (SIPP), which provides a longitudinal sample, albeit smaller than the NLSY and with some states not uniquely identified for confidentiality reasons. Blumberg, Dubay, and Norton (2000) examined changes in health insurance coverage among children who gained eligibility from Medicaid expansions and concluded that, compared to those who gained public insurance, only 4 percent as many lost private insurance. Shore-Sheppard (2008), using the CPS (the same data set used by Gruber and Cutler 1996) but a longer time frame (1987–1995) and a model specification that allowed child responses to program expansions to vary across states and by age and year, found little evidence of crowding-out. She also found that later expansions appeared to generate evidence of much lower Medicaid take-up rates and private insurance crowd-out. Her findings highlight the importance of business cycle conditions since rising national output and declining unemployment characterized the latter part of her time frame.

Hudson, Selden, and Banthin (2005) investigated the impact of SCHIP on children's insurance coverage using the 1996–2002 Medical Expenditure Panel Survey. Using both IV and difference-in-difference models, they found SCHIP to have an important positive impact on increasing insurance rates among children targeted by both SCHIP and Medicaid. However, their attempts to estimate crowd-out effects were highly unstable, very sensitive to changes in specification, and very imprecise. They concluded that "it is difficult to draw economic and policy significance from estimates of crowd-out" and they cautioned policymakers "from interpreting any measure of crowd-out as a definitive measure" (248).

More recently, Gruber and Simon (2008), using the SIPP and model specifications similar to those of Shore-Sheppard, found evidence of considerable crowding-out. They revisited the earlier work by Cutler and Gruber (1996) but instead used the longitudinal 1996–2002 SIPP. They used the same measure of crowd-out as Cutler and Gruber and an additional measure: [one minus (the change in probability of private coverage/the change in probability of public insurance expansion)]. The latter was aimed at avoiding a problem that plagued previous studies: that some Medicaid recipients report both Medicaid and private insurance during the same recall or reporting period. Gruber and Simon argued that the latter measure is more appropriate if it is assumed that most people in this "overlap" group are moving from private to public insurance and not the other way around. They estimated Medicaid crowd-out effects that range from 47 to 92 percent, which conflicts rather dramatically with Shore-Sheppard's (2008) finding of no crowd-out.

Another potential caveat of the Gruber and Simon study is their implausible finding that state anti-crowd-out regulations (such as requiring privately insured individuals and families to be uninsured for some minimum amount of time—two months—before they can qualify for Medicaid) actually produce *more* crowding-out. A more likely explanation is that their instrument, the same used in the 1996 study, is not uncorrelated with state-specific traits that influence Medicaid expansions beyond those mandated at the federal level or to state-specific macroeconomic trends that influence state adoption of anti-crowd-out restrictions. If anti-crowd-out legislation is endogenous (more likely to be passed in states where the near-poor are more likely to be losing private insurance at high or increasing rates), and if Gruber and Simon's simulated instrument is correlated with state sentiments that favor anti-crowd-out legislation, this could account for waiting periods appearing to increase take-up of Medicaid.

Dave and colleagues (2008) used 1985–1996 National Hospital Discharge Survey data to investigate the impact of Medicaid expansions on infant health. They employed a state-specific measure of Medicaid eligibility that is like that of Cutler and Gruber, except it is normed to a state-specific sample rather than a national sample. Using a variety of specifications and functional forms, they estimated crowd-out effects that are quite similar to those of Cutler and Gruber, on the order of 50 percent. They confirmed previous findings that estimates are sensitive to inclusion of state-specific trends. They also found that crowd-out effects are most pronounced among white women and at higher levels of eligibility.

The problem with many of the studies to date is that they rely on instrumental variables or difference-in-difference estimates to establish causal estimates of the magnitude of substitution of public for private insurance (like person 5 in table 11.1). When confronted with a sizable portion of families or individuals who report both public and private insurance, the assumption seems to be that all are moving from private to public, and doing so voluntarily. Unfortunately, the only way to be truly certain about the proportion of individuals who drop private insurance in response to expanded availability of public insurance while holding other economy-wide trends constant is to employ longitudinal data sets that include accurate income and insurance variables accompanied by information about reasons for changing insurance. Such a data set is not available. Therefore, researchers have been forced to impute such things as pregnancy status and to assume that those who move from private to public insurance are doing so voluntarily. A few credible efforts to examine the issue using longitudinal data indicate low levels of crowd-out, but even these are not perfect studies, mainly because of data limitations.

Discussion

What are we to make of the equivocal findings from many studies that for the most part represent sound econometric methods applied to less than ideal data? Is public sector crowd-out of the private sector an important problem when public safety-net programs are expanded? The one consistent finding is that, if there is private sector crowd-out, it appears to occur most frequently and most importantly from a policy perspective among individuals and families who are above the federal poverty line but not too far above it. This seems plausible since individuals and families below the FPL do not participate in private health insurance markets in significant enough numbers to result in substantial crowd-out. The results also seem plausible because they suggest that the farther above poverty a family or individual rises, the less likely it is that they will find public insurance an attractive substitute for private insurance. Stigma and inconvenience, time costs, and other barriers have been suggested as reasons for this (Cutler and Gruber 1996; Card and Shore-Sheppard 2004). Ham, Li, and Shore-Sheppard (2009) and Shore-Sheppard's (2008) findings that fluctuations in take-up and crowd-out appear to be somewhat cyclical (Medicaid) and countercyclical (private insurance) with business cycle fluctuations suggest that care must be taken in assuming that any change in insurance status is voluntary and runs only one way (from private to public). Moreover, given the strong link between health insurance and employment in the United States, crowd-out, if any, is most likely to be observed in those income groups affected by eligibility expansions and that are most vulnerable to output contractions and the accompanying growth in unemployment. Since affected income groups and sectors may vary from recession to recession (Boushey 2010), any crowd-out that results is also likely to vary.

What is the likely magnitude of such crowd-out among individuals and families who teeter on the edge of poverty and topple as the business cycle waxes and wanes? Estimates of the crowd-out in this group range from 0 to 16 percent, but possibly go as high as 25 percent. Three studies (Cutler and Gruber 1996; Dave et al. 2008; Gruber and Simon 2008) put the estimates higher. It is hard to reconcile the higher estimates of these studies with lower estimates from all other studies except to note that work by Yazici and Kaestner (2000) and Shore-Sheppard (2008), in combination with the counterintuitive waiting period results in the Gruber and Simon (2008) study, suggest that the instrument used in two of the high-estimate studies may not have been uncorrelated with state or regional business cycle fluctuations. If this were the case, it would tend to bias the IV estimates of crowd-out and could lead to the large-in-magnitude results from these two studies. This is perhaps not surprising.

While theoretically sound, IV estimates have been much less reliable in practice (Bollen, Guilkey, and Morz 1995; Bound, Jaeger, and Baker 1995; Staiger and Stock 1997). Results from Hudson, Selden, and Banthin (2005) provide further evidence that IV estimates may be unreliable in formulating policy aimed at improving insurance rates. The empirical problems with IV estimators may be further exacerbated by measurement error induced by sometimes multiple imputations of key covariates that do not accurately identify survey respondents who are or who might become eligible for Medicaid (such as pregnancy status, income, and other state-level eligibility determinants).

Because of the considerable uncertainty regarding the size of substitution and the danger that large but imprecise or, worse, biased estimates may divert policymakers from efforts to close the access gap, it might make sense to follow the advice of Hudson, Selden, and Banthin (2005) and focus the policy debate on changes in *net benefits* that result from program expansions and public–private substitution, rather than on the magnitude of crowd-out alone. Current studies appear to assume implicitly that any crowd-out diminishes public or social welfare, even when narrowly defined as bang per public buck. However, it may be that even large amounts of substitution do not represent a large societal loss when all aspects and consequences of public expansions are considered. Holahan (1997) estimates that even at the fairly high crowd-out rates estimated by Cutler and Gruber (1996), only about 1 percent of Medicaid spending is attributable to crowd-out.

Among the group in which crowd-out appears to be most prevalent— families with income between 100 and 200 percent of the FPL—other micro- and macroeconomic trends must also matter. Over the period of the reviewed studies, other trends besides Medicaid expansion almost certainly influenced individual and family choices about health insurance. Increasing price (Chernew, Cutler, and Keenan 2005) and declining comprehensiveness (Reschovsky, Strunk, and Ginsburg 2006) in private insurance along with improved under-writing screens no doubt altered the optimization calculus among the near-poor who were trading off an increasingly higher-priced, less-comprehensive, lower-quality private product against higher time price, uncertain eligibility, and other barriers to obtaining public insurance (Baicker et al. 2010).

In 1988 a family of four making $11,650 was at 100 percent of the FPL. By 2005 the threshold had risen an average of 4 percent per year to $19,350, reflecting the roughly 65 percent increase in the consumer price index over that time period (Department of Health and Human Services 2010). However, over the same period, health insurance premiums increased by an average of 10.4 percent per year, outpacing increases in workers' earnings and general price inflation. More recently the rate of increase in health insurance premiums has exceeded the rate at which the FPL has increased by a factor of four or more (Kaiser Family Foundation 2010). These price changes alone would be expected to cause declining private coverage even in the absence of public program expansions (Kronick and Gilmer 1999; Gilmer and Kronick 2005).

Against the backdrop of business cycle fluctuations, rising private price, and declining private comprehensiveness, it is hard to imagine that any families strategically substituting public for private coverage are necessarily made worse off, at least if we believe in sovereign consumers making rational choices about how to allocate scarce dollars. While such substitution may erode a policy goal of reducing the rate of uninsured and may also transfer insurance costs from low-income individuals and families to taxpayers, its impact on overall welfare is complex and not easily evaluated. To make such an evaluation, it would be necessary to evaluate the nature and magnitude of potential societal losses as well as any gains that such crowding-out might represent.

In the most common sense of the term "crowd-out," the concern would be that public provision of health services and insurance crowds out private provision of the same, thereby incurring efficiency losses. This concern presupposes that the private sector is able to provide services more efficiently in terms of quality, mix, and amounts than the public sector. Yet it is doubtful that the private health insurance sector is more efficient than the public sector given the many market failures that characterize these private markets. For a variety of well-documented reasons having to do with price setting, information asymmetries, and agency problems, private health insurance markets and private medical care markets do not have the characteristics of perfectly competitive markets. Moreover, many private insurers have managed over time to capture what many would regard as monopolistic shares in some markets (GAO 2002; Furnas and Buckwalter-Poza 2009). Of course, this is not surprising, nor is it necessarily inefficient, since smaller firm size would increase risk variances, placing them at higher risk for medical losses. However, in light of their large size and market shares, they cannot be assumed to be constrained by a competitively determined market demand curve that determines the price at which they can sell their products.

Nor can we be confident that consumer surplus, the traditional Paretian measure that underlies efficiency arguments aimed at improving welfare, is maximized. Evidence of inefficiency is readily available. We know that US health care costs twice as much per capita as any other developed country (Kaiser Family Foundation 2007), delivers lower population health outcomes (ibid.), and—until full phase-in of the ACA in 2014, if it occurs—leaves a substantial proportion of Americans uninsured. Underwriting costs for private health insurance cause private administrative costs to exceed those of public health insurance (Medicare) by a factor of at least three to four (Social Security and Medicare Boards of Trustees 2009). In addition, financial incentives created by private (and to some extent public) health insurance reimbursement policies distort resource allocation away from prevention and chronic disease management and toward complex, high-tech (and in many cases marginally beneficial) rescue and end-of-life care. Increased moral hazard associated with expanded health insurance coverage may also represent a welfare loss. However, if expanded coverage moves consumers to demand an amount and mix of health care that is closer to the socially optimal amount and mix, then that assumed loss may be overstated (Nyman 2008; Frick and Chernew 2009). Moreover, there may be other side effects of expanded coverage, such as increased labor force participation, that should be taken into account in evaluating welfare gains and losses associated with any crowding-out (Yelowitz 1995).

Crowding-Out of Private Sector Providers
or Insurers by Safety-Net Providers

The ACA, if not subsequently repealed, will lead to a large and important expansion in Medicaid eligibility. At present, the proportion of Americans without health insurance has risen from forty-six to fifty-one million as a result of the 2007 economic downturn (DeNavas-Walt, Proctor, and Smith 2010). This is largely the result of a roughly three-percentage-point decline between 2008 and 2009, from 58.5 to 55.8 percent, in employer-provided insurance that has left the proportion covered by such plans at its lowest level since 1987 when the statistic was first recorded. Over the same time, the proportion of people covered by government health insurance increased from 29 to 30.6 percent. Full enactment of ACA in 2014 is expected to provide health insurance coverage to roughly 70 percent of the currently uninsured (Wilen-Berg 2010). This means that there will still be a role for safety-net providers: for undocumented workers, the homeless, and for those ineligible for Medicaid and who opt to face a relatively low-priced penalty rather than purchase subsidized, but still more expensive, mandated private insurance.

Two studies have attempted analyses of safety-net crowd-out. Rask and Rask (2000) find that the availability of a local public hospital reduces by 3.5 to 8.6 percent the probability that families with incomes between 100 and 400 percent of the federal poverty level will have private insurance. They observed income effects similar to those observed in studies of public insurance crowd-out, with higher income individuals less likely to view publicly supplied hospital care as a close substitute for private insurance. Unfortunately, the authors do not control for the potential reverse causality (sometimes called endogeneity) between the supply of public hospital beds and the supply of private insurance in local areas.

Herring (2005) provides the most econometrically heroic of these two studies. In a manner similar to that of Cutler and Gruber (1996), he attempts to construct an instrument that is uncorrelated with local area supply of private insurance but correlated with local area "altruism" (or preferences for charity care), as manifested by the ease with which uninsured local area residents report being able to access affordable care. As with most IV estimates, something of a leap of faith is required. The leap is that the variable he constructs is truly correlated with local preferences for charity care provision and that those preferences are not influenced by local area supply of private insurance (or demand for charity care). My confidence in the constructed instrument is weakened by its strong negative correlation with provision of private insurance in the bivariate probit results and its weak correlation with individual uptake of private insurance. Assuming the instrument is sound, the results suggest a very small crowd-out effect. A 10 percent expansion in the variable purported to capture local altruism (independent of the amount of safety-net care actually provided) results in only about a 1 percent contraction in the demand for private insurance. Like other researchers, Herring finds a stronger substitution effect for families who are <300 percent of the federal poverty level, compared to their more affluent counterparts. He fails to reject the null hypothesis despite a difference between income groups that may be important. The high income uninsured group is much smaller, which may account for the failure to achieve statistical significance. Herring rightly notes that a number of other factors, including stigma, price, and quality of care, none of which are included in his model or in his empirical estimation, may also be influencing individual take-up of private insurance, particularly among the higher income group. He concludes by noting that without some knowledge of the incremental effects of different sources of health care on health outcomes, it is difficult to assess the true public and private gains and losses from any substitution away from the private sector.

How the ACA will change the tradeoffs made by individuals and families remains to be seen. The relative appeal of the public sector, and especially of safety-net providers, will depend on incentives created by the law. The individual mandate and noncompliance penalty may provide incentives to surmount enrollment barriers, such as red tape, if an individual or family is

Medicaid-eligible. Similarly, the mandate and penalty increase incentives to remain enrolled in or to obtain private insurance if Medicaid-ineligible. How this plays out will be an important topic for future research and policy development.

There is also some uncertainty about how safety-net providers will fare under health reform (Siegel, Shin, and Regenstein 2004; Katz 2010). Expansion of Medicaid eligibility should enhance provider finances, thereby enabling safety-net providers to become more competitive. However, they might also be forced to compete with private health care providers to retain or gain market share among Medicaid eligibles (Siegel, Shin, and Regenstein 2004). The mix of patients within market share will also matter. If the private sector is able to entice the healthiest of the currently uninsured, leaving safety-net providers with the sickest and without some means of recovering the higher costs of such patients, safety-net providers will fail. On the other hand, if safety-net providers successfully compete by providing high-quality, integrated medical care and chronic disease management that result in better health outcomes, they may become a more attractive option for near-poor individuals and families, enticing them away from private insurers and providers.

If safety-net providers were to induce crowd-out, it could well be with both Medicaid and the private sector, given the safety net's historical mission to deliver low-cost, high-quality care to vulnerable populations. As with Medicaid crowd-out examined earlier, I would expect this phenomenon to be most prevalent among the near-poor. It will be exacerbated if barriers to obtaining either private or Medicaid coverage, such as money price, time price, and bureaucratic red tape, are high. Whether or not this represents a welfare loss will depend on whether safety-net providers are better or worse at delivering preventive care and chronic disease management. If they are better, then the individuals who choose to use them may be much better off in terms of health, well-being, and disposable income. If this translates into higher labor force productivity and reduced emergency care use and hospital admissions, then the larger society, facing an ethical constraint to provide and pay for such care either directly or indirectly, may also be better off or at least not as badly off as an analysis that does not take account of these gains would suggest.

In light of safety-net providers' dependence on state and federal aid, any crowd-out of the private sector will impact taxpayers. However, the welfare effects will depend on whether the net societal benefits from safety-net care exceed the net societal benefits from private sector care. If the private sector is more fragmented and less efficient at providing care to chronically ill and disadvantaged populations, it may be more cost-beneficial to have the care delivered by safety-net providers. It is also possible that competition with more efficient and effective safety nets could improve private sector care. This could be seen as a form of "crowding-in" in which private sector provision of care becomes more efficient and expands coverage over time.

Perhaps the most serious potential problem associated with safety-net crowding-out of private health insurance could be its impact on private risk pools that the ACA attempts to create through mandated coverage. If the young and healthy opt for safety-net care, then the safety-net will siphon low-risk individuals from risk pools that require their participation in order to manage risk and costs efficiently.

Conclusion

Passage of the ACA in 2010 could mean that the issue of Medicaid crowding-out is less salient than it was in a more fragmented system with a large proportion of uninsured. But if all or parts of the ACA are repealed, then the financing and provision of care to the uninsured and to low-income families will continue to command both moral and economic center stage in any discussion of US health care costs. However, even if the ACA remains intact and funded, the tension between public and private financing of health insurance is likely to remain acute, if only because of ideological differences about government's role in what some believe are or should be quasi-private, quasi-competitive markets. In addition, there will be some families and individuals who fall through the ACA's gaps because they are undocumented and the law does not cover them; they live on the fringes of society, whether in homeless shelters or under bridges, where they may escape the individual mandate for a variety of reasons; or they simply opt to risk the penalty of defying the mandate.

For these reasons, we need a more critical examination of what to date has been a rather simplistic conceptualization of crowding-out and, implicitly, of the welfare losses and gains associated with the substitution of public for private health insurance or care. This will require us to ask and to answer more complex questions. For example, if public insurance expansions result in lower-priced, higher-quality, more-comprehensive coverage for the near-poor than they can obtain in private markets, does this represent a welfare loss or a welfare gain? If private insurers cannot compete successfully with publicly funded and provided insurance on these three dimensions, is this evidence of market failure? Why is private provision taken to be the preferred method for structuring and obtaining health insurance if consumer surplus is larger for some when health insurance is publicly financed? If all or part of the final "price" will be paid by taxpayers and private insurers who to some extent underwrite the costs of charity care, then should we not evaluate that price in light of the likely costs to taxpayers of untreated contagion, expensive primary-care-preventable emergency care, poorly managed chronic disease, reduced health outcomes, and higher costs? As long as there is a moral imperative to treat the ill and injured, surely sound economic analysis requires us to consider cost minimization (subject to quality and ethical constraints) from a societal perspective rather than from the perspective of a single interest group, whether it is taxpayer, insurer, or Medicaid recipient? The ethical and economic aspects of timely disease prevention and health promotion almost certainly figure in this calculation.

As part of a new perspective, we need also to determine how we should weigh the obvious gains to poor and near-poor families when income previously spent on higher-priced, less-comprehensive private policies is freed up through publicly provided care. These freed resources could be allocated to other privately produced goods and services that provide better nutrition, education, and health, and other attributes of welfare. Is an allocation away from privately but possibly *inefficiently* produced goods and toward other privately but *efficiently* produced goods a welfare gain or a welfare loss? What about when those gains translate into higher labor force participation and reduced welfare rolls? Should we not include those social and individual benefits in the utilitarian calculation of the value of publicly provided coverage or access?

If the marginal utility of income diminishes with increasing income, then the reduction in utility that results from payment of high private health insurance premiums is much higher for the poor or near-poor than it is for those further up the economic and social pyramid. If the utilitarian goal is to increase total happiness, then so-called crowd-out may be welfare enhancing. In purely monetary terms, monopoly rents to insurers and physicians shrink an already small market basket and they crowd out goods and services that are also necessary for health and human capital production and investment. If this leads to higher social immobility, reduced future productivity, and slowed economic growth, we all lose. As health reform continues to evolve, it is critical that discussions about public–private crowd-out take a broader and more informed perspective, one that recognizes the disparity between the efficiency posited by economic welfare theory and the real potential waste of diverting resources to failed private markets and away from hard-working families who live at or near poverty. At a minimum, future theoretical and empirical research should be directed to answering empirically some of the questions posed here, before we act unequivocally as though public crowd-out of private health insurance is always and everywhere a net loss.

Acknowledgments

Funding for this chapter was provided by the Robert Wood Johnson Foundation. The author wishes to thank Keshia Maughn for invaluable research assistance in the preparation of this manuscript. All errors are my own.

References

Aizer, A. 2007. "Public Health Insurance, Program Take-Up, and Child Health." *Review of Economics and Statistics* 89, no. 3: 400–415.

Aizer, A., and J. Grogger. 2003. "Parental Medicaid Expansions and Health Insurance Coverage." NBER Working Paper 9907. Cambridge, MA: National Bureau of Economic Research. http://www.nber.org/papers/w9907.

Baicker, K., B. J. Wright, S. Taubman, H. Allen, and A. Finkelstein. 2010. "What the Oregon Health Study Can Tell Us About Expanding Medicaid." *Health Affairs* 29, no. 8: 1498.

Blumberg, L., L. Dubay, and S. A. Norton. 2000. "Did the Medicaid Expansions for Children Displace Private Insurance? An Analysis Using the SIPP." *Journal of Health Economics* 19, no. 1: 33–60.

Bollen, K., D. K. Guilkey, and T. A. Morz. 1995. "Binary Outcomes and Endogenous Explanatory Variables: Tests and Solutions with an Application to the Demand for Contraceptive Use in Tunisia." *Demography* 32: 111–131.

Bound, J., D. A. Jaeger, and R. M. Baker. 1995. "Problems with Instrumental Variables Estimation When the Correlation between the Instruments and the Endogenous Explanatory Variable Is Weak." *Journal the American Statistical Association* 90, no. 430: 443.

Boushey, H. 2010. "This Has Been an Equal Opportunity Recession When It Comes to Job Losses Across Industries." *Think Progress: The Wonk Room.* Center for American Progress in Action Fund. http://thinkprogress.org/economy/2010/07/29/173424/boushey-equal/.

Buchmueller, T., K. S. Cooper, and J. Vistnes. 2005. "The Effect of SCHIP Expansions on Insurance Decisions by Employers." *Inquiry* 42, no. 3: 218–231.

Card, D., and L. D. Shore-Sheppard. 2004. "Using Discontinuous Eligibility Rules to Identify the Effects of the Federal Medicaid Expansions on Low-Income Children." *Review of Economics and Statistics* 86, no. 3: 752–766.

Chernew, M., D. Cutler, and P. S. Keenan. 2005. "Charity Care, Risk Pooling, and the Decline in Private Healthy Insurance." *American Economic Review* 95, no. 2: 209–213.

Currie, J., and J. Gruber. 1996a. "Health Insurance Eligibility, Utilization of Medical Care, and Child Health." *Quarterly Journal of Economics* 111, no. 2: 431–466.

———. 1996b. "Saving Babies: The Efficacy and Cost of Recent Changes in the Medicaid Eligibility of Pregnant Women." *Journal of Political Economy* 104, no. 6: 1263–1296.

Cutler, D. M., and J. Gruber. 1996. "The Effect of Medicaid Expansions on Public Insurance, Private Insurance, and Redistribution." *American Economic Review* 86, no. 2: 378–383.

Dafny, L., and J. Gruber. 2000. "Does Public Insurance Improve the Efficiency of Medical Care? Medicaid Expansions and Child Hospitalization." NBER Working Paper 7555. Cambridge, MA: National Bureau of Economic Research.

Dave, D. M., S. Decker, R. Kaestner, and K. I. Simon. 2008. "Re-examining the Effects of Medicaid Expansions for Pregnant Women." NBER Working Paper 14591. Cambridge, MA: National Bureau of Economic Research. http://www.nber.org/papers/w14159.

DeNavas-Walt, C., B. D. Proctor, and J. C. Smith. 2010. "Income, Poverty, and Health Insurance Coverage in the United States: 2009." Washington, DC: US Census Bureau.

Department of Health and Human Services. 2005. "Prior HHS Poverty Guidelines and Federal Register References." Accessed Dec. 1, 2010, http://aspe.hhs.gov/poverty/figures-fed-reg.shtml.

Dubay, L., and G. Kenney. 1996. "Revisiting the Issues: The Effects of Medicaid Expansions on Insurance Coverage of Children." *Future of Children* 6, no. 1: 152–161.

———. 1997. "Did Medicaid Expansions for Pregnant Women Crowd Out Private Coverage?" *Health Affairs* 16, no. 1: 185.

Federal Reserve. 2010. 97th Annual Report, "Minutes of the Federal Open Market Committee." Washington, DC.

Frick, K. D., and M. E. Chernew. 2009. "Beneficial Moral Hazard and the Theory of the Second Best." *Inquiry* 46, no. 2: 229–240.

Furnas, B., and R. Buckwalter-Poza. 2009. "Health Care Competition: Insurance Market Domination Leads to Fewer Choices." Washington, DC: Center for American Progress. http://www.americanprogress.org/issues/2009/06/pdf/health_competitiveness.pdf.

Gilmer, T., and R. Kronick. 2005. "It's the Premiums, Stupid: Projections of the Uninsured through 2013." *Health Affairs* Web Exclusive, W-5–143–151.

Government Accountability Office (GAO). 2002. "Private Health Insurance: Number and Market Share of Carriers in the Small Group Health Insurance Market." Report to US Senator Christopher Bond. Washington, DC. http://www.gao.gov/new.items/d02536r. pdf.

Gruber, J., and K. Simon. 2008. "Crowd-Out 10 Years Later: Have Recent Public Insurance Expansions Crowded Out Private Health Insurance?" *Journal of Health Economics* 27, no. 2: 201–217.

Ham, J., and L. Shore-Sheppard. 2005. "Did Expanding Medicaid Affect Welfare Participation?" *Industrial and Labor Relations Review* 58, no. 3: 452–470.

Ham, J. X. Li, and L. D. Shore-Sheppard. 2009. "Public Policy and the Dynamics of Children's Health Insurance, 1986–1999." *American Economic Review* 99, no. 2: 522–526.

Heckman, J. 1997. "Instrumental Variables: A Study of Implicit Behavioral Assumptions Used in Making Program Evaluations." *Journal of Human Resources* 32, no. 3: 441.

Herring, B. 2005. "The Effect of the Availability of Charity Care to the Uninsured on the Demand for Private Health Insurance." *Journal of Health Economics* 24:225–252.

Holahan, J. 1997. "Crowding Out: How Big a Problem?" *Health Affairs*, 16, no. 1: 204–206.

———. 2010. "The 2007–09 Recession and Health Insurance Coverage." *Health Affairs* 30, no. 1: 145–152.

Hudson, J. L., T. M. Selden, and J. S. Banthin. 2005. "The Impact of SCHIP on Insurance Coverage for Children." *Inquiry* 42, no. 3: 232–254.

Kaiser Family Foundation. 2007. "Health Care Spending in the United States and OECD Countries." *Snapshots: Health Care Costs.* Menlo Park, CA. http://www.kff.org/insurance/snapshot/chcm0103070th.cfm.

———. 2010. "Cumulative Change in Single and Family Health Insurance Premiums and Federal Poverty Level, 1996–2009." *Kaiser Fast Facts.* Menlo Park, CA. Accessed Jan. 3, 2010, http://facts.kff.org/chart.aspx?ch=157.

Katz, M. H. 2010. "Future of the Safety Net under Health Reform." *Journal of the American Medical Association* 304, no. 6: 679.

Kronick, R., and T. Gilmer. 1999. "Explaining the Decline in Health Insurance Coverage, 1979–1995." *Health Affairs* 18, no. 2: 30–47.

Krugman, P., and R. Wells. 2006. *Macroenconomics*. New York: Worth Publishing.

Lipsey, R. G., and K. Lancaster. 1956. "The General Theory of Second Best." *Review of Economic Studies* 24, no. 1: 11–32.

Long, S. K., and K. Stockley. 2009. "Massachusetts Health Reform: Employer Coverage from Employees' Perspective." *Health Affairs* 28, no. 6: W1079–87.

LoSasso, A., and T. Buchmueller. 2004. "The Effect of the State Children's Health Insurance Program on Health Insurance Coverage." *Journal of Health Economics* 23: 1059–1082.

Marquis, S. M. 2005. "The Role of the Safety Net in Employer Health Benefit Decisions." *Medical Care Research and Review* 62, no. 4: 435–457.

Nyman, J. 2008. "Health Insurance Theory: The Case of the Missing Welfare Gain." *European Journal of Health Economics* 9:369–380.

Rask, K. N., and K. J. Rask. 2000. "Public Insurance Substituting for Private Insurance: New Evidence Regarding Public Hospitals, Uncompensated Care Funds, and Medicaid." *Journal of Health Economics* 19, no. 1: 1–31.

Reschovsky, J. D., B. C. Strunk, and P. Ginsburg. 2006. "Why Employer-Sponsored Insurance Coverage Changed, 1997–2003." *Health Affairs* 25, no. 3: 774.

Shore-Sheppard, L. D. 2008. "Stemming the Tide? The Effect of Expanding Medicaid Eligibility on Health Insurance Coverage." *B.E. Journal of Economic Analysis and Policy: Advances in Economic Analysis and Policy* 8, no. 2: 1–33.

Shore-Sheppard, L. D., T. C. Buchmueller, and G. A. Jensen. 2000. "Medicaid and Crowding Out of Private Insurance: A Re-examination Using Firm Level Data." *Journal of Health Economics* 19, no. 1: 61–91.

Siegel, B., P. Shin, and M. Regenstein. 2004. "Health Reform and the Safety Net: Big Opportunities, Major Risks." *Journal of Law, Medicine & Ethics* 32, no. 3: 426–432.

Social Security and Medicare Boards of Trustees. 2009. "Status of the Social Security and Medicare Programs." *Social Security Online Actuarial Publications*. Washington, DC. http://ssa.gov/OACT/TRSUM/index.html.

Staiger, D. S., and J. H. Stock. 1997. "Instrumental Variables Regression with Weak Instruments." *Econometrica* 65:557–586.

Swartz, K. 1996. "Medicaid Crowd Out and the Inverse Truman Bind." *Inquiry* 33:5–8.

Thorpe, K. F., and C. Florence. 1998. "Health Insurance Coverage among Children: The Role of Expanded Medicaid Coverage." *Inquiry* 35, no. 4: 369–379.

Wilen-Berg, J. 2010. "What Is Left of Charity Care after Health Reform?" *Hasting Center Report* 40, no. 4: 12.

Yazici, E. Y., and R. Kaestner. 2000. "Medicaid Expansions and the Crowding Out of Private Health Insurance." *Inquiry* 36, no. 1: 23–32.

Yelowitz, A. S. 1995. "The Medicaid Notch, Labor Supply, and Welfare Participation: Evidence from Eligibility Expansions." *Quarterly Journal of Economics* 110, no. 4: 909–939.

About the Contributors

Gloria J. Bazzoli, PhD, is the Bon Secours Professor with the Department of Health Administration, Virginia Commonwealth University. She has published more than eighty articles in peer-reviewed journals, including *Journal of Health Economics*, *Journal of the American Medical Association*, *Health Services Research*, *Health Affairs*, *Medical Care Research and Review*, and *Inquiry*. She has been lead investigator in various research projects, including studies of financial pressures affecting the hospital safety net, relationships between hospital financial condition and the quality of hospital care, and the effects of hospital mergers and closures on health care markets and consumers. She received her doctorate in economics from Cornell University.

Judith G. Calhoun, PhD, MBA, is senior research investigator at the University of Michigan Medical School, specializing in health professions education, outcomes-based learning and assessment, and leadership development programming, evaluation, and research. She has held faculty positions in both public health and medicine at the university and has served as an executive leader in strategic planning, communications, and physician services at three academic health care centers. She has authored more than seventy juried articles and chapters in health care management and education. Recently she served as a faculty consultant to the Association of Schools of Public Health and the National Center for Healthcare Leadership regarding the development of competency-based educational programs and models across the health professions.

Byron J. Crouse, MD, is professor of family medicine in the School of Medicine and Public Health, University of Wisconsin. He serves as associate dean for rural and community health, and he directs the Wisconsin Academy for Rural Medicine, an initiative to increase the number of physicians practicing in rural Wisconsin. In addition to his work in rural medical education and the health care workforce, he is chair of the National Advisory Committee of the National Health Service Corps and serves on the advisory committee of the Technical Assistance and Services Center, a program of the National Rural Health Resource Center.

John G. Frohna, MD, MPH, is professor of pediatrics and medicine at the University of Wisconsin School of Medicine and Public Health. He serves as vice chair for education and residency program director for the Department of Pediatrics. Dr. Frohna completed a residency in internal medicine-pediatrics at the University of Michigan. He is a past president of the national Med-Peds Program Directors Association. In addition to maintaining an active primary care practice, Dr. Frohna's research interests include substance abuse and infant health, med-peds training outcomes, professionalism in residency, and evidence-based medicine.

Sheryl L. Garland, MHA, is vice president of health policy and community relations for the Virginia Commonwealth University Health System. In this role, she coordinates efforts to expand the health system's legislative services and establishes activities to coordinate health system initiatives. Additionally, she is leading efforts to prepare for health reform, including novel educational programs and grant opportunities. Formerly, she was vice president of community outreach for the VCU Health System and administrative director for the VCU Center on Health Disparities. In this role, she developed relationships at the federal, state, and local levels to address access and funding needs for vulnerable populations.

Michael K. Gusmano, PhD, is associate professor of health policy and management at New York Medical College and a research scholar at the Hastings Center. Dr. Gusmano's research interests include health policy, comparative health systems, health inequalities, and normative theories of policy analysis. In addition to his doctorate in political science from the University of Maryland at College Park, he holds a master's in public policy from the State University of New York at Albany. He was also postdoctoral fellow in the Robert Wood Johnson Foundation Scholars in Health Policy program at Yale University.

Mark A. Hall, JD, is the Fred D. and Elizabeth L. Turnage Professor of Law and Public Health at Wake Forest University. Professor Hall specializes in health care law and public policy, with a focus on economic, regulatory, and ethical issues. His present research interests include consumer-driven health care, insurance regulation, the doctor–patient relationship, conflicts of interest in research, and genetics. He is the author or editor of thirteen books on health care law and policy, including *Making Medical Spending Decisions*, and *Health Care Law and Ethics* (8th ed.).

Peter D. Jacobson, JD, MPH, is professor of health law and policy, and director, Center for Law, Ethics, and Health, at the University of Michigan School of Public Health. He teaches courses on health law, public health law, and health care regulations. Jacobson's current research includes projects on public health entrepreneurship, safety net services, and how state and federal law influence public health preparedness. Jacobson's most recent books are *Law and the Health System* (coauthored with Lawrence O. Gostin), and *False Hope vs. Evidence-Based Medicine: The Story of a Failed Treatment for Breast Cancer* (coauthored).

Michelle Ko, MD, is a PhD candidate in the Department of Health Services, UCLA School of Public Health. She graduated from the UCLA/Drew Medical Education Program in 2004. Her research interests include healthcare workforce education, access to care for underserved populations, and the intersection of community social context with health, and healthcare disparities. Her current work addresses the impact of social stratification on local safety-net infrastructure, particularly the stability of public hospitals and community health centers.

Dayna Bowen Matthew, JD, holds a joint appointment as a professor of law at the University of Colorado Law School and the Colorado School of Public Health's Center for Bioethics and Humanities. She teaches evidence, civil procedure, health law, and public health law and ethics and from 2004 to 2011 she served as the law school's associate and, later, vice dean. Professor Matthew earned a BA in economics from Harvard-Radcliffe and a JD from the University of Virginia, where she was an editor of the *Virginia Law Review*. Professor Matthew's most recent scholarship focuses on addressing racial, ethnic, and gender disparities in American health care. She is the author of a forthcoming book concerning the impact of implicit bias on disparate health and health outcomes.

Robert W. Mickey, PhD, is associate professor of political science and research associate at the Center for Political Studies at the University of Michigan. He is the author of the forthcoming *Paths Out of Dixie: The Democratization of Authoritarian Enclaves in America's Deep South, 1944–1972*. Mickey is very grateful for the support of the Robert Wood Johnson Foundation's Scholars in Health Policy Research Program, and especially its University of California–Berkeley site.

Valerie Myers, PhD, MA, MSW, is assistant professor of management and organizations at the University of Michigan, School of Public Health Department of Health Management and Policy and the Ross School of Business Department of Management and Organizations, where she is affiliated with the Center for Positive Organizational Scholarship. Dr. Myers earned her dual doctorate in organizational psychology and social work (policy) from the University of Michigan, Ann Arbor. Her research interests include organizational culture and performance outcomes; healthcare; leadership, diversity management, and employee engagement; and work ethics and dignity in organizations. She has private sector experience in management and consulting.

Jack Needleman, PhD, FAAN, is professor of health services at the UCLA School of Public Health. He also is director of the Health Services Department's PhD and research master's programs, and associate director of the UCLA Patient Safety Institute. His research on nurse staffing and quality won the first AcademyHealth Health Services Research Impact Award, and his research on quality, staffing, and health care organizations has appeared in the *New England Journal of Medicine*, *Health Affairs*, *Health Services Research*, and *Medical Care*.

Thomas R. Oliver, PhD, MHA, is professor of population health sciences at the University of Wisconsin School of Medicine and Public Health. He serves as director of the UW Master of Public Health program and the Wisconsin Center for Public Health Education and Training. Professor Oliver's research examines critical issues in health policy, politics, and system reform. His most recent work includes studies of state and national health care reforms; the use of county health rankings and multisector partnerships to stimulate and guide population health improvement; and comparative analysis of health policy development and governance in the United States and European Union.

Jodyn E. Platt, MPH, is a doctoral student in the Health Services Organization and Policy Program at the University of Michigan School of Public Health. She received her MPH in health policy from the University of Michigan in 2005. Her research interests include science and technology studies, public health and health services systems, and public health genetics.

Richard E. Rieselbach, MD, is professor emeritus of medicine, University of Wisconsin School of Medicine and Public Health, and past president of the Association of Program Directors in Internal Medicine. He is a health policy consultant for the UW Foundation, with a major area of interest in the development of CHAMP Medicaid and Medicare accountable care organizations, as currently described in a recent *New England Journal of Medicine* Perspective article. He is a former dean and chair of medicine at the UW Medical School–Milwaukee and former vice chair of medicine at the UW Medical School–Madison.

Sara Rosenbaum, JD, is the Hirsh Professor of Health Law and Policy and founding chair of George Washington University's Department of Health Policy. She has devoted her career to issues of health law and policy affecting low income and medically underserved populations. An author of a leading health law textbook and more than 350 articles and studies focusing on the medically underserved, Professor Rosenbaum has received numerous awards for her scholarship and service and serves on numerous boards, including the CDC Director's Advisory Committee, the CDC Advisory Committee on Immunization Practices, and the Medicaid and CHIP Payment and Access Commission, which advises Congress on Medicaid policy.

Alison Snow Jones, PhD, died in January 2011. She was associate professor of health management and policy in the Drexel University School of Public Health. As a health economist, Dr. Snow Jones conducted research on alcohol use and abuse and its impact on labor force outcomes and children's health; intimate partner violence; women's health; and tobacco control. She served as a consultant on a number of cost-effectiveness evaluations of programs that targeted children's health and taught courses in health economics, research methods and statistics, mathematical methods for economics, and cost–benefit/cost-effectiveness analysis. In addition, she taught courses about ethics and the economics of social justice to theologians and MBA students.

Frank J. Thompson, PhD, is professor in the School of Public Affairs and Administration at Rutgers University–Newark and an affiliated faculty member with the Rutgers Center for State Health Policy in New Brunswick. Previously, he served as dean of the Rockefeller College at the University at Albany, SUNY. Thompson has published extensively on issues of politics and administration, public management, and health policy. He currently has a Robert Wood Johnson Investigator Award to study Medicaid, federalism, and health reform during the Clinton, G. W. Bush, and Obama administrations. He is a fellow of the National Academy of Public Administration.

Index

Figures in the text are designated by f; tables by a t.

Available titles in the Critical Issues in Health and Medicine series:

1866024

CPSIA information can be obtained at www.ICGtesting.com
Printed in the USA
BVOW041338250612

293591BV00002B/4/P